A Comprehensive Manual for Drug Prescribing in Dentistry

nova
Medicine & Health
New York

Dentistry and Oral Sciences Series

The New Challenges of Dentistry: Advances and Innovations
Roshan Melwani-Sadhwani, PhD, DHSc, Ana Isabel Contreras-Madrid, Vinicius Coelho Carrard, PhD, David Pérez-Jorge, PhD and Juliana Cassol Spanemberg, PhD
ISBN: 979-8-89530-480-8
eBook ISBN: 979-8-89530-510-2

Bio-Functional Dentistry: Principles, Material Designs and Applications
Victoria Tamara Perchyonok, PhD
ISBN: 979-8-89530-024-4
eBook ISBN: 979-8-89530-079-4

Regenerative Endodontics: Biological Foundation, Protocols and Future Directions
Alexandre Henrique dos Reis-Prado, MSc
ISBN: 979-8-89530-027-5
eBook ISBN: 979-8-89530-091-6

Digital Implant Planning and Guided Implant Surgery
Niveditha S. Prasad, MDS, Sheejith Madapathi, MDS, Sarath Raj, DMRD, DNB, and Nivea T. Francis, MDS
ISBN: 979-8-89113-324-2
eBook ISBN: 979-8-89113-375-4

More information about this series can be found at

Nilay Aksoy

A Comprehensive Manual for Drug Prescribing in Dentistry

nova
Medicine & Health
New York

DOI: https://doi.org/10.52305/OLPK8753

Library of Congress Cataloging-in-Publication Data
Library of Congress Control Number: 2026930281
ISBN: 979-8-90134-135-3 (Hardcover)
ISBN: 979-8-90134-193-3 (eBook)

Published by Nova Science Publishers, Inc. † New York

For my husband, Dr. Ihab Abunahlah. You left us far too early and could not see this achievement, but your love, strength and quiet wisdom guided every page. Rest in peace. You will always be here beside us.

Contents

Preface

The safe and effective use of medications is a cornerstone of modern dental practice, directly impacting patient outcomes, satisfaction, and overall oral health. In recent years, advances in pharmacology, evolving clinical guidelines, and the growing complexity of patient populations have made drug prescribing in dentistry more challenging and more important than ever. Recognizing the need for a comprehensive, up-to-date resource, this book was developed to provide dental professionals, students, and educators with a clear and practical guide to pharmacological principles and prescribing practices in dentistry.

This book covers the fundamental concepts of drug action, selection, and administration, as well as the management of common dental conditions and emergencies. Special attention is given to the needs of vulnerable patient groups, the prevention of adverse drug reactions, and the ethical and legal responsibilities of prescribers. Each chapter is informed by the latest research and clinical guidelines, ensuring that readers are equipped with current, evidence-based knowledge.

Our aim is to support dental practitioners in making informed, patient-centered decisions, and to foster a culture of safety, responsibility, and lifelong learning in dental pharmacotherapy. We hope this book will serve as a valuable reference and inspire continued professional development in this vital area of dental care.

Acknowledgments

I acknowledge the use of artificial intelligence technologies for language editing and grammar refinement during the preparation of this book. The author gratefully acknowledges Nur Ozturk for designing the book's final version and for her invaluable assistance throughout the publication process.

Chapter 1

The Importance and Principles of Rational Drug Use in Dentistry

Abstract

Rational prescribing in dentistry is essential for effective patient care and public health, ensuring medications are chosen and used based on clinical evidence and individual patient needs. This chapter reviews the significance of rational prescribing in dental practice, particularly given the frequent use of antibiotics and analgesics. It discusses the principles and benefits of rational prescribing, such as improved patient outcomes, reduced adverse effects, and the prevention of antibiotic resistance. Key challenges including practitioner knowledge gaps, patient pressure, and ethical dilemmas are examined, alongside practical strategies like education, guideline adoption, and prescription audits to promote best practices. The chapter also provides clear guidelines for safe prescription writing and presents a case study illustrating the positive impact of educational interventions on prescribing habits. By following rational prescribing principles, dental professionals can enhance care quality, ensure patient safety, and support the responsible use of medications in dentistry.

Keywords: rational prescribing, prescription writing, patient safety, clinical guidelines, ethical dilemmas

1.1. An Overview of the Importance of Rational Prescribing in Dentistry

Rational prescribing of medicine is a critical component of effective patient care and public health. It refers to a systematic approach that includes formulating a differential diagnosis, assessing prognosis, defining therapeutic objectives, choosing the most suitable treatment, and evaluating treatment outcomes (Maxwell, 2016). Rational prescribing is a key aspect of rational drug use (RDU), ensuring that medication selections are evidence-based, appropriate for the patient's condition, and tailored to optimize therapeutic outcomes while minimizing risks (Quick et al., 1997). The World Health Organization (WHO) has established indicators to assess the implementation of RDU in healthcare facilities. The most common indicators are prescribing, health facility, and patient care indicators (WHO, 1993). Prescribing indicators assess how medications are prescribed by healthcare providers; health facility indicators evaluate the resources available within healthcare systems; and patient care indicators measure various aspects of patient care. The WHO has reported that incorrect prescribing and dispensing of medications account for over 50% of all pharmaceuticals available on the market (WHO, 2010).

In dentistry, rational prescribing is of particular importance due to the frequent use of antibiotics and analgesics. Dentists are responsible for prescribing 6–12% of all antibiotics in outpatient settings, which translates to millions of antibiotic courses annually (Thompson et al., 2022; Walsh et al., 2021; Hubbard et al., 2021). However, evidence indicates that more than 70% of these prescriptions may be inappropriate (Chate et al., 2006; Chopra et al., 2014; Rodríguez-Fernández et al., 2023). In the realm of analgesia, research has shown that between 25% and 50% of opioids prescribed to adult dental patients in the United States of America (USA) are overprescribed (Suda et al., 2020). Despite a notable decrease in opioid prescription rates in dentistry for Medicaid enrollees in USA from 2012 to 2019, the overall rate remains high, with many prescriptions issued unnecessarily (Chua et al., 2021; Okunev et al., 2021). Prescription opioids are widely recognized as some of the most frequently misused and abused medications worldwide (Thornhill et al., 2019).

Nonsteroidal Anti-Inflammatory Drugs (NSAIDs) are highly effective for managing acute dental pain due to their anti-inflammatory and analgesic properties. Nonetheless, they are often prescribed in excess or inappropriately, sometimes without considering patient-specific risk factors such as gastrointestinal, renal, or cardiovascular conditions. There is also a tendency to use NSAIDs even when milder analgesics, such as acetaminophen, would suffice, particularly when inflammation is not the main issue. Such prescribing practices can result in unnecessary complications, including gastrointestinal bleeding and renal impairment, highlighting the need for more careful and patient-focused prescribing in dental care (Dionne & Berthold,2001; Barkin et al., 2010).

1.2. What is Rational Prescribing?

Rational prescribing involves selecting and using drugs based on clinical evidence, patient-specific factors, and a clear understanding of the associated risks and benefits. This approach ensures that the right drug is prescribed for the right condition, with careful attention to the appropriate dose, route, and duration of treatment. Ultimately, rational prescribing aims to provide effective therapy that is as safe and harmless as possible for the patient.

In dentistry, rational prescribing is of particular importance, since dental practitioners are often called upon to manage conditions such as infections, pain, and inflammation, which require specific and targeted pharmacological interventions (Maxwell, 2009).

1.3. Implications of Rational Prescribing for Patient Outcomes

In dentistry, rational prescribing leads to positive outcomes. By ensuring the use of the appropriate drug for the correct diagnosis, rational prescribing enhances treatment outcomes and reduces the risk of treatment failure (Kaufmann et al., 2014). It also lowers the likelihood of drug-related adverse effects and medication errors (Mokrzecki et al., 2023). Additionally, rational prescribing aims to provide services at the lowest possible cost by standardizing medication prescription practices (Bates, 1997; Terzi & Yilmaz, 2021). Patients are more likely to adhere to their treatment regimens when they receive appropriate and clear instructions along with suitable medications.

Rational antibiotic prescribing is particularly important in combating antibiotic resistance. Prescribing antibiotics only, when necessary, helps prevent the development of resistant bacterial strains, a significant public health concern. Rational prescribing practices also promote the use of medical evidence and reliable information sources among dentists, leading to decisions that adhere to the best available clinical guidelines and improve the quality of care (Cope & Chestnutt, 2014; Theodorou et al., 2009; WHO, 2002a; WHO, 2002b; Terzi & Yilmaz, 2021).

1.4. Key Principles of Rational Prescribing in Dentistry

The key principles of rational prescribing in dentistry include appropriateness of medication, correct dosage and duration, cost-effectiveness, minimizing polypharmacy, ongoing education, and patient involvement. By following these principles, dentists can improve the quality of care, minimize the risk of medication errors, and support the overarching goal of rational drug use in healthcare (Terzi & Yilmaz, 2021). Additionally, dentists have an ethical obligation to prioritize patient welfare and public health. Rational prescribing aligns with this responsibility by ensuring that medications are used appropriately and responsibly.

1.5. Challenges to Rational Prescribing in Dentistry

A major challenge to rational prescribing in dentistry is insufficient knowledge among practitioners. Both undergraduate and postgraduate dental students often lack adequate understanding of appropriate antibiotic use, leading to improper prescribing practices. This knowledge gap is also present in the broader dental community, with a significant proportion of dentists reporting insufficient understanding of antibiotics and related conditions, contributing to overprescription. Many dental students consider it ethical to prescribe antibiotics unnecessarily, reflecting a concerning attitude toward appropriate medication use. A large majority of dentists recognize overprescription as a significant barrier to rational antibiotic use (Roganović & Barać, 2024; Kadu et al., 2024).

Pressure from patients is another significant challenge. Dentists frequently encounter requests from patients or their families for antibiotics, even when such prescriptions are not clinically warranted. Studies have shown that a notable percentage of dental students consider it ethical to prescribe antibiotics to family members without proper assessment, and many practitioners admit to prescribing antibiotics primarily to satisfy patient comfort. This practice contributes to the misuse of antibiotics and the growing problem of resistance (Roganović & Barać, 2024; Oberoi et al., 2015; Özdemir et al., 2024).

Ethical dilemmas also pose significant challenges. According to Roganović & Barać (2024), around 70% of participants consider giving a placebo instead of an antibiotic to be an ethical practice. However, the use of placebos in place of antibiotics when they are not clinically indicated raises concerns about honesty and the integrity of the dentist-patient relationship. These ethical challenges can complicate decision-making and undermine trust in dental care (Roganović & Barać, 2024).

1.6. Recommendations to Promote Rational Prescribing

Effective strategies for rational prescribing include adopting consensus-based treatment protocols and guidelines that are regularly updated to reflect the latest evidence. It is crucial to educate prescribers in clinical pharmacology, therapeutics, and problem-solving to help them resist external pressures and avoid irrational influences. Utilizing structured tools, such as the WHO Guide to Good Prescribing, ensures a systematic approach to all aspects of rational prescribing.

Promoting shared decision-making and respecting patient values and preferences are also essential for achieving optimal, individualized care. Educating patients about the appropriate use of medications can help align their expectations with clinical necessity and reduce demand-driven prescribing. Integrating comprehensive ethical training into dental education can better prepare practitioners to handle dilemmas such as placebo use and reinforce their role in combating antibiotic resistance.

Implementing policies to monitor and regulate antibiotic and medication prescriptions, encouraging prescription audits to identify and correct inappropriate practices, supporting research on the safety and effectiveness of dental medications, and developing new diagnostic tools to accurately identify infections requiring antibiotics are all important steps. By focusing on these areas, dental practice can advance toward more rational and responsible antibiotic prescribing, minimizing unnecessary use and contributing to the global effort against antibiotic resistance (WHO, 1994; Aronson, 2004; Roganović & Barać, 2024; Donker et al., 2024).

1.7. Case Studies: Implications of Rational Prescribing for Patient Outcome

A multimodal interventional pilot study evaluated the impact of educational initiatives and a dentistry-specific prescribing website on prescribing behaviors. Twenty-six dentists participated in this 12-week pre–post study, during which they self-recorded their prescriptions for antibiotics, analgesics, and anxiolytics over an initial 6-week period. Following the introduction of educational resources and access to the prescribing website, dentists continued to document their prescribing for another 6 weeks. The intervention led to a significant 44.6% reduction in inappropriate antibiotic prescriptions and a 40.5% decrease in the overall number of antibiotics prescribed (Teoh et al., 2021).

1.8. How to Write a Prescription: Detailed Guidelines for Safe and Effective Medication Use

Writing a prescription is a fundamental responsibility of healthcare providers, requiring precision, clarity, and adherence to legal and clinical standards. A well-crafted prescription ensures that patients receive the correct medication, dosage, and instructions, minimizing the risk of errors and enhancing therapeutic outcomes.

Every prescription must begin with clear patient identification details, including the full name, address, age, and sometimes gender. This information helps avoid confusion and ensures that the medication is dispensed to the correct individual. The date of the prescription is crucial, as it determines the validity period.

The medication should be written clearly, preferably using the generic name to avoid confusion and reduce costs. Brand names may be used when necessary (but with the scientific name mentioned to minimise error), but the prescriber must indicate if substitution with a generic is allowed. The strength of the medication must be explicitly stated, for example, "Amoxicillin 500 mg," to ensure the pharmacist dispenses the correct potency.

The dosage form, such as tablets, capsules, suspension, or solution, must be specified. For example, "28 capsules" or "100 ml suspension." This is important because the same medication can come in multiple forms, and the form affects how the medication is administered and absorbed.

The quantity is indicated using the "#" symbol followed by the number, e.g., "Dispense #12," which instructs the pharmacist to provide twelve units of the medication. Sometimes the term "Disp" is used before the quantity. This helps the pharmacist know exactly how much medication to prepare or dispense.

The "Sig" section provides detailed instructions on how the patient should take the medication. "Sig" is derived from the Latin word "signa," meaning "write on the label." This section must be clear and unambiguous, specifying the route, dose, frequency, and duration of treatment. For example, "Take one capsule orally every 12 hours for 10 days."

It is highly recommended to avoid Latin abbreviations that can be misinterpreted. Instead, use plain language to reduce errors. However, if abbreviations are used, they should be standardized and well understood. Despite the existence of these abbreviations, it is safer to write instructions in full English to avoid misinterpretation. For example, instead of "tid," write "three times daily."

The length of treatment must be clearly stated, such as "for 7 days" or "10 days." This helps ensure the patient completes the full course, which is especially important for antibiotics and other time-sensitive medications.

The number of refills allowed should be clearly indicated. If no refills are permitted, write "NR" (no refills) or spell out "none." Controlled substances often have strict limits on refills, sometimes none at all, depending on the drug schedule and local laws.

The prescription must be signed manually by the prescriber on the date it is written. Pre-signing prescriptions is prohibited, especially for controlled substances. Electronic prescriptions are increasingly accepted and can reduce errors, but they must comply with regulatory standards and may not be permitted for all medication types in every jurisdiction (Volpe et al., 2016; Connor et al., 2011).

1.9. Additional Important Considerations

Prescriptions should always be typed or printed whenever possible to ensure legibility; if handwritten, the writing must be clear and easily readable to prevent any risk of dispensing errors. It is important to avoid ambiguity in instructions; vague phrases such as "take as directed" or "take as needed" should not be used without further clarification, as they can lead to confusion for both the patient and the pharmacist.

Before prescribing any medication, clinicians must always check for patient allergies and potential drug interactions. This process is essential for ensuring patient safety and preventing adverse events. For example, failure to recognize a patient's allergy to penicillin could result in the prescription of an antibiotic, such as amoxicillin, potentially leading to severe allergic reactions like anaphylaxis. Similarly, overlooking possible drug interactions may cause reduced therapeutic efficacy or dangerous side effects, especially in patients taking multiple medications for chronic conditions.

Additionally, the prescriber should indicate whether generic substitution is permitted; if the brand name drug is specifically required, this should be clearly stated by writing "DAW" (Dispense as Written) on the prescription. For controlled substances, it is essential to adhere strictly to all relevant regulations regarding prescribing, refills, and documentation, as these medications are subject to additional legal and safety requirements.

1.10. An Example of a Proper Prescription

Patient Name: Jack Sassen. Date: 07/27/2025.

Rx: Amoxicillin Clavulanic Acid 500 mg / 125 mg tablets.

Dispense: #20 (twenty).

Sig: Take one tablet orally every 8 hours for 7 days for bacterial infection.

Refills: None.

Prescriber Signature: Dr. X.

This example clearly states the medication, strength, dosage form, quantity, detailed instructions, duration, and refill status, ensuring safe and effective use. This detailed approach to prescription writing helps healthcare providers minimize errors, comply with legal requirements, and promote patient safety and treatment efficacy.

Chapter 2

Principles of Pharmacology

Abstract

This chapter provides a comprehensive overview of pharmacokinetics and pharmacodynamics, the two foundational branches of pharmacology that govern the fate and effects of drugs within the body. Pharmacokinetics explores the processes of absorption, distribution, metabolism, and excretion (ADME), detailing how drugs are introduced, transported, transformed, and eliminated. The chapter examines the influence of drug administration routes, bioavailability, and patient-specific factors on drug disposition and therapeutic outcomes. Pharmacodynamics is discussed in terms of drug receptor interactions, efficacy, potency, and the mechanisms underlying drug action and variability in response. The chapter also addresses the clinical significance of adverse drug reactions (ADRs), their classification, mechanisms, diagnosis, management, and prevention, as well as the principles of pharmacovigilance. Finally, it delves into drug interactions—pharmacodynamic, pharmacokinetic, and pharmaceutical—highlighting their detection, clinical implications, and management strategies. By integrating these concepts, the chapter underscores the importance of individualized drug therapy, patient safety, and the optimization of therapeutic efficacy in clinical practice.

Keywords: pharmacokinetics, pharmacodynamics, adverse drug reactions, individualized therapy, patient Safety

2.1. Fundamental Concepts of Pharmacology

Pharmacology is the scientific field dedicated to the study of medications and therapeutic agents (Vallance & Smart, 2006). It encompasses an extensive analysis of drugs, including their origins, physical and chemical properties, formulation, biochemical and physiological effects, pharmacodynamics (mechanisms of action), pharmacokinetics (absorption, distribution, biotransformation, and excretion), as well as their therapeutic and supplementary uses (Emmett et al., 2019).

2.1.1. Pharmacokinetics

Pharmacokinetics is a branch of pharmacology that focuses on what happens to substances such as drugs, hormones, nutrients, and toxins after they are introduced into a living organism. It examines how the body influences these substances. Pharmacokinetics encompasses four main processes absorption, distribution, metabolism, and excretion collectively known as ADME (Doogue & Polasek, 2013). The ADME process is critical in determining the concentration of a drug at its site of action and its overall therapeutic effect.

2.1.1.1. Absorption

Absorption refers to the passage of a drug or xenobiotic through membranes, skin, or injection sites into the systemic circulation (blood and/or lymph) (Tran et al., 2013). Drugs can be transported across biological membranes via several mechanisms, including passive (simple) diffusion, filtration/pore/paracellular transport, facilitated diffusion, active transport, electrochemical/ionic diffusion, ion pair transport, and endocytosis/pinocytosis. However, most drugs are absorbed into the systemic circulation via passive diffusion (Buxton, 2023).

2.1.1.1.1. Route of Drug Administration

The route of drug administration refers to the path by which a drug is introduced into the body to achieve its desired therapeutic effect. The choice of route depends on various factors, including the drug's properties, the condition being treated, patient compliance, and the pharmacokinetics and pharmacodynamics of the drug. Each route has its own advantages, disadvantages, and specific considerations.

The enteral route involves delivering drugs through the gastrointestinal (GI) tract. The oral route is the most widely used due to its convenience and cost-effectiveness. Drugs are primarily absorbed in the small intestine, and their bioavailability is influenced by the first-pass effect, where the drug is metabolized in the liver before reaching systemic circulation. The oral route is easy, non-invasive, cost-effective, widely accepted by patients, and suitable for self-administration. However, it has disadvantages such as variable absorption influenced by food, pH, and GI motility; degradation of certain drugs by stomach acid or enzymes; reduced bioavailability due to first-pass metabolism; and unsuitability for patients experiencing nausea, vomiting, or difficulty swallowing.

The sublingual and buccal routes involve placing the drug under the tongue (sublingual) or against the cheek (buccal), allowing absorption directly through the oral mucosa. These methods bypass the first-pass effect and offer rapid absorption and onset of action, making them suitable for patients with swallowing difficulties. Disadvantages include limitation to small doses, potential for unpleasant taste or irritation, and the need for patient cooperation to prevent swallowing the medication.

The rectal route involves absorption through the highly vascularized rectal mucosa, partially bypassing the first-pass effect. This route is useful for patients unable to take oral medications (e.g., vomiting, unconscious), bypassing stomach acid and enzymes, and is suitable for both local and systemic effects. However, absorption can be inconsistent, may cause rectal irritation, and is not always acceptable to patients due to discomfort or cultural factors (George, 2010).

- Parenteral routes deliver drugs directly into the body, bypassing the GI tract. These methods are often used for rapid drug action or when oral administration is not feasible.
- The intravenous (IV) route delivers drugs directly into the bloodstream, providing immediate systemic effects, rapid onset of action, precise control over drug levels, and suitability for large volumes and irritant drugs. However, IV administration requires trained personnel, carries risks of infection, thrombosis, and extravasation, and may cause pain and discomfort at the injection site.
- The intramuscular (IM) route involves injection into muscle tissue, where drugs are absorbed into the bloodstream. IM administration is suitable for depot formulations for sustained release, offers faster absorption than subcutaneous injections, and is useful for patients unable to take oral medications. However, it can cause pain, carries a risk of nerve or blood vessel injury, is limited to smaller volumes, and may result in local complications such as abscesses or hematomas (Hedaya, 2024).
- The subcutaneous (SC) route involves injection into the fatty tissue beneath the skin, allowing for slow and sustained absorption. SC administration is easy, suitable for self-administration, and provides sustained drug release, but absorption can be slow and unpredictable, is limited to small volumes, and carries a risk of local irritation or tissue damage.

- The intra-arterial route involves injecting drugs directly into an artery, typically for localized treatment such as chemotherapy for tumors. It delivers high drug concentrations to a specific area but is technically challenging, rarely used, and carries risks of arterial damage and complications.
- The intraosseous route involves injecting drugs into the bone marrow, often used in emergencies when IV access is not available. It offers rapid absorption and onset of action, is useful in neonates and critically ill patients, but requires specialized training and carries risks of infection and bone damage (Soar et al., 2009; Ruiz & Scioli, 2024).

Other routes used for specific drugs or conditions, often bypassing the GI tract, include:

- Inhalational route: Drugs are delivered as aerosols or gases and absorbed through the respiratory tract. This route offers rapid absorption due to the large surface area of the lungs, avoids first-pass metabolism, and is suitable for local and systemic effects. However, it requires proper technique, is limited to drugs that can be aerosolized, and carries risks of local irritation or systemic side effects.
- Transdermal route: Drugs are delivered through the skin using patches, gels, or ointments. This route provides sustained drug release, avoids first-pass metabolism, and is non-invasive and convenient. However, it is limited to lipophilic drugs, can cause skin irritation, and has a slow onset of action.
- Intranasal route: Drugs are absorbed through the nasal mucosa, bypassing the first-pass effect. This route offers rapid absorption and onset of action and is easy to administer, but is limited to small doses and may cause nasal irritation or congestion (Erdő et al., 2018).
- Vaginal route: Drugs are administered into the vagina for local or systemic effects. This route bypasses first-pass metabolism and is suitable for local treatments (e.g., infections, hormone therapy), but has limited patient acceptance and risk of local irritation (Neves et al., 2021).
- Ophthalmic route: Drugs are administered to the external eye, offering rapid action and systemic absorption, but absorption is

variable, requires special delivery systems, and may irritate ocular mucosa.

The selection of a drug administration route depends on multiple factors, including the drug's characteristics (solubility, stability, bioavailability), patient-related considerations (age, health status, ability to tolerate specific routes), therapeutic objectives, required onset and duration of action, convenience, and patient compliance. Each route carries potential risks and complications, such as pain, irritation, infection at the site, systemic side effects, allergic reactions, and technical challenges. Healthcare professionals must carefully assess the risks and benefits of each route and monitor patients for adverse effects.

2.1.1.1.2. Bioavailability

Bioavailability refers to the extent and rate at which the active moiety (drug or metabolite) enters the systemic circulation, thereby accessing the site of action (Currie, 2018; Herkenne et al., 2008). For drugs administered intravenously, bioavailability is 100%. However, drugs administered orally or by other non-intravenous routes may reach a maximum blood concentration significantly lower than the administered dose; this is called "fractional bioavailability" (Buxton, 2023). Two important parameters related to absorption are the degree of absorption (the percentage of the administered dose that reaches systemic circulation) and the rate of absorption. Bioavailability is a crucial pharmacokinetic parameter, as it determines whether the expected therapeutic response from systemically effective drugs can be achieved. Many factors can affect drug bioavailability, including both patient- and medication-related factors (Caldwell et al., 1995; Martinez & Amidon, 2002).

Patient-related factors include individual variances, genetic variations, and genetic polymorphisms, particularly of liver enzymes. Even a small genetic change at a single locus may result in intra- or interindividual differences in therapeutic efficacy. The gastric emptying rate, characterized by rapid gastric emptying, enhances the absorption rate of drugs from the small intestine. Elevated blood flow to the absorption site facilitates medication absorption by sustaining a concentration gradient, while inadequate perfusion, as seen in shock or certain illnesses, may diminish bioavailability. Factors associated with the GI tract, such as perfusion, are crucial for the absorption of lipophilic drugs, which typically undergo simple diffusion. Reduced intestinal motility extends transit time, enhancing solubility and absorption for poorly soluble drugs. The pH of the GI system influences absorption by modifying the ionization rate and, therefore, lipophilicity; nonionized drugs are absorbed more readily. GI enzymes can break down medications prior to absorption, and gut flora may metabolize certain drugs, influencing bioavailability. The presence of food may delay gastric emptying, modify pH, and interact with medications, potentially increasing or decreasing absorption. For instance, lipid-rich meals enhance the absorption of lipophilic drugs such as griseofulvin and piperaquine (Ogunbona et al., 1985; Sim et al., 2005). Disease states such as celiac disease, Crohn's disease, or gastric bypass surgery can diminish the surface area for absorption, limiting bioavailability, while liver disorders may hinder first-pass metabolism, thereby enhancing bioavailability. Drug interactions with other medications or foods can occur because some drugs inhibit or activate enzymes and transporters, altering the bioavailability of other drugs taken at the same time. Grapefruit juice suppresses CYP3A4, enhancing the bioavailability of drugs such as felodipine. Some foods may chelate medications (e.g., calcium binding to tetracyclines), diminishing absorption (Buxton, 2023). In dentistry, such interactions are also clinically relevant, for example, tetracyclines used for periodontal infections interact with dairy products, metronidazole (used for anaerobic dental infections) interacts adversely with alcohol, and NSAIDs such as ibuprofen, commonly prescribed for dental pain, may cause gastric irritation when taken on an empty stomach.

The degree of ionization influences solubility and membrane permeability. Non-ionized forms are more lipophilic and better absorbed. Reduced particle size and improved formulations, such as nanoparticles, enhance solubility and absorption. Drug stability is essential, as drugs must survive the acidic conditions of the stomach and withstand enzymatic breakdown in the GI system to ensure adequate absorption. Enteric coatings are often used to protect acid-sensitive medications such as omeprazole. Additional medication-related properties include the route of administration and pharmaceutical formulation, as oral dosage forms (tablets, capsules, solutions) vary in their dissolution and absorption rates. Controlled-release formulations may delay absorption while maintaining consistent levels. Parenteral routes, such as intravenous administration, bypass absorption obstacles, ensuring 100% bioavailability. Other routes, such as intramuscular or subcutaneous, may exhibit inconsistent absorption. The sublingual and buccal routes bypass first-pass metabolism, enhancing the bioavailability of certain drugs. The dose and dosing regimen of Active Pharmaceutical Ingredients (API) pertain to the fraction of the dosage that reaches systemic circulation, influencing effectiveness. Therefore, a drug's bioavailability must be considered when designing a treatment and dose. Effective dosage adjustment requires understanding the API's absorption, transport processes, metabolism, and systemic elimination (Olivares et al., 2014; Doogue & Polasek, 2013). Transport mechanisms also affect bioavailability. Most drugs are absorbed via passive diffusion, which depends on concentration gradients and lipophilicity, while others depend on carrier proteins for absorption via active transport (e.g., levodopa via amino acid transporters). For example, lipophilic local anesthetics such as lidocaine are absorbed through passive diffusion across oral and mucosal tissues. Other proteins, such as P-glycoprotein, may extrude drugs back into the intestinal lumen, diminishing bioavailability. The first-pass effect is a critical physiological component that may influence drug bioavailability. Orally administered drugs may be degraded in the GI lumen or metabolized before entering systemic circulation, a process referred to as the first-pass effect. This phenomenon can markedly diminish the bioavailability of drugs, particularly those with high extraction ratios, as they undergo considerable hepatic metabolism before entering the circulatory system. Labetalol, an antihypertensive agent, has significant hepatic first-pass metabolism, resulting in an absolute bioavailability of around 25%, similarly, morphine, sometimes used for severe dental pain, undergoes extensive first-pass hepatic metabolism, resulting in an oral bioavailability of approximately 19–47% (MacCarthy & Bloomfield, 1983; Christrup, 1997; Buxton, 2023).

2.1.1.2. Distribution

Once absorbed, the drug is distributed throughout the body. The volume of distribution (Vd) is a key parameter that relates the amount of drug in the body to its concentration in the blood or plasma. Factors influencing distribution include blood flow to tissues, the drug's affinity for tissue binding, and its ability to cross cell membranes. There are two phases of drug distribution: the first phase involves distribution to well-perfused organs such as the liver, kidney, heart, and brain; the second phase is slower, taking minutes to hours, and involves distribution to less-perfused tissues such as muscle, skin, fat, and bone. Highly lipophilic drugs may have a larger volume of distribution as they penetrate more readily and preferentially accumulate in fatty tissues. Only unbound drug molecules can distribute into tissues, making the fraction unbound (fu) an important consideration. Barriers such as the blood-brain barrier (BBB) can affect drug distribution. The BBB is composed of tightly connected cells in the brain, forming a selective barrier. Penetration of the

BBB depends on the lipid solubility and ionization of the drug; non-ionized, lipid-soluble drugs cross more easily. Conditions such as edema can compromise the integrity of the BBB, making it more permeable (Buxton, 2023; Dong, 2018; Feucht & Patel, 2011).

The Volume of Distribution (Vd) is a pharmacokinetic parameter representing the theoretical volume required to contain the total amount of drug in the body at the same concentration as in the plasma. It is not a physical volume but indicates the proportion of drug in tissues versus plasma. Factors such as lipid solubility and plasma protein binding affect the volume of distribution. For example, warfarin has a Vd of 10 L/70 kg, reflecting a high degree of plasma protein binding (Holford, 1986), while the antimalarial drug chloroquine has a Vd of 200 to 800 L/kg, indicating highly lipophilic molecules that are extensively distributed and sequestered into total body fat (Ducharme & Farinotti, 1996). Clindamycin, with a Vd of about 0.9 L/kg, is favored for its excellent diffusion into oral and maxillofacial spaces, particularly in penicillin-allergic patients. The clinical significance of Vd lies in its influence on drug dosing, plasma concentrations, and therapeutic effects, especially across different age groups and physiological states.

Total body water (TBW) decreases with age, but intracellular water remains relatively stable from infancy through adulthood. TBW typically comprises about 75% of an infant's body weight, compared to 50–60% in older persons (Luckey & Parsa, 2003). Younger children require higher doses of drugs per kilogram of body weight because they have a higher percentage of water. The decrease in body water content with age significantly impacts medication dosing in the elderly, primarily due to a reduction in lean body mass and an increase in body fat. This change in body composition affects drug distribution. Water-soluble drugs, which distribute primarily in the body's water, will have a smaller Vd in older adults, resulting in a higher initial drug concentration in the plasma. Lipophilic drugs tend to concentrate in areas with high lipid content. Body fat distribution varies with age, gender, and genetics, influencing drug distribution. Lipid-soluble drugs will have a larger Vd in older adults due to the increased proportion of body fat, leading to a prolonged elimination half-life and a longer duration of effect (Luckey & Parsa, 2003). Many drugs bind to plasma proteins, particularly albumin and globulins. Plasma protein levels are affected by age, nutritional status, and disease. Understanding protein binding is critical for clinicians to predict drug distribution and pharmacokinetics. In dental practice, this concept is clinically relevant because highly protein-bound drugs such as ibuprofen and warfarin may compete for albumin binding sites, increasing the risk of bleeding when co-administered (Guzzi & Bartucci, 2022) .

Only unbound (free) drugs can cross the blood/tissue barrier and engage with receptors. Numerous factors may influence binding, including protein content, pH levels, metabolic circumstances (e.g., hyperglycemia, uremia), and the presence of competing chemicals. The volume of distribution is used to calculate the desired loading dose (D): $D = Ct \times Vd$, where Ct is the desired concentration and Vd is the volume of distribution. The main goal of dose loading is to reach an effective target steady-state concentration (Css) earlier, resulting in a faster clinical response (Brunton, 2011). Loading doses are higher than maintenance doses and are often provided in a single bolus; however, certain medicines (such as amiodarone or digoxin) may require multiple loading doses over several hours to days (Miniaci & Gupta, 2023). Drugs can compete for plasma protein binding sites. For example, valproate displaces phenytoin from plasma proteins, resulting in an increased concentration of free phenytoin, which may amplify medication effects and increase phenytoin toxicity (Bourgeois, 1988). Additionally, drugs that cross the placenta must be chosen carefully to avoid harm to the fetus. In dental settings, this interaction is clinically relevant because phenytoin, used in seizure control, may cause gingival hyperplasia, and displacement by other drugs can heighten its adverse effects. Likewise, NSAIDs such as ibuprofen, frequently prescribed for dental pain, can displace warfarin from albumin binding sites, potentiating anticoagulant effects and increasing the risk of bleeding during dental procedures. Additionally, drugs that cross the placenta, such as tetracyclines, sometimes used in dental infections, must be avoided during pregnancy to prevent tooth discoloration and fetal bone defects (Niebyl, 2003; Droździk& Droździk, 2023; Teoh et al., 2020).

2.1.1.3. Metabolism

Metabolism, primarily occurring in the liver, transforms drugs into more water-soluble compounds for easier excretion. The process is divided into two phases: Phase I and Phase II. Phase I involves oxidation, reduction, and hydrolysis, introducing or exposing a functional group to prepare for Phase II. This process is carried out mainly by the CYP family of enzymes. Phase II reactions conjugate a molecule such as glucuronic acid, sulfate, or glutathione to create a more polar (water-soluble) molecule. Other organs such as the GI tract, kidneys, and lungs can also metabolize drugs. Clearance is the rate at which a drug is removed from the body, defined as the volume of blood or plasma cleared of the drug per unit of time. Clearance can refer to blood clearance, plasma clearance, or clearance based on the unbound (active) drug. The total systemic clearance is the sum of clearances from all organs, mainly the liver and kidneys. Both organs remove drugs from the body, and the extraction ratio (ER) is the extent to which an organ removes a drug from the blood, i.e., the fraction of the drug removed by the organ per unit time. High extraction ratio drugs (ER > 0.7) are removed quickly and extensively by the organ, usually the liver. Drugs with an ER < 0.3 are considered low extraction ratio drugs, cleared slowly and more susceptible to influences such as plasma protein binding and enzymatic activity. The extraction ratio is an important factor in determining hepatic clearance (CL_h), which is the volume of blood cleared of the drug by the liver per unit time. Hepatic clearance is influenced by three main factors: hepatic blood flow (Q), intrinsic clearance (CLint), and the fraction of unbound drug (fu). High extraction ratio drugs like morphine (ER > 0.7) are often limited by liver blood flow, while low extraction ratio drugs like warfarin (ER < 0.3) are more influenced by intrinsic clearance and plasma protein binding (Hsu et al., 2021).

Understanding drug metabolism is crucial for clinicians to ensure safe and effective prescribing. Drug metabolism determines how a drug is processed in the body, influencing its therapeutic effects, duration of action, and potential for adverse effects. Key clinical considerations include:

- Metabolism affects the bioavailability of a drug, i.e., the fraction of the administered dose that reaches systemic circulation in an active form. Some drugs, such as prodrugs (e.g., codeine), require metabolic activation to become therapeutically effective. Without proper metabolism, these drugs may fail to produce the desired effect (Dayer et al., 1988).
- Metabolism can convert drugs into inactive forms for excretion, but in some cases, it produces toxic metabolites. For example, acetaminophen is metabolized into a toxic compound N-acetyl-p-benzoquinone imine (NAPQI) in high doses, which can cause liver damage. Understanding metabolic pathways helps clinicians anticipate and prevent such toxic effects, especially in patients with compromised liver function (Mazaleuskaya et al., 2015).
- Genetic variations in drug-metabolizing enzymes (e.g., CYP450 enzymes) can lead to differences in drug metabolism among individuals. Poor metabolizers may experience drug accumulation and toxicity, while ultra-rapid metabolizers may clear the drug too

quickly, reducing its efficacy. Pharmacogenetic testing can guide dose adjustments and drug selection to optimize therapy for individual patients (Malsagova et al., 2020).

- Many drugs are metabolized by the same enzymes, leading to competition and potential interactions. For example, co-administration of alprazolam and erythromycin can increase alprazolam effects and toxicities (e.g., sedation, lethargy), as erythromycin is a moderate CYP3A4 inhibitor (Yasui et al., 1996). In contrast, coadministration of carbamazepine with apixaban can significantly decrease the anticoagulant effect of apixaban and increase the risk for stroke and pulmonary embolism, as carbamazepine is a strong inducer of CYP3A4 and P-glycoprotein (Gronich et al., 2021).
- Factors such as age, liver function, and comorbidities can alter drug metabolism. Elderly patients often have reduced liver enzyme activity, leading to slower drug clearance. Neonates have immature metabolic pathways, requiring careful dose adjustments. Patients with liver disease may have impaired metabolism, increasing the risk of drug accumulation and toxicity; thus, the dose of certain drugs should be adjusted based on liver function values (Tam, 1993).
- Knowledge of metabolism allows clinicians to determine appropriate dosing intervals and routes of administration. For drugs with extensive first-pass metabolism (e.g., nitroglycerin), alternative routes like intravenous or sublingual administration may be necessary to achieve therapeutic levels (Robertson, 2017). Patients with renal or hepatic impairment require tailored drug regimens based on metabolic considerations.

2.1.1.4. Excretion

Excretion is the final step in the pharmacokinetic process. Drugs are eliminated either unchanged or as metabolites, with the kidney being the most important organ for excretion. Other excretory pathways include the liver (via bile), feces, lungs, sweat, saliva, and breast milk. The efficiency of excretion depends on the polarity of the compounds, as polar substances are eliminated more readily than lipid-soluble ones, which often require metabolism to more hydrophilic forms before excretion (Zhang et al., 2021).

Renal excretion involves three main processes:

- Glomerular filtration: Drugs are filtered from the blood into the renal tubules at the glomerulus. Only unbound drugs (not bound to plasma proteins) are filtered, as protein-bound drugs are too large to pass through the glomerular membrane. The rate of filtration depends on the glomerular filtration rate (GFR) and the concentration of unbound drug in the plasma.
- Active tubular secretion: In the proximal tubule, drugs are actively secreted into the tubular fluid by carrier-mediated transport systems. There are specific transporters for acidic drugs (e.g., penicillin, furosemide) and basic drugs (e.g., dopamine, histamine). Tubular secretion is an energy-dependent process and can be saturated or competitively inhibited by other drugs.
- Passive tubular reabsorption: In the distal tubule, non-ionized forms of weak acids and bases can be reabsorbed back into the bloodstream by passive diffusion (Masereeuw & Russel, 2001). The extent of reabsorption depends on the drug's lipid solubility and the pH of the tubular fluid, which influences the ionization state of the drug. Alkalinization of urine (e.g., with sodium bicarbonate) can enhance the excretion of weak acids like aspirin, while acidification of urine can increase the excretion of weak bases.

The liver plays a significant role in drug excretion by secreting drugs and their metabolites into bile. Active transporters in the hepatocyte canalicular membrane facilitate the secretion of drugs into bile. Drugs excreted in bile may undergo enterohepatic recycling, where they are reabsorbed from the intestine back into the bloodstream, prolonging their presence in the body. Interrupting enterohepatic recycling (e.g., with bile acid sequestrants) can enhance drug elimination. Drugs that are not absorbed after oral administration or are secreted into bile are excreted in feces. Conjugated metabolites, such as glucuronides, may require enzymatic hydrolysis by intestinal bacteria before being reabsorbed or excreted (Hagenbuch, 2010).

The lungs are important for the excretion of volatile substances, such as anesthetic gases. Excretion via the lungs is rapid and depends on the drug's solubility in blood and its partial pressure gradient between blood and alveolar air (Varughese & Ahmed, 2021). Other routes, such as sweat, saliva, and breast milk, are quantitatively minor but can contribute to drug elimination. Lipid-soluble drugs may be excreted in sweat, potentially causing skin irritation. Drugs excreted in breast milk can affect nursing infants, especially those with immature metabolic systems. Basic drugs tend to concentrate in breast milk due to its slightly acidic pH compared to plasma (Arbitman et al., 2024; Pichai & Lakshmanan, 2019).

Half-life is defined as the time it takes for the concentration of the drug in the plasma to be reduced by 50%. The formula for half-life is:

$$T1/2 = \ln 2 \times V / CL$$

where ln2 is the natural log of 2, V is the volume of distribution, and CL is clearance. The elimination half-life (T1/2) is used to determine how long it takes for the body to clear the drug or for the concentration to reach half its original value (Andrade, 2022). The half-life is also used to calculate dosing frequency and predict how long a drug will remain in the body. A drug with a long half-life will take longer to reach steady-state concentration than a drug with a short half-life; however, the drug with the longer half-life may only need to be dosed once every 24 hours, while a drug with a short half-life reaches steady state quickly but requires more frequent dosing (Koen et al., 2008).

Understanding drug elimination has profound clinical implications for optimizing therapeutic outcomes, minimizing toxicity, and tailoring drug regimens to individual patient needs. Drug elimination directly influences the time required to reach steady-state concentrations. Steady-state concentration is defined as the dynamic equilibrium in which drug concentrations consistently stay within therapeutic limits for long, potentially indefinite periods. For most drugs, steady-state is achieved after approximately 4–5 half-lives (Ito, 2011). This knowledge helps clinicians design appropriate dosing intervals and loading doses, particularly for medications such as antibiotics, where maintaining effective plasma concentrations is essential for therapeutic success. The maintenance dose is the dose administered throughout a dosage regimen to maintain effective drug concentrations. The rate of drug elimination determines the maintenance dose required to sustain therapeutic drug levels. For example, drugs with high clearance rates require more frequent or higher doses to maintain efficacy (William & Sams, 2009). Drugs with long half-lives or reduced clearance (e.g., due to renal or hepatic impairment) can accumulate in the body, leading to toxicity. For instance, in elderly patients with declining renal function, antibiotics like gentamicin require dose adjustments to prevent adverse effects (Bailey et al., 1997). Measuring drug concentrations at steady-state allows clinicians to refine dosing regimens, especially for drugs with narrow therapeutic windows (e.g., phenytoin, tacrolimus) (Jain et al., 2021). Genetic variations in drug-metabolizing enzymes (e.g., CYP450 isoforms) can alter drug elimination rates. For example, variations in 2C9 metabolism lead to high interpatient variability in dosing requirements for anticoagulants like warfarin (Black et al., 1996; Pinto & Eileen, 2011). Conditions such as liver cirrhosis or renal failure can significantly impair drug elimination.

Understanding these effects allows for individualized dose adjustments to maintain therapeutic efficacy while minimizing harm. In situations requiring rapid therapeutic effects (e.g., arrhythmias treated with lidocaine), a loading dose can quickly achieve target drug concentrations. However, care must be taken to avoid toxicity, especially for drugs with small central volumes of distribution. For example, the coadministration of probenecid with penicillin or cephalosporins in the treatment of sexually transmitted diseases results in increased antibiotic concentrations due to probenecid inhibition of the OAT1/3 transporter, which is necessary for penicillin renal elimination (Craft et al., 1979). The elimination of weak acids (e.g., aspirin) or weak bases can be enhanced by altering urine pH. Alkalinizing the urine with sodium bicarbonate promotes the excretion of weak acids, a strategy used in aspirin overdose management (Proudfoot et al., 2002; Prescott et al., 1983). Lipid-soluble drugs like thiopental can redistribute into fat stores, prolonging their elimination and effects. Increased adipose tissue in obese patients increases the volume of distribution of thiopental sodium (Jung et al., 1982). Increased volume of distribution means lower drug plasma concentrations but a longer elimination time. Thus, the induction dose of thiopental is adjusted according to ideal body weight. Neonates have immature renal and hepatic systems, leading to slower drug elimination (Ruggiero et al., 2019). Conversely, elderly patients often experience reduced renal clearance, necessitating dose adjustments for renally excreted drugs (Ebert et al., 2017). Enhanced renal clearance during pregnancy can increase the elimination of certain drugs (e.g., cefazolin), requiring higher doses to maintain therapeutic levels, especially in obese patients (Davison & Dunlop, 1980; ACOG 2018; Dallmann et al., 2019).

2.1.2. Pharmacodynamics

Pharmacodynamics is the study of the biochemical, cellular, and physiological effects of drugs and their mechanisms of action. It focuses on how drugs interact with specific targets such as receptors, enzymes, ion channels, and transporters to produce therapeutic or adverse effects. Rather than creating new biological effects, drugs typically modify the rate or magnitude of existing cellular or physiological processes. These targets can be located on the cell surface, within the cytoplasm, or in the extracellular space. Receptors, including G protein-coupled receptors (GPCRs), ligand-gated ion channels, enzyme-linked receptors, and nuclear receptors, recognize signaling molecules (ligands) and translate this recognition into cellular responses (Rosenbaum et al., 2020; Hauser et al., 2017). In addition to receptors, drug targets may include enzymes, which can be inhibited or activated to alter metabolic or signaling pathways; ion channels, which regulate ion flow and cellular excitability; and transporters, which control the movement of substances across membranes.

2.1.2.1. Drug-Receptor Interactions

Drug-receptor interactions can be classified based on how different agents affect receptor activity. Agonists bind to receptors and mimic the action of endogenous ligands, thereby producing a biological response. Partial agonists also bind to receptors but elicit a weaker response compared to full agonists. Antagonists attach to receptors without activating them, effectively blocking the action of endogenous ligands or other agonists. Inverse agonists bind to the same receptors as agonists but induce the opposite effect, reducing the receptor's baseline activity. Additionally, allosteric modulators bind to sites on the receptor distinct from the active site and can either enhance or inhibit the receptor's response to its primary ligand (Barbosa et al., 2024; Śliwa et al., 2024).

2.1.2.2. Efficacy and Potency

Efficacy refers to the maximum effect that a drug is capable of producing, regardless of dose. In contrast, potency describes the concentration or dose of a drug needed to achieve 50% of its maximum effect, commonly expressed as EC50 or ED50. While efficacy indicates the upper limit of a drug's action, potency reflects how much of the drug is required to reach a specific level of response (Simon et al., 2024).

2.1.2.3. Concentration-Response Relationships

Drugs exhibit a dose-response relationship, which can be plotted as a curve to show the relationship between drug concentration and effect. The curve's shape depends on factors such as receptor affinity, spare receptors, and cooperative effects. Quantal dose-response curves are used to evaluate drug effects in populations, while graded dose-response curves focus on individual responses (Aronson, 2007).

2.1.2.4. Mechanisms of Drug Action

Drugs can act by activating or inhibiting signaling pathways, altering gene expression, or modulating physiological processes. Examples include β-adrenergic receptor antagonists reducing heart rate, or calcium channel blockers inhibiting calcium influx to relax vascular smooth muscle (Mitchell et al., 2023).

2.1.2.5. Pharmacodynamic Variability

Drug responses can differ greatly among individuals due to genetic, physiological, and environmental variables. This variability can lead to differences in drug efficacy, potency, or the likelihood of adverse effects, even when the same dose is administered to different individuals. Key factors contributing to pharmacodynamic variability include genetic polymorphisms (Roden et al., 2011), differences in receptor sensitivity and density (Gordon & Marianela, 2010), age (Lamy, 1991), gender and hormonal differences (Soldin & Mattison, 2009), disease states (Keller & Hann, 2018), drug interactions (Niu et al., 2019), tolerance and sensitization (William, 2015), immune responses, placebo (positive) and nocebo (negative) effects (Colloca & Miller, 2011; Modell & Garrett, 1960), and environmental and lifestyle factors (Vesell, 1991).

2.1.2.6. Drug Tolerance and Sensitization

A reduced response to a drug over time, often due to receptor desensitization or downregulation, is called drug tolerance (Altman et al., 1996). Drug tolerance differs significantly from drug resistance, which describes the innate or baseline magnitude of drug responsivity. For example, prolonged use of opioids or alcohol can lead to tolerance, requiring higher doses for the same effect. Tolerance may be classified into two types: pharmacokinetic (metabolic) tolerance and pharmacodynamic (functional) tolerance. In pharmacokinetic tolerance, alterations in drug metabolism and/or distribution lead to a reduced response because less of the medication reaches the target organ. In contrast, pharmacodynamic tolerance occurs due to diminished sensitivity or responsiveness at the target site of action (e.g., receptors, signaling molecules in the brain) (Howard et al., 2013).

Sensitization, conversely, is the opposite of tolerance. Sensitization refers to an increased response to a drug after repeated exposure, often due to upregulation of receptors. Repeated use of methamphetamine, for example, can lead to increased behavioral responses, such as hyperactivity or stereotyped behaviors, with the same dose (Pierce & Kalivas, 1997).

2.1.2.7. Hysteresis in Drug Response

Hysteresis refers to a time-dependent relationship between drug concentration and effect. In counterclockwise hysteresis, the effect is greater at a later time for the same concentration, often due to delayed drug distribution to the site of action or accumulation of active metabolites. In clockwise hysteresis, the effect diminishes over time for the same concentration, often due to tolerance or the accumulation of antagonistic metabolites (Louizos et al., 2014).

2.1.2.8. Pharmacodynamic Drug Interactions

Pharmacodynamic drug-drug interactions (DDIs) arise when the pharmacological effect of one drug is modified by the presence of another drug in combination therapy. Drugs can interact to provide additive, synergistic, or antagonistic effects. In additive effects, the total impact is the sum of individual effects; in synergistic effects, the total effect exceeds the sum of individual effects; in antagonistic effects, one drug diminishes or inhibits the effect of another (Niu et al., 2019). Examples of pharmacodynamic interactions include the simultaneous administration of an NSAID and phenprocoumon (additive interaction), or aspirin and ibuprofen (antagonistic interaction) (Cascorbi, 2012).

2.1.2.9. Clinical Significance of Understanding Drug Pharmacodynamics

Understanding the pharmacodynamics (PD) of drugs is of immense clinical significance, as it provides the foundation for optimizing drug therapy, improving therapeutic outcomes, and minimizing adverse effects. Pharmacodynamics focuses on the relationship between drug concentration and the resulting effect, which is critical for tailoring drug therapy to individual patients. Variability in drug response among individuals can arise from differences in receptor sensitivity, genetic factors, age, disease states, and concurrent drug use. For example:

- Genetic polymorphisms in drug targets, such as receptors or enzymes, can alter drug efficacy or safety. For instance, the upregulation of dihydrofolate reductase (DHFR) in cancer cells can lead to resistance to methotrexate, necessitating alternative therapies (Meng et al., 2024).

- Pharmacodynamic parameters can differ significantly in neonates, children, and the elderly. For example, elderly patients may exhibit altered receptor sensitivity, requiring dose adjustments to avoid toxicity (Drenth et al., 2020).
- Advances in pharmacogenomics allow clinicians to predict drug responses based on genetic biomarkers, such as the HER2/neu receptor for trastuzumab in breast cancer (Seidman et al., 2008) or the V600E mutation in melanoma for vemurafenib (Chapman et al., 2011). This ensures that the right drug is given to the right patient at the right dose.
- Pharmacodynamics provides critical insights into the dose-response relationship, which helps clinicians determine the appropriate dose to achieve the desired therapeutic effect while minimizing toxicity. Understanding the maximum effect a drug can produce (efficacy) and the concentration required to achieve half of this effect (potency) allows for rational drug selection. For example, a drug with a lower EC50 is more potent and may require a lower dose to achieve the same effect.
- The therapeutic window represents the range of drug concentrations that provide efficacy with minimal toxicity. Drugs like warfarin, which have a narrow therapeutic window, require careful monitoring of pharmacodynamic markers (e.g., International Normalized Ratio, INR) to avoid complications such as bleeding or clot formation (Burns, 1999). Incorporating baseline physiological values (e.g., blood pressure, heart rate) into pharmacodynamic models ensures that drug effects are accurately measured and adjusted for individual patients (Colburn & Lee, 2003).

Pharmacodynamic drug interactions can significantly impact clinical outcomes, either by enhancing therapeutic effects or increasing the risk of adverse effects. Examples include:

- Combining drugs with similar mechanisms of action can lead to additive or synergistic effects. For instance, combining nitroglycerin (a nitric oxide donor) with sildenafil or tadalafil (Phosphodiesterase type 5 inhibitors) can cause profound vasodilation and catastrophic hypotension, highlighting the need for careful drug selection (Webb et al., 2000).

- Co-administration of drugs that prolong the corrected QT(QTc) interval increases the risk of life-threatening arrhythmias, such as torsades de pointes. Understanding these interactions helps clinicians avoid harmful combinations (Li & Ramos, 2017).
- Drugs like warfarin are highly sensitive to dietary vitamin K intake (de Carvalho Minighini et al., 2020) and interactions with other drugs (e.g., NSAIDs), which can enhance the risk of bleeding (Choi et al., 2010). Pharmacodynamic knowledge allows for appropriate dose adjustments and monitoring.
- Pharmacodynamic principles explain phenomena such as tolerance, resistance, and supersensitivity, which are critical for long-term drug therapy. Repeated drug exposure can lead to reduced efficacy due to receptor desensitization or downregulation. For instance, prolonged use of opioids frequently leads to tolerance, meaning higher doses are needed to achieve the same level of pain relief. In antimicrobial and cancer therapy, resistance mechanisms (e.g., altered drug targets, enhanced efflux, or alternative pathways) can render drugs ineffective (Lei et al., 2023). Understanding these mechanisms allows clinicians to modify treatment strategies, such as using combination therapies to overcome resistance. Abrupt withdrawal of antagonists, such as β-blockers, can lead to supersensitivity and rebound effects, such as increased heart rate and blood pressure. Gradual tapering of the drug can prevent these adverse outcomes (Reidenberg, 2011).
- Pharmacodynamic models, such as the Emax and sigmoid Emax models, help clinicians predict drug effects at different concentrations and guide dose adjustments. For example:
- Monitoring the area under the curve (AUC) for vancomycin ensures that drug concentrations remain within the therapeutic range (400–600 mg*hr/L) to maximize efficacy against Methicillin-Resistant *Staphylococcus aureus* (MRSA) while minimizing nephrotoxicity (Rybak et al., 2020).
- Drugs like β-blockers, ACE inhibitors, and calcium channel blockers target different pathways to lower blood pressure. Understanding their pharmacodynamic effects allows for combination therapy to achieve optimal blood pressure control while minimizing side effects.

- Pharmacodynamic knowledge is essential for identifying and managing adverse drug reactions (ADRs), which can result from off-target effects or excessive drug action. Drugs like sotalol, which is a racemic mixture, exhibit different pharmacodynamic properties for each enantiomer. The L-enantiomer is a potent β-blocker, while both enantiomers block K+ channels, increasing the risk of QT prolongation (Funck, 1993). Active metabolites, such as NAPQI (a toxic metabolite of acetaminophen), can cause severe toxicity (Bender et al., 2004). Pharmacodynamic understanding helps clinicians anticipate and mitigate these risks.
- Pharmacodynamics plays a crucial role in antimicrobial therapy by targeting unique microbial structures and pathways, ensuring selective toxicity. For example, combining antimicrobial drugs with different mechanisms of action can enhance efficacy and prevent resistance. Selection of drugs should depend on local susceptibility patterns, clinical experience, site of infection, potential toxicities, and cost (Rybak et al., 1996).
- Pharmacodynamics is central to the development of precision medicine, which aims to optimize drug therapy based on individual patient characteristics. For example, genetic biomarkers, such as the Philadelphia chromosome in chronic myelogenous leukemia, guide the use of targeted therapies like nilotinib (Sampaio et al., 2021). Advances in gene therapy, such as the use of adeno-associated virus (AAV) vectors engineered to deliver DNA to target cells, rely on pharmacodynamic principles to achieve therapeutic effects while minimizing off-target actions (Naso et al., 2017).

2.1.3. Adverse Drug Reactions

Adverse drug reactions (ADRs) are a significant concern in clinical practice, as they can lead to patient harm, increased healthcare costs, and reduced trust in medical treatments.

2.1.3.1. Definition of Adverse Drug Reactions

The World Health Organization (WHO) defines an adverse drug reaction as "a response to a drug that is noxious and unintended and occurs at doses normally used in humans for the prophylaxis, diagnosis, or therapy of disease, or for modification of physiological function" (WHO, 1972). This definition excludes reactions caused by overdose, drug abuse, or medication errors. A more precise definition by Edwards and Aronson describes an ADR as "an appreciably harmful or unpleasant reaction resulting from an intervention related to the use of a medicinal product, which predicts hazard from future administration and warrants prevention, specific treatment, alteration of the dosage regimen, or withdrawal of the product." This definition emphasizes the clinical significance of ADRs and their potential to impact future treatment decisions (Edwards & Aronson, 2000).

It is important to differentiate between ADRs and adverse drug events (ADEs). ADRs are harmful and unintended reactions caused by drugs at normal doses, while ADEs include all untoward events during drug use, regardless of causality. Similarly, side effects are predictable and often less severe than ADRs, and are related to the drug's pharmacological action (Edwards & Aronson, 2000).

2.1.3.2. Classification of Adverse Drug Reactions

ADRs are classified into six main types, often remembered using the mnemonic ABCDE:

- Type A (Augmented): Dose-related, predictable, and related to the pharmacological action of the drug. For example, hypoglycemia caused by insulin or hypotension caused by beta-blockers. These reactions can often be managed by reducing the dose or withdrawing the drug.
- Type B (Bizarre): Non-dose-related, unpredictable, and often immunological or idiosyncratic in nature. Examples include anaphylaxis caused by penicillin or aplastic anemia caused by chloramphenicol. Management involves discontinuing the drug and avoiding re-exposure.
- Type C (Chronic): Dose-related and time-related, occurring due to cumulative drug exposure. For example, corticosteroids can suppress the hypothalamic-pituitary-adrenal (HPA) axis, which can be managed by gradually tapering the drug or reducing the dose.
- Type D (Delayed): Time-related, occurring after prolonged use or even after the drug has been discontinued. For example, thalidomide can cause teratogenic effects, and some anticancer drugs are

associated with carcinogenesis. Prevention is key, as these reactions are often intractable.

- Type E (End of Use): Withdrawal reactions occurring after discontinuation of a drug. Examples include opiate withdrawal syndrome and rebound hypertension following the discontinuation of beta-blockers. These conditions can be managed by reintroducing the drug and then gradually tapering the dose.
- Type F (Failure of Therapy): The unexpected inability of a drug to produce its intended therapeutic effect. For example, inadequate contraception can occur when drug interactions with enzyme inducers reduce the effectiveness of contraceptive medications. Management involves adjusting the dose or considering alternative therapies (Hartigan & Wong, 2018; Zazzara et al., 2021).

2.1.3.2.1. Allergic Reactions (Drug Allergy)

An allergic reaction is an immunologically mediated response to a drug that is unrelated to its pharmacological action (Khan & Solensky, 2010). These reactions are unpredictable, not dose-related, and can occur even with small doses (e.g., anaphylaxis caused by penicillin). Allergic drug reactions are classified as Type B (bizarre) ADRs, which are unpredictable and immunologically mediated. There are four main types:

- Type I (Immediate hypersensitivity): IgE-mediated reactions that occur rapidly after drug exposure, resulting in symptoms such as urticaria, angioedema, bronchospasm, and anaphylaxis (e.g., anaphylaxis from penicillin, angioedema from angiotensin converting enzyme inhibitors) (Warrington & Silviu, 2011; Edwards & Aronson, 2000).
- Type II (Cytotoxic hypersensitivity): Involves IgG or IgM antibodies targeting drug-bound cells, leading to cell destruction and conditions such as hemolytic anemia, thrombocytopenia, and neutropenia (e.g., hemolysis from methyldopa, thrombocytopenia from quinine) (Bajwa & Mohammed, 2023).
- Type III (Immune complex-mediated hypersensitivity): Characterized by the formation of immune complexes that deposit in tissues and cause inflammation, resulting in symptoms like serum sickness, vasculitis, fever, and arthralgia (e.g., serum sickness from

antitoxins or monoclonal antibodies, vasculitis from hydralazine) (Usman & Annamaraju, 2023).
- Type IV (Delayed hypersensitivity): T-cell-mediated reactions that occur days to weeks after drug exposure, manifesting as contact dermatitis, Stevens-Johnson syndrome (SJS), or toxic epidermal necrolysis (TEN), with SJS often associated with sulfonamides and TEN with carbamazepine (Marwa et al., 2025).

2.1.3.3. Mechanisms of Adverse Drug Reactions
ADRs can occur through various mechanisms, including:

- Exaggeration of the drug's intended therapeutic action (e.g., excessive anticoagulation with warfarin)
- Unintended effects unrelated to the primary therapeutic action (e.g., diarrhea caused by antibiotics)
- Immunological reactions (e.g., anaphylaxis or drug-induced rash)
- Idiosyncratic reactions (genetically determined abnormal responses, such as hemolysis in Glucose-6-Phosphate Dehydrogenase -deficient individuals)
- Drug interactions that alter the pharmacokinetics or pharmacodynamics of another drug, leading to enhanced toxicity or reduced efficacy
- Genetic factors, such as polymorphisms in drug-metabolizing enzymes (e.g., CYP450), which can predispose individuals to ADRs (Kommu et al., 2024).

2.1.3.4. Diagnosis of Adverse Drug Reactions
Diagnosing ADRs requires a systematic approach, utilizing established ADR reporting systems through which healthcare providers assess the likelihood that a drug caused an adverse reaction. This evaluation is often guided by standardized tools such as the *Naranjo Causality Scale*, which helps determine the probability of a causal relationship between the suspected drug and the observed effect (Naranjo et al., 1981; Misra et al., 2025). The diagnostic process typically includes:

- A thorough medication history (including prescription drugs, over-the-counter medications, herbal products, and supplements)

- Determining the temporal relationship between drug administration and symptom onset
- Comparing the observed response to established ADR patterns for the suspected medication
- Laboratory testing (e.g., liver or kidney function tests) to assess organ damage
- In some cases, allergy testing or drug rechallenge may be necessary.

2.1.3.5. Management of Adverse Drug Reactions

Management of ADRs involves several steps:

- Discontinue the suspected drug if possible
- Provide symptomatic treatment (e.g., antihistamines for allergic reactions, corticosteroids for severe inflammation)
- Administer antidotes when available (e.g., naloxone for opioid overdose, acetylcysteine for paracetamol toxicity)
- Provide supportive measures (e.g., intravenous fluids, oxygen, mechanical ventilation) as needed
- If the drug is essential, consider reintroducing it at a lower dose or using an alternative drug
- Monitor the patient closely for recurrence or progression of symptoms (Kommu et al., 2024).

2.1.3.6. Prevention of Adverse Drug Reactions

Preventing ADRs is a critical aspect of patient safety and can be achieved by:

- Educating patients about potential side effects and the importance of adherence to prescribed doses
- Using the lowest effective dose for the shortest duration
- Avoiding polypharmacy whenever possible
- Regularly monitoring patients on high-risk drugs (e.g., anticoagulants, immunosuppressants)
- Considering genetic testing for drugs with known genetic predispositions to ADRs (e.g., HLA-B*5701 testing for abacavir hypersensitivity)
- Encouraging healthcare professionals to report ADRs to pharmacovigilance programs to improve drug safety data (Kommu et al., 2024).

2.1.3.7. Pharmacovigilance and ADR Reporting

Pharmacovigilance is the science of detecting, assessing, understanding, and preventing ADRs. It plays a vital role in ensuring drug safety. Reporting ADRs helps identify new safety concerns and improves the safe use of medicines. WHO's Adverse Reaction Terminology (WHO-ART) and MedDRA are widely used for ADR reporting (Brown, 2002). In India, the Pharmacovigilance Programme of India (PvPI) collects and analyzes ADR data (Gupta, 2010). In Türkiye, the pharmacovigilance center TÜFAM operates under the Regulation on the Safety of Drugs (Güner & Ekmekci, 2019; Ozcan et al., 2016).

Underreporting and lack of awareness among healthcare professionals remain significant barriers. Advances in technology and pharmacogenomics hold promise for improving ADR prediction and prevention. Key advancements include the use of artificial intelligence to analyze large datasets and detect patterns of adverse drug reactions, the customization of drug therapy according to genetic profiles to reduce ADR risk, and the enhancement of pharmacovigilance systems for real-time monitoring and improved surveillance of ADRs (Serrano et al., 2024). While adverse drug reactions are an inevitable aspect of drug therapy, their impact can be minimized through careful prescribing, patient education, and robust pharmacovigilance systems. By understanding the mechanisms, classifications, and management strategies for ADRs, healthcare professionals can improve patient safety and optimize therapeutic outcomes.

2.1.4. Drug Interactions

Drug interactions are a critical aspect of pharmacology and clinical practice, as they can significantly impact the efficacy and safety of medications. A drug interaction occurs when the pharmacological or clinical effects of one drug are altered by the presence of another drug, food, disease, or environmental factor.

2.1.4.1. Drug-Food Interactions

Drug-food interactions occur when the consumption of certain foods or beverages affects the pharmacokinetics or pharmacodynamics of a drug. For example, grapefruit juice is a well-documented inhibitor of the cytochrome P450 enzyme CYP3A4, leading to increased plasma concentrations of drugs like statins, calcium channel blockers, and immunosuppressants, which can result in toxicity. Similarly, high-protein diets can increase the metabolism of drugs like propranolol, while foods rich in vitamin K (such as spinach and kale) can antagonize the effects of warfarin, reducing its anticoagulant efficacy.

2.1.4.2. Drug-Disease Interactions

Drug-disease interactions occur when a drug exacerbates an existing medical condition or when the disease alters the drug's pharmacological effects. For instance, nonsteroidal anti-inflammatory drugs (NSAIDs) can worsen chronic kidney disease by reducing renal perfusion, while beta-blockers may exacerbate symptoms in patients with asthma or chronic obstructive pulmonary disease (COPD) by causing bronchoconstriction. Chronic conditions like diabetes, heart failure, and depression are particularly prone to drug-disease interactions, as highlighted in the United Kingdom National Institute for Health and Care Excellence (NICE) guidelines, where comorbidities such as chronic kidney disease often necessitate dose adjustments or alternative therapies. Understanding these interactions is essential for optimizing drug therapy, minimizing adverse effects, and ensuring patient safety (Dumbreck et al., 2015; Bushra et al., 2011).

2.1.4.3. Types of Drug-Drug Interactions

Drug-drug interactions are broadly classified into three categories: pharmacodynamic interactions, pharmacokinetic interactions, and pharmaceutical incompatibilities. Each type has distinct mechanisms and clinical implications.

2.1.4.3.1. Pharmacodynamic Interactions

Pharmacodynamic interactions occur when two drugs influence each other's effects at the site of action. These interactions can be classified into three subtypes:

- Interactions at the same receptor site: Drugs compete for the same receptor, leading to either antagonistic or synergistic effects. For example, naloxone reverses the effects of opioids by competitively binding to opioid receptors, and flumazenil antagonizes benzodiazepines at gamma-aminobutyric acid (GABA) receptors (Sivilotti, 2016).

- Interactions at different receptor sites: Drugs act on different receptors but produce additive or opposing effects. For example, beta-blockers (e.g., propranolol) and calcium channel blockers (e.g., verapamil) can both reduce heart rate, leading to bradycardia (Wołowiec et al., 2023). Beta-agonists (e.g., salbutamol) and beta-blockers (e.g., atenolol) may counteract each other's effects.
- Non-specific interactions: Drugs interact through undefined mechanisms, often leading to additive or synergistic effects. For example, thiopentone and midazolam exhibit synergy during anesthesia induction, reducing the required dose of each drug. Nitrous oxide and volatile anesthetics show summation, where their combined effects are additive (Knuf & Maani, 2025).

2.1.4.3.2. Pharmacokinetic Interactions

Pharmacokinetic interactions occur when one drug affects the absorption, distribution, metabolism, or excretion of another. Examples include:

- Drugs may modify stomach pH, motility, or enzyme activity, impacting the absorption of other drugs. For example, antacids inhibit tetracycline absorption by generating insoluble complexes, while metoclopramide accelerates gastric emptying, improving the absorption of drugs like paracetamol.
- Drugs can compete for plasma protein binding sites, raising the free concentration of one drug. For example, aspirin displaces warfarin, increasing the risk of bleeding.
- Medications can stimulate or inhibit liver enzymes, affecting the metabolism of other drugs. Enzyme inducers (such as rifampicin and phenytoin) decrease the effectiveness of warfarin by increasing its metabolism, while enzyme inhibitors (e.g., amiodarone, erythromycin) raise the plasma levels of drugs like warfarin, causing toxicity.
- Drugs can impact renal clearance by influencing glomerular filtration, tubular secretion, and reabsorption. Probenecid decreases penicillin's renal excretion, extending its half-life. Sodium bicarbonate alkalizes urine, increasing the excretion of weak acids such as aspirin (Torrent Rodríguez et al., 2024).

2.1.4.3.3. Pharmaceutical Incompatibilities

Pharmaceutical interactions can arise from physical or chemical incompatibilities between drugs, which may cause precipitation or loss of drug activity. For instance, combining thiopentone with suxamethonium leads to the formation of a precipitate (Khan et al., 2011). Similarly, mixing calcium chloride with sodium bicarbonate produces insoluble calcium carbonate (Bentley et al., 2015).

2.1.4.4. Detection of Drug Interactions

Identifying drug interactions is essential for preventing adverse consequences. Common methods include:

- Comprehensive assessment of the patient's medication history, including prescription drugs, over-the-counter medications, and supplements. For example, recognizing a patient on warfarin and aspirin, which increases the risk of hemorrhage.
- Identifying patterns in established drug interactions based on pharmacological properties, such as recognizing that combining beta-blockers and calcium channel blockers may induce bradycardia.
- Monitoring drug levels, organ function, and biomarkers to facilitate the identification of interactions. For example, INR assessment in warfarin patients to evaluate the impact of enzyme inducers or inhibitors.
- Utilizing resources such as Lexi-comp, Micromedex, and Medscape, which provide extensive information on drug interactions. Lexi-comp and Micromedex have shown the best performance (Kheshti et al., 2016).
- Temporary discontinuation of a suspected drug (dechallenge) followed by its reintroduction (rechallenge) to confirm an interaction. For example, discontinuing a suspected drug that induces bradycardia and monitoring for symptom remission.

2.1.4.5. Management of Drug Interactions

Managing drug interactions involves several strategies to mitigate risks and enhance therapeutic outcomes:

- Avoid prescribing medications with known severe interactions unless absolutely necessary (e.g., avoid co-administering monoamine oxidase inhibitors (MAOIs) with sympathomimetics to prevent hypertensive crises).

- Modify the dosage of one or both medications to minimize interaction risks (e.g., decrease the dosage of warfarin when starting amiodarone therapy).
- Consistent monitoring of drug concentrations and clinical indicators to identify and manage interactions (e.g., monitoring potassium levels in patients on potassium-sparing diuretics and ACE inhibitors).
- Stagger the administration of conflicting medications to minimize the chance of interactions (e.g., administer antacids and tetracyclines at separate intervals to prevent chelation).
- Substitute one medication with a safer alternative that does not interact (e.g., use a selective serotonin reuptake inhibitor (SSRI) instead of a tricyclic antidepressant in patients on antihypertensive therapy).
- Educate patients about possible interactions and the importance of adhering to recommended treatments (e.g., advise patients on warfarin to avoid over-the-counter NSAIDs).

Conclusion

Drug interactions present a considerable challenge in clinical practice, especially among patients undergoing polypharmacy. Understanding the types of interactions, using effective detection techniques, and implementing appropriate management strategies are crucial for ensuring patient safety and treatment effectiveness. Clinicians must remain vigilant and utilize available resources, such as drug interaction databases, to mitigate the risks associated with drug interactions (Corrie & Hardman, 2020; Kheshti et al., 2016).

Chapter 3

Commonly Prescribed Medications in Dentistry

Abstract

This chapter presents a comprehensive overview of the principal medications prescribed in dental practice, emphasizing their pharmacological properties, clinical uses, and safety profiles. Analgesics including non-steroidal anti-inflammatory drugs (NSAIDs) and opioids are examined for their mechanisms, efficacy, and adverse effects in managing dental pain, with attention to evidence-based prescribing and regulatory considerations. The chapter also details the use of corticosteroids for their anti-inflammatory and immunosuppressive actions, discussing indications, contraindications, monitoring, and dose tapering. Antibiotics are reviewed for their role in preventing and treating oral infections, while local and general anesthetics, as well as sedatives, are discussed in the context of pain control and patient comfort during dental procedures. Additionally, the chapter covers topical agents for oral conditions and prescription-strength oral hygiene products for disease prevention and management. Emphasis is placed on individualized drug selection, patient education, and adherence to clinical guidelines to ensure optimal and safe dental care.

Keywords: analgesics, non-steroidal anti-inflammatory drugs, opioids, corticosteroids, antibiotics, local anesthetics, general anesthesia, sedation, topical agents, oral hygiene products

3.1. Analgesics and Anti-Inflammatories

3.1.1. Introduction to Pain and Its Causes

Pain is a complex and multidimensional experience that serves as a protective mechanism, alerting the body to potential or actual tissue damage. It is defined as an unpleasant sensory and emotional experience associated with actual or potential tissue damage (Świeboda et al., 2013). Pain can be classified into acute and chronic pain. Acute pain, such as that experienced after dental procedures, is typically short-lived and resolves as the underlying cause is treated. Chronic pain, on the other hand, persists for at least three months and may result from conditions such as temporomandibular joint disorders or neuropathic pain (Cohen et al., 2021).

In dentistry, pain is a common reason for patients to seek treatment. Orofacial pain, which includes pain in the teeth, gums, jaw, and surrounding structures, can arise from various causes, including dental infections (e.g., caries, pulpitis, periodontal disease), trauma (e.g., dental injuries, temporomandibular joint injuries), neoplastic conditions (e.g., oral cancer), and craniofacial procedures (e.g., tooth extractions, implant placement). Phantom tooth pain is a condition resulting from peripheral nerve damage, central sensitization, and cortical reorganization. Other causes include nerve-related conditions such as trigeminal neuralgia and systemic diseases like diabetes or viral infections (Ing, 2017; Conti et al., 2021; Evans & McCahon, 2019; Pergolizzi et al., 2020; Gambeta et al., 2020; Treede et al., 2015; Joseph et al., 2000).

The mechanisms of pain involve four stages: transduction, transmission, modulation, and perception. Transduction refers to the conversion of a damaging stimulus into an electrical impulse. Transmission involves the conduction of this impulse to the central nervous system. Modulation includes the amplification or inhibition of pain signals, while perception is the conscious awareness of pain, often accompanied by emotional and psychological responses (Porreca & Navratilova, 2017).

Dental pain is unique due to the anatomy and physiology of the oral cavity. The pulp–dentin complex, a richly innervated and vascularized structure, plays a central role in dental pain. Pain in this region can be classified into two types based on the nerve fibers involved: A-fibers and C-fibers. A-fibers are responsible for sharp, localized pain, such as dentin hypersensitivity, while C-fibers mediate dull, throbbing pain associated with pulpitis (Jain et al., 2013). Common types of dental pain include dentin hypersensitivity, which is characterized by sharp, acute pain triggered by thermal, chemical, or mechanical stimuli and is often experienced during restorative procedures (Davari et al., 2013). Pulpal and periapical pain results from inflammation of the dental pulp or surrounding tissues and can present as either acute or chronic discomfort (Estrela et al., 2011). Postoperative pain frequently follows dental surgeries such as extractions or implant placements. Neuropathic pain, such as that seen in trigeminal neuralgia, arises from nerve inflammation or damage. Additionally, pain from oral mucosal diseases, including conditions like aphthous ulcers, oral lichen planus, or fungal infections, can cause significant discomfort (Renton, 2011).

3.1.2. Pharmacological Management of Pain in Dentistry

The management of dental pain involves a combination of diagnosis, dental treatment, and pharmacological intervention. Analgesics are the cornerstone of pharmacological pain management and are broadly classified into opioid and non-opioid analgesics. Non-opioid analgesics, particularly NSAIDs, are the most commonly used drugs in dentistry due to their efficacy in managing mild to moderate pain and inflammation.

3.1.2.1. Non-Steroidal Anti-Inflammatory Drugs (NSAIDS)

NSAIDs are a diverse group of drugs with analgesic, anti-inflammatory, and antipyretic properties. They work by inhibiting cyclooxygenase (COX) enzymes, which are responsible for the synthesis of prostaglandins. Prostaglandins play a key role in pain and inflammation by sensitizing nociceptors and promoting vasodilation and edema.

3.1.2.1.1. Mechanism of Action of NSAIDS

There are two main isoforms of COX enzymes: COX-1 and COX-2. COX-1 is constitutively expressed and involved in maintaining physiological functions such as gastric mucosal protection and platelet aggregation. COX-2, on the other hand, is inducible and primarily involved in the inflammatory response. Most NSAIDs inhibit both COX-1 and COX-2, leading to their therapeutic effects as well as adverse effects. Selective COX-2 inhibitors, such as celecoxib and etoricoxib, have been developed to minimize gastrointestinal side effects associated with COX-1 inhibition. Some NSAIDs, such as diclofenac and meloxicam, exhibit antioxidant properties and inhibit nuclear factor kappa B (NF-κB), further reducing inflammation. NSAIDs also reduce leukocyte migration and adhesion, contributing to their anti-inflammatory effects (Kotowska et al., 2023).

3.1.2.1.2. Classification of NSAIDs

NSAIDs are grouped into major chemical classes based on their molecular structure: salicylic acid derivatives such as acetylated salicylates (aspirin) and non-acetylated salicylates (diflunisal, salsalate); aryl and heteroaryl acetic acid derivatives (ibuprofen, fenoprofen, naproxen); indole and indene acetic acid derivatives (indomethacin, sulindac, etodolac); anthranilic acid derivatives (diclofenac, mefenamic acid); and enolic acid derivatives (piroxicam, meloxicam) (Bindu et al., 2020).

There is another classification for NSAIDs based on the type of prostaglandin-endoperoxide synthase (PGHS) interaction and selectivity. The bioconversion of arachidonic acid into inflammatory prostanoids (prostaglandins and prostacyclin) is facilitated by cyclooxygenase (COX), officially named PGHS enzymes (PGHS-1 and PGHS-2; COX-1 or COX-2), which are inhibited by NSAIDs. NSAIDs have different selectivity to these enzymes. Non-selective NSAIDs include ibuprofen, naproxen, diclofenac, and aspirin; they inhibit both COX-1 and COX-2. Selective COX-2 inhibitors (coxibs), including celecoxib, etoricoxib, and parecoxib, preferentially inhibit COX-2, reducing the risk of gastrointestinal side effects. Preferential COX-2 inhibitors include meloxicam, etodolac, and nabumetone. The classification of NSAIDs based on COX selectivity provides a framework for understanding their therapeutic effects and adverse event profiles. Nonselective NSAIDs are versatile but carry higher risks of GI and renal toxicity. Preferential and selective COX-2 inhibitors offer safer alternatives for specific patient populations, particularly those at risk of GI complications, but require caution in patients with cardiovascular risks. The choice of NSAID should be individualized based on patient-specific factors, including comorbidities and concurrent medications (Bindu et al., 2020; Arfeen et al., 2024).

Lastly, NSAIDs may be categorized as short-acting (plasma half-life under 6 hours), including aspirin, diclofenac, and ibuprofen, and long-acting (half-life beyond 10 hours), such as naproxen and celecoxib. Substances with a short half-life, such as ibuprofen, demonstrate rapid onset of action, making them appropriate for acute pain management. Naproxen has a prolonged half-life and is beneficial in managing chronic diseases (Conaghan, 2012).

3.1.2.1.3. Pharmacokinetics of NSAIDs

Pharmacokinetics refers to the absorption, distribution, metabolism, and excretion of drugs. NSAIDs share several pharmacokinetic properties, but they also exhibit significant differences that influence their clinical use. Most NSAIDs are rapidly absorbed after oral administration, with peak plasma concentrations typically reached within 1–3 hours; while food may delay absorption, it does not significantly affect the overall bioavailability of most NSAIDs (Verbeeck et al., 1983). Topical NSAIDs, such as diclofenac gels or mouthwashes, are absorbed locally in the oral cavity, resulting in lower systemic concentrations and a reduced risk of systemic side effects (Mishra et al., 2017). NSAIDs are highly protein-bound (primarily to albumin), with binding rates exceeding 90% (Davies & Skjodt, 2000), which limits their free, active form in plasma but ensures prolonged action. Their distribution to inflamed tissues is critical for their therapeutic effects; for example, lysine acetylsalicylate demonstrates superior dentin permeability, making it effective for pulp inflammation (Lin et al., 2019). NSAIDs are primarily metabolized in the liver via cytochrome P450 enzymes, and variations in metabolism can lead to differences in efficacy and toxicity among individuals. Diclofenac, for instance, undergoes hepatic first-pass metabolism, which lowers its bioavailability, while certain medications, including parecoxib and sulindac sulfide, are prodrugs that require hepatic metabolism to generate their active metabolites (Wongrakpanich et al., 2018). Most NSAIDs are excreted via the kidneys, either as unchanged drug (less than 5%) or as metabolites; however, renal impairment can prolong the half-life of NSAIDs, necessitating dose adjustments (Verbeeck et al., 1983). An overview of NSAID pharmacokinetics, pharmacodynamics, dosage forms, and precautions is provided in Table 1.

3.1.2.1.4. Clinical Applications of NSAIDs in Dentistry

NSAIDs are used in almost every field of dentistry (Kotowska et al., 2023). In restorative dentistry and endodontics, they are effective in managing pain associated with pulpitis and periapical inflammation and are often used as premedication to enhance the efficacy of local anesthetics. In dental surgery, NSAIDs are commonly prescribed for postoperative pain following extractions, implant placements, and other surgical procedures, with ibuprofen and diclofenac frequently recommended due to their efficacy and safety profile. In periodontology, NSAIDs help reduce inflammation and bone destruction in periodontal diseases, and topical formulations are particularly useful for localized gingivitis and mucositis. In orthodontics, NSAIDs alleviate pain associated with orthodontic tooth movement, although their long-term use is discouraged as they may interfere with bone remodeling. For oral mucosal diseases, topical NSAIDs are effective in managing pain and inflammation in conditions such as aphthous ulcers and oral lichen planus. Additionally, in head and neck oncology, NSAIDs are used to manage pain in patients undergoing radiotherapy for head and neck cancers and also exhibit potential anti-cancer properties by inhibiting tumor growth and metastasis (Singgih et al., 2020; Kotowska et al., 2023). Table 2 outlines the indications of NSAIDs for managing dental pain.

3.1.2.1.5. Differences among NSAIDS and Their Advantages and Disadvantages in Dental Pain Management

NSAIDs differ in their COX selectivity, potency, half-life, and safety profiles, which influence their clinical applications in dentistry (see Tables 1–3). Non-selective NSAIDs such as ibuprofen, naproxen, and diclofenac inhibit both COX-1 and COX-2, providing effective pain relief but with a higher risk of gastrointestinal side effects. Ibuprofen is the most commonly used NSAID in dentistry due to its favorable safety profile and efficacy in managing mild to moderate pain and inflammation. However, flurbiprofen is noted to have a longer duration of action compared to ibuprofen, which may make it more suitable for conditions requiring sustained pain relief. Additionally, flurbiprofen has been shown to have a stronger inhibitory effect on bone destruction in periodontal disease compared to ibuprofen, as it significantly reduces prostaglandin E2 (PGE2) levels, which are key mediators of inflammation and bone resorption. A study demonstrated that flurbiprofen significantly reduced bone mass loss in patients with periodontitis compared to placebo (Jeffcoat et al., 1988). This suggests that flurbiprofen may have a superior role in managing periodontal inflammation and preventing bone destruction. Ibuprofen, while effective in reducing inflammation, does not show the same level of impact on bone metabolism as flurbiprofen. Both ibuprofen and flurbiprofen are effective in managing postoperative dental pain, such as after tooth extractions or periodontal surgeries. However, flurbiprofen's longer half-life may reduce the need for frequent dosing, which can improve patient compliance. Moreover, flurbiprofen has been studied for its topical application in conditions like pericoronitis. In one study, topical flurbiprofen was as effective as oral NSAIDs (including ibuprofen) in improving oral health–related quality of life (OHQoL) scores. Flurbiprofen may have certain advantages over ibuprofen in specific dental contexts, particularly in managing periodontal disease and conditions requiring sustained anti-inflammatory effects. However, for general dental pain management, ibuprofen remains the preferred choice due to its widespread availability, proven efficacy, and safety profile (Alam et al., 2024).

Selective COX-2 inhibitors such as celecoxib and etoricoxib preferentially inhibit COX-2, reducing the risk of gastrointestinal complications. However, they may increase cardiovascular risks. Etoricoxib is effective for managing pain during orthodontic treatment and postoperative pain (Kuswandani et al., 2023).

Topical NSAIDs like diclofenac mouthwash and benzydamine are used for localized pain and inflammation in the oral cavity, such as mucositis and aphthous ulcers. They have minimal systemic absorption, reducing the risk of adverse effects.

3.1.2.1.6. Dosage and Administration of NSAIDS

The dosage of NSAIDs varies depending on the drug and the severity of pain. For example, ibuprofen is typically prescribed at 200–600 mg every 4–6 hours, with a maximum daily dose of 2400 mg (Motov et al., 2019). Topical NSAIDs are applied directly to the affected area and are associated with fewer systemic side effects (Meretskyi et al., 2024) (See Table 2).

3.1.2.1.7. Adverse Effects and Precautions

While NSAIDs are generally safe, they can cause adverse effects, particularly with long-term use or high doses. Common side effects include gastrointestinal irritation, ulceration, and bleeding due to COX-1 inhibition. Other potential adverse effects include renal impairment, cardiovascular complications, and hypersensitivity reactions. Selective COX-2 inhibitors have a better gastrointestinal safety profile but may increase the risk of cardiovascular events. Therefore, the choice of NSAID should be individualized based on the patient's medical history and risk factors (Arnal et al., 2021; Panchal et al., 2023). The adverse effects of the most commonly used NSAIDs are listed in Table 3.

3.1.2.1.8. Future Directions

Research is ongoing to develop NSAIDs with improved selectivity and safety profiles. Topical formulations are being explored to enhance drug delivery to the site of action while minimizing systemic side effects. Additionally, the role of NSAIDs in modulating oxidative stress and inflammatory pathways offers potential for new therapeutic applications in dentistry (Kotowska-Rodziewicz et al., 2023).

Conclusion

NSAIDs are indispensable in the management of dental pain and inflammation. Their widespread use across various dental specialties underscores their importance in improving patient comfort and quality of life. However, their use should be guided by a thorough understanding of their pharmacology, clinical indications, and potential adverse effects. Future research and clinical guidelines will further optimize the use of NSAIDs in dentistry, ensuring safe and effective pain management for patients.

3.1.1.2. Opioid Analgesia in Dentistry

Opioid analgesics have been widely used in dentistry for the management of acute and postoperative pain. However, their role in dental practice has come under scrutiny due to the ongoing opioid crisis, which has highlighted the risks of dependence, misuse, and addiction associated with these medications. Dentists are among the top prescribers of opioids, particularly for procedures such as tooth extractions, including third molar (wisdom tooth) surgeries. Opioids are often combined with non-opioid analgesics, such as acetaminophen or ibuprofen, to enhance analgesic effects through synergistic mechanisms. This section explores the pharmacology, clinical applications, risks, and alternatives to opioids in dentistry, emphasizing evidence-based practices to optimize pain management while minimizing harm.

3.1.1.2.1. Mechanism of Action of Opioid Analgesia

Opioids are a class of drugs that act on the central nervous system (CNS) by binding to opioid receptors (mu, kappa, and delta) (Pathan & Williams, 2012). These receptors modulate pain perception, producing analgesia, sedation, and euphoria. Common opioids used in dentistry include codeine, hydrocodone, oxycodone, and tramadol. Opioids inhibit the transmission of pain signals by reducing neurotransmitter release in the CNS and activating descending inhibitory pathways (Corder et al., 2018).

3.1.1.2.2. Pharmacokinetics of Opioid Analgesia

Most opioids are metabolized in the liver and excreted via the kidneys. Their half-life and potency vary, influencing their duration of action and risk of side effects (Mercadante, 2015). The pharmacokinetic properties of the most commonly described opioids in dentistry are summarized in Table 4.

3.1.1.2.3. Clinical Indications of Opioids in Dentistry

Opioids are primarily prescribed in dentistry for the short-term management of moderate to severe pain following surgical procedures. Common indications include third molar extractions, which are among the most frequent dental procedures associated with opioid prescriptions; studies have shown that opioids are often prescribed as a precautionary measure, even when non-opioid alternatives may be adequate (Harbaugh et al., 2018). Opioids are also occasionally used for managing postoperative pain after invasive procedures, such as dental implant placement or periodontal surgeries, particularly when NSAIDs or acetaminophen are contraindicated or insufficient (Hersh et al.,

2020). In rare cases, opioids may be prescribed for acute dental pain caused by conditions such as pulpitis or abscesses, especially when immediate dental treatment is not feasible and when post-visit pain control using NSAIDs in combination with acetaminophen is inadequate or contraindicated (Carrasco et al., 2024). Morphine Milligram Equivalent (MME) is a standardized value used to represent the relative potency of various opioids compared to morphine. For instance, 200 mg of codeine, 30 mg of hydrocodone, and 20 mg of oxycodone are considered equipotent oral doses, each providing an analgesic effect equivalent to the conventional opioid standard of 10 mg intramuscular (IM) or 30 mg oral (PO) morphine. When transitioning a patient from one opioid to another, it is essential for the dentist to consult an appropriate opioid conversion table to ensure safe and effective dosing (Becker, 2010). Table 4 presents the key parameters of opioid and combination products commonly prescribed in dental practice.

3.1.1.2.4. Efficacy of Opioids in Dental Pain Management

Numerous studies have questioned the efficacy of opioids compared to non-opioid analgesics in managing dental pain. Randomized controlled trials have consistently demonstrated that NSAIDs, such as ibuprofen, are more effective than opioids in managing dental pain. NSAIDs address the inflammatory component of pain, which is a key factor in dental procedures. Additionally, the combination of ibuprofen and acetaminophen has been shown to provide superior pain relief compared to opioids or opioid–acetaminophen combinations. For example, Moore et al., (2018) found that 400 mg of ibuprofen combined with 1000 mg of acetaminophen was more effective than any opioid-containing regimen for postoperative dental pain (Moore et al., 2018).

3.1.1.2.5. Risks and Adverse Effects of Opioids

The use of opioids in dentistry is associated with several risks. One major concern is dependence and addiction, as opioids have a high potential for misuse. Studies have shown that dental opioid prescriptions, particularly for adolescents and young adults, can serve as a gateway to persistent opioid use (Schroeder et al., 2019). Persistent use is another risk; Harbaugh et al., (2018) reported that opioid-naive patients prescribed opioids after wisdom tooth extraction were at increased risk of developing long-term opioid use. In large studies, the risk of prolonged opioid use after a 1–3-day supply is typically less than 1%, while prescriptions of 7 days or more are associated with a much higher risk (up to 4-6%) (Young et al., 2021). Opioids also carry the risk of adverse effects, including nausea, vomiting, constipation, sedation, and respiratory depression, all of which can impair recovery and quality of life (Benyamin et al., 2008). Additionally, leftover pills from dental prescriptions contribute to the reservoir of drugs available for misuse, with Maughan et al., (2016) finding that over 50% of opioids prescribed for dental procedures went unused, highlighting the need for smaller prescription quantities. Finally, dentists may be targeted by individuals seeking opioids for non-medical use, a risk that can be mitigated through real-time prescription monitoring programs (Weiner et al., 2015).

3.1.1.2.6. Regulatory Changes and Guidelines for Opioid Analgesia

In response to the opioid crisis, several regulatory and professional guidelines have been introduced to curb opioid prescribing in dentistry. In Australia, codeine was rescheduled to a prescription-only medication in 2018, leading to a reduction in its misuse; however, this also resulted in an increase in dental prescriptions for stronger opioids, such as oxycodone (Cairns, 2020). Oral and dental guidelines recommend that opioids should only be prescribed when NSAIDs and acetaminophen are contraindicated or ineffective. When opioids are necessary, the lowest effective dose should be prescribed for the shortest duration (e.g., a maximum of three days). In the US, the American Dental Association (ADA) and CDC encourage short-term opioid prescriptions, and many states require the use of Prescription Drug Monitoring Programs (PDMPs), contributing to reductions in opioid use (Townsend et al., 2021). In Canada, the Canadian Dental Association (CDA) advises short-term opioid use, emphasizing the effectiveness of non-opioid strategies. The UK government encourages non-opioid options for pain management and enforces stricter controls on opioid prescriptions, resulting in fewer prescriptions. European countries, including Germany and France, have tightened opioid prescribing and promote non-opioid analgesia, further reducing use (Encinosa et al., 2021; Manchikanti et al., 2017; Schoenfeld et al., 2024). The Pharmaceutical Benefits Advisory Committee (PBAC) has recommended reducing the pack sizes of immediate-release opioids to minimize leftover pills and the risk of misuse (Scheme et al., 2020; Teoh et al., 2020; Teoh, 2020).

3.1.1.2.7. Alternatives to Opioids in Dentistry

Given the risks associated with opioids, non-opioid analgesics are the preferred first-line treatment for dental pain. NSAIDs such as ibuprofen and naproxen are highly effective for managing dental pain due to their anti-inflammatory properties and are particularly useful for postoperative pain following extractions or surgeries. Acetaminophen is another effective analgesic and antipyretic with a favorable safety profile, and it is often combined with NSAIDs for enhanced pain relief. Topical analgesics, including topical NSAIDs like diclofenac gels, can be used for localized pain with minimal systemic side effects. Additionally, non-pharmacological methods such as acupuncture, behavioral therapy, and preoperative patient education can help reduce pain perception and decrease the need for opioid use (Feldman et al., 2022).

3.1.1.2.8. Patient Education and Risk Mitigation

Dentists can educate patients about the risks of opioids. Examples include pre-surgical counseling to set expectations for pain and recovery goals, which can reduce the need for opioids and the risk of dependence. Education on safe storage and disposal is crucial to reduce misuse; patients should store extra pills securely and dispose of them properly to prevent unauthorized access. Identifying high-risk patients—such as those with substance use disorders, chronic pain, or mental health conditions—is important, and dentists should be cautious when prescribing opioids to these patients (Denisco et al., 2011).

3.1.1.2.9. Future Directions

Research and policy efforts should prioritize the development of safer analgesics, such as biased opioid agonists, which are being investigated as alternatives to traditional opioids due to their reduced abuse potential. Additionally, improving prescribing practices through real-time prescription monitoring systems and continuing education for healthcare providers, including dentists, can help minimize inappropriate opioid use. Enhancing public awareness is equally critical, with educational campaigns informing the public about the risks associated with opioid use and the availability of effective, non-opioid alternatives for pain management. These combined efforts can significantly contribute to reducing opioid misuse and its associated harms (Volkow et al., 2019; Denisco et al., 2011).

Conclusion

Opioids have a limited role in modern dental practice, given the availability of safer and more effective alternatives. Dentists must prioritize active dental treatment and the use of NSAIDs and acetaminophen for pain management. When opioids are necessary, they should be prescribed judiciously, with careful consideration of the risks and benefits. By adopting evidence-based practices and educating patients, dentists can help reduce the burden of the opioid crisis while ensuring optimal pain management. Table 5 presents the guidelines for drug prescription in dental pain management.

3.1.1.3. Corticosteroids

Corticosteroids are widely used in dentistry due to their potent anti-inflammatory and immunosuppressive properties (Satpathi et al., 2024). These drugs have revolutionized the management of various oral and maxillofacial conditions, particularly those involving inflammation, immune-mediated diseases, and postoperative complications. Corticosteroids are broadly classified into two main types: glucocorticoids (such as dexamethasone, prednisolone, and hydrocortisone), which primarily exert anti-inflammatory and immunosuppressive effects, and mineralocorticoids (such as aldosterone and fludrocortisone), which mainly regulate electrolyte and water balance. In dental practice, glucocorticoids are most commonly used. Further classification is based on their duration of action short-acting (e.g., hydrocortisone), intermediate-acting (e.g., prednisolone, methylprednisolone), and long-acting (e.g., dexamethasone, betamethasone). The order of potency generally increases from hydrocortisone (least potent) to dexamethasone and betamethasone (most potent). However, their use requires careful consideration of dosage, duration, and potential side effects. This chapter provides a detailed overview of the applications, mechanisms, contraindications, side effects, and guidelines for the use of corticosteroids in dentistry.

3.1.1.3.1. Mechanism of Action of Corticosteroids

Corticosteroids, particularly glucocorticoids, act by inhibiting the production of inflammatory mediators such as prostaglandins, leukotrienes, and cytokines. They suppress the migration of leukocytes to the site of inflammation and reduce capillary permeability, thereby controlling swelling and pain. Additionally, corticosteroids inhibit the hypothalamic–pituitary–adrenal (HPA) axis, which can have systemic effects when used for prolonged periods (Satpathi et al., 2024; Kallali et al., 2011; Venkatech et al., 2010; Saravanan et al., 2014).

3.1.1.3.2. Adverse Effects of Corticosteroids

The side effects of corticosteroids depend on the dosage, duration, and route of administration. Common systemic side effects include cushingoid features, hypertension, hyperglycemia, osteoporosis, adrenal suppression, and increased susceptibility to infections. Local side effects may include skin atrophy, hypopigmentation, oral thrush, and mucosal atrophy. Psychological effects can manifest as euphoria, insomnia, and, in severe cases, psychosis. Additionally, corticosteroids can lead to delayed wound healing, peptic ulcers, and growth retardation in children (Peppa et al., 2011).

3.1.1.3.3. Contraindications of Corticosteroids

Corticosteroids are contraindicated in patients with hypersensitivity to any component of the formulation; with concurrent administration of live or live-attenuated vaccines (when using immunosuppressive dosages); and in systemic fungal infections, significant osteoporosis, uncontrolled hyperglycemia or diabetes mellitus, glaucoma, joint infections, uncontrolled hypertension, herpes simplex keratitis, and active varicella infection. Relative contraindications include peptic ulcer disease, congestive heart failure, and viral or bacterial infections that are not adequately controlled by anti-infective therapy (Hodgens & Sharman, 2024).

3.1.1.3.4. Indication of Corticosteroids in Dentistry

Corticosteroids are commonly used to manage postoperative inflammation and edema following oral surgical procedures, such as third molar extractions and implant surgeries (Ngeow & Lim, 2016). Dexamethasone is often administered preoperatively or immediately postoperatively to reduce swelling and pain. However, a recent study demonstrated that administering dexamethasone before surgery results in better management of swelling, pain, and mouth opening post-procedure, compared to giving it postoperatively (Kalita et al., 2024). The dose of dexamethasone used in this study was 8 mg intramuscularly one hour before the surgery, compared to the same dose given immediately after the surgery in the postoperative phase.

The most commonly used corticosteroids in dentistry are dexamethasone and methylprednisolone. Dexamethasone can be given in doses between 4–8 mg intramuscularly (IM) or intravenously (IV), or 4–10 mg as a submucosal form, while methylprednisolone is used in a dose of 20–40 mg IM or 1.5 mg/kg to 3 mg/kg IV. Both are administered 30–60 minutes before surgery or immediately after surgery, or within the first few hours (Larsen et al., 2018; Micó-Liorens et al., 2006; Ustün et al., 2003; Chaurand-Lara & Facio, 2013).

Oral Lichen Planus: Corticosteroids are a mainstay in the management of Oral Lichen Planus (OLP), a chronic inflammatory disease of the oral mucosa characterized by painful lesions. Topical corticosteroids, such as clobetasol propionate (0.05%), fluocinonide, and triamcinolone acetonide, are typically the first-line treatment due to their effectiveness in reducing pain and inflammation with minimal systemic side effects (Lodi et al., 2020). These agents are usually applied in the form of gels, pastes, or mouthwashes. A gingival tray can be used to deliver the medication effectively. Systemic corticosteroids, such as oral prednisone, are reserved for severe or refractory cases, particularly those with extensive mucocutaneous involvement (Didona et al., 2022). However, the use of systemic corticosteroids is associated with more significant side effects, including immunosuppression and metabolic disturbances, and should be used cautiously (Wongpakorn et al., 2024). Recent studies have shown that the effectiveness of corticosteroids can vary based on factors such as the patient's age and the duration of treatment. For instance, older patients and those with longer treatment durations are more likely to experience incomplete remission (Wongpakorn et al., 2024). Despite their efficacy, corticosteroids do not provide a permanent cure for OLP, and many patients experience relapses after discontinuation of treatment (Lodi et al., 2020). Therefore, long-term management and regular follow-up are essential for optimal control of the disease.

Oral Submucous Fibrosis: Corticosteroids play a significant role in the management of Oral Submucous Fibrosis (OSF), a chronic and potentially malignant disorder characterized by inflammation and progressive fibrosis of the oral submucosa. The primary goals of corticosteroid therapy in OSF are to reduce inflammation, prevent fibrosis, and improve mouth opening. In a study by Tilakaratne et al., (2016), intralesional corticosteroid injections were found to significantly improve mouth opening in patients with OSF, demonstrating the anti-inflammatory benefits of corticosteroids. Corticosteroids inhibit the proliferation of fibroblasts and the deposition of collagen, which are key processes in the development of fibrosis. By reducing these processes, corticosteroids can help prevent the formation of fibrous bands and the subsequent restriction of mouth opening. A study by Shanbhag highlighted the use of intralesional steroids such as dexamethasone, which are injected submucosally into the fibrotic bands. This treatment was effective in improving mouth opening and reducing the burning sensation (Shanbhag, 2015). Another study by Deepak et al., compared the efficacy of curcumin and topical steroids in the treatment of OSF. While both treatments were effective, curcumin was found to be more efficient in improving mouth opening and reducing burning sensation (Deepak et al.,2021). Corticosteroids are often used in combination with other agents such as hyaluronidase, antioxidants, and multivitamins to enhance their therapeutic effects. Hyaluronidase, for example, can help in the breakdown of hyaluronic acid, which is increased in fibrotic tissues, thereby improving the penetration and effectiveness of corticosteroids. Jiang et al., study reported that the combination of salvianolic acid B and triamcinolone acetonide was effective in treating OSF, with significant improvements in mouth opening and other clinical parameters (Jiang et al.,2013). Forty mg of methylprednisolone is commonly used for intralesional injections. Injections are typically administered monthly for 6 consecutive months (Tilakaratne et al., 2016). 0.01% triamcinolone acetonide is commonly used for topical application, applied three times daily for 3 months (Deepak et al., 2021).

Oral Pemphigus Vulgaris: (PV) is a rare, potentially fatal, autoimmune disease characterized by the presence of flaccid intraepithelial bullae and erosions in the oral mucosa. Early diagnosis and treatment by dentists are crucial to prevent the progression of the disease and improve the patient's quality of life. Corticosteroids play a significant role in the management of oral PV. Oral PV often presents as painful, flaccid blisters that rupture easily, leaving areas of denuded and hemorrhagic erosions. Common sites include the buccal mucosa, palate, and tongue (Al-Harbawee et al., 2021). Conditions like recurrent aphthous ulcers, Behçet's disease, erosive lichen planus, and oral candidiasis can mimic oral PV. Accurate diagnosis requires a thorough clinical examination and diagnostic tests (Kala et al., 2018). Topical corticosteroids can be used as a first-line treatment for mild to moderate oral PV. They help in reducing inflammation and promoting healing of the lesions (Davis et al., 2024). Agents such as 0.1% triamcinolone acetonide in Orabase, 0.05% clobetasol propionate, or 0.05% halobetasol can be applied directly to the affected areas multiple times daily. For extensive oral ulceration or when topical treatment is insufficient, systemic corticosteroids are necessary (Mezzour et al., 2024). Prednisolone at a dose of 0.5–1 mg/kg/day is commonly recommended. The dose is gradually reduced to the lowest effective dose to minimize side effects. Regular follow-up is essential to monitor the response to treatment and adjust the dose as needed. Additionally, maintaining strict oral hygiene is crucial. This includes regular brushing, flossing, and the use of antiseptic mouthwashes (Kala et al., 2018). Periodontal health should be monitored, and scaling and root surface debridement may be necessary. Soft, bland diets can help reduce irritation and promote healing. Furthermore, patients on long-term steroids may require anti-candida medications to prevent oral candidiasis (Harman et al., 2017).

Bullous Pemphigoid: (BP) is an autoimmune subepidermal blistering disorder that primarily affects elderly patients. Corticosteroids play a crucial role in the management of BP, both as systemic and topical treatments. Systemic corticosteroids, particularly oral prednisolone, are the mainstay of treatment for BP. They are effective in controlling the disease and reducing inflammation. The initial dose is typically 0.5 to 1.0 mg/kg per day. This dose is usually sufficient to control the disease within 2 weeks. The dose is gradually tapered over 6 to 9 months or longer to minimize side effects. Systemic corticosteroids are highly effective in achieving rapid disease control, but they are associated with significant side effects, especially in elderly patients (Fung, 2024). Topical corticosteroids are often used as a first-line treatment for mild to moderate BP. They help in reducing inflammation and promoting healing of the lesions. Super-potent topical corticosteroids such as clobetasol propionate 0.05% and triamcinolone acetonide 0.1% in orabase are commonly used. These agents are applied directly to the affected areas several times a day. Topical corticosteroids are effective in controlling localized disease and can be used to avoid or reduce the need for systemic corticosteroids, thereby minimizing systemic side effects (Joly & Tedbirt, 2022). For difficult-to-treat cases, such as relapsing, corticosteroid-dependent, or corticosteroid-resistant BP, combination therapy with biologics like dupilumab can be used. Dupilumab, which targets the IL-4 and IL-13 pathways, has shown promising results in reducing disease severity and allowing corticosteroid tapering (Liang et al., 2024).

Endodontic treatment: Corticosteroids play a crucial role in endodontic treatment by managing pain, inflammation, and post-treatment complications. They are effective in reducing acute periapical inflammation and postoperative pain and swelling. Systemic corticosteroids, such as oral prednisone, are often prescribed for a short duration to manage these conditions (Hargreaves & Cohen, 2011). Intralesional corticosteroid injections can also be used to reduce the size of chronic periapical lesions and improve clinical outcomes (Koch & Brave, 2013). Additionally, corticosteroids are beneficial in endodontic surgery, such as apicoectomy, to reduce postoperative inflammation and pain (Cohen & Hargreaves, 2014). They are also effective in managing trismus and swelling, enhancing patient comfort and function (Fouad, 2012). Corticosteroids are included in intracanal medicaments, such as Ledermix paste, to reduce pulpal inflammation and root resorption. Ledermix paste contains an antibiotic (demeclocycline-HCl) and a corticosteroid (triamcinolone acetonide) in a polyethylene glycol base. The corticosteroid component helps control pain and inflammation related to pulp and periapical diseases, while the antibiotic component helps manage bacterial infections. This combination is effective in reducing inflammation and preventing root resorption, making it a valuable tool in endodontic treatment. Corticosteroids are also used in cavity liners, often mixed with chloramphenicol and gum camphor, to alleviate postoperative thermal sensitivity. These liners are applied to the dentin surface before the placement of a restoration to reduce inflammation and sensitivity. The corticosteroid component helps to control inflammation and pain, while chloramphenicol provides antibacterial properties, and gum camphor has a soothing effect. This combination is effective in reducing postoperative thermal sensitivity and enhancing patient comfort (Bansal & Jain, 2014).

Corticosteroids, such as hydrocortisone, have been shown to reduce root resorption associated with orthodontic tooth movement in experimental studies (Verna et al., 2006; Michelogiannakis et al., 2018). They play a role in managing post-treatment inflammation and pain. Corticosteroids can be used to reduce the inflammatory response and discomfort associated with orthodontic procedures, such as bracket placement and archwire adjustments. Topical corticosteroids, often in the form of gels or pastes, can be applied to the oral mucosa to alleviate irritation and promote healing (Kumar, 2016). Systemic corticosteroids may also be prescribed in cases of severe inflammation or to manage allergic reactions to orthodontic materials (Alajlan et al., 2024). Their anti-inflammatory properties help improve patient comfort and adherence to orthodontic treatment.

Systemic corticosteroids are used to reduce pain and inflammation in patients with post-herpetic neuralgia (Jiang et al., 2023).

Erythema Multiforme: (EM) is an acute, self-limiting, immune-mediated hypersensitivity reaction that typically presents with target lesions on the skin and mucous membranes (Sokumbi & Wetter, 2012). The use of corticosteroids in EM is controversial (Rasmussen, 1976). Corticosteroids play a significant role in the management of EM, particularly in cases with mucosal involvement or severe symptoms. For acute EM, topical corticosteroids are often used to reduce inflammation and alleviate symptoms such as pruritus and discomfort. In cases of herpes simplex virus (HSV)-associated EM, some experts recommend early intervention with oral corticosteroids, such as methylprednisolone, to reduce disease duration and symptom severity, although the evidence supporting this approach is limited (Soares & Sokumbi, 2021). For severe cases with extensive mucosal involvement, systemic corticosteroids, such as prednisone (40–60 mg/d), may be necessary. Corticosteroids are typically tapered over 2–4 weeks to prevent rebound inflammation and to manage symptoms effectively (Soares & Sokumbi, 2021). In recurrent EM, corticosteroids are used less frequently as first-line therapy due to the risk of side effects and the potential for disease rebound upon discontinuation. However, they can be considered in refractory cases or as part of a combination therapy with antiviral agents (Soares & Sokumbi, 2021). Overall, the use of corticosteroids in EM should be individualized based on the severity of the condition and the presence of mucosal involvement.

Bell's Palsy: is an idiopathic, acute, unilateral facial nerve paralysis (Tiemstra & Khatkhate, 2007). Corticosteroids are commonly used in the treatment of Bell's Palsy to reduce inflammation and improve recovery. A Cochrane review by de Almeida et al., found that corticosteroids significantly improve the rate of complete recovery at 3 months compared to placebo. The review also suggested that the combination of corticosteroids and antiviral agents may be more effective than corticosteroids alone, although the evidence is not conclusive (de Almeida et al., 2009). The timing of corticosteroid administration is crucial. Studies have shown that corticosteroids are most effective when started within 72 hours of symptom onset. Early treatment can significantly improve recovery rates (Rim et al., 2023). Prednisolone (60–80 mg daily for 5 days, tapered over the next 5 days) is used to reduce inflammation and improve recovery in patients with Bell's palsy.

Corticosteroids play a significant role in the treatment of Central Giant Cell Granuloma (CGCG) as a less invasive alternative to surgical methods (Gülcan & Gülşen, 2021). Intralesional corticosteroid injections are a viable and effective alternative to surgery for the treatment of CGCG, especially in non-aggressive cases. They offer a less invasive approach with good long-term outcomes. However, careful monitoring and consideration of potential side effects are essential to ensure the best possible treatment outcomes (de Mendonça et al., 2020).

Post-Herpetic Neuralgia: (PHN) is a painful condition that can occur after an episode of herpes zoster (shingles) (Schmader et al., 2008). Corticosteroids are often used in the acute phase of herpes zoster to reduce inflammation and the risk of developing PHN. The use of oral corticosteroids to prevent PHN is uncertain, with little to no difference in adverse events. A multidisciplinary approach is recommended for managing PHN, and several investigational drugs are showing promise (Jiang et al., 2023).

Melkersson-Rosenthal Syndrome: Corticosteroids are the mainstay of treatment for Melkersson-Rosenthal Syndrome (MRS), particularly for managing acute episodes of facial paralysis and orofacial swelling. Oral corticosteroids, such as prednisone, are typically administered in short courses (50 to 60 mg per day for 5 to 7 days, followed by a taper over 2 weeks). Intralesional corticosteroids, such as triamcinolone acetonide (1–1.5 mL of a 10–20 mg/mL solution), can be used for localized swelling, particularly in the lips, to reduce inflammation and improve cosmetic appearance. These treatments help reduce inflammation and prevent the progression of edema to chronic fibrosis, leading to significant improvement in symptoms in 50–80% of patients and reducing relapse frequency by 60–75%. Short courses of prednisolone (1–1.5 mg/kg/day) are used to reduce swelling and persistent edema. Tapering is done over 3–6 weeks based on the severity and response (Dhawan et al., 2020; Chatzistefanou et al., 2015).

3.1.1.3.5. Monitoring Patients on Corticosteroid Therapy

Patients receiving long-term corticosteroid therapy require careful monitoring for adrenal suppression, osteoporosis, and other systemic side effects. To minimize risks, corticosteroids should always be prescribed at the lowest effective dose and for the shortest possible duration. Whenever feasible, topical or localized administration is preferred over systemic use to reduce systemic exposure. Probiotics may be considered to lower the risk of candidiasis during corticosteroid treatment. Vigilant monitoring for signs of infection and delayed wound healing is essential, as these are common complications. Tapering corticosteroids is crucial to prevent disease relapse and avoid adrenal insufficiency. Tapering should be considered for patients who have been on corticosteroids for more than 2–3 weeks, those receiving high doses, or those at risk for adrenal suppression. The process should begin once the underlying condition is controlled or if adverse effects outweigh the benefits. Slow, gradual tapering is especially important for patients on prolonged therapy (over 6 months), those with a history of severe disease exacerbations, or those struggling to reach a safe maintenance dose (Suehs et al., 2020).

Conclusion

Corticosteroids are a double-edged sword in dentistry. While they offer significant benefits in managing inflammation and immune-mediated conditions, their use must be judicious to avoid potential side effects. Dentists should adhere to established guidelines and consider the patient's medical history before prescribing corticosteroids.

Table 1. Key properties and precautions of NSAIDs: Pharmacokinetics, pharmacodynamics, and dosage forms (Motov et al., 2019; Laursen et al., 2025; Costa et al., 2017)

Drug	Pharmacokinetics (PK)	Pharmacodynamics (PD)	Forms (Topical/Systemic)	Precautions
Paracetamol	Bioavailability is dose -dependent: it increases from 63% for 500 mg dose to 89% for 1000 mg dose, Hepatic metabolism (conjugation pathways), Renal excretion of metabolites	Inhibiting central prostaglandin synthesis, modulating serotonergic and endocannabinoid pathways, and has minimal peripheral anti-inflammatory effects. Analgesic/antipyretic, weak anti-inflammatory activity	Oral /Tablets/Liquid Rectal IV in some settings	Avoid exceeding 4 g/day in adults or 75 mg/kg/day in children to prevent hepatotoxicity. Check total dose for combination products
Aspirin	Rapid GI absorption. Aspirin is a prodrug, which is transformed into salicylate in the stomach, in the intestinal mucosa, in the blood and mainly in the liver. Salicylate metabolized by the liver. Renal excretion.	Irreversible COX-1 and COX-2 inhibitors. Inhibits formation of prostaglandin derivative Thromboxane A2 (Antiplatelet effect). Analgesic, Antipyretic and anti-inflammatory	Oral tablets (buffered, enteric-coated, chewable)/Capsule (extended release). Rectal	Avoid in children (Reye's syndrome risk). Risk of prolonged bleeding; caution in dental surgery. Avoid using in patients with dehydration, heavy ethanol use, gastrointestinal disease, severe hepatic failure.
Ibuprofen	Rapid GI absorption. Bioavailability %80 Hepatic metabolism into hydroxylated and carboxylated compounds. Renal excretion and 1% of the original drug is excreted unchanged	Nonselective COX-1 and COX-2 inhibition. Analgesic, Antipyretic and anti-inflammatory	Oral tablet/Chewable tablet/capsules/ liquids. IV	GI irritation, gastritis, ulcer risk. Caution with renal and hepatic impairment. Ibuprofen injections must be diluted prior to administration as hemolysis can occur. It is recommended to discontinue ibuprofen at least 4 to 6 half-lives before major dental surgical procedures to minimize the risk of perioperative bleeding.

Drug	Pharmacokinetics (PK)	Pharmacodynamics (PD)	Forms (Topical/Systemic)	Precautions
Ketorolac	Rapid and complete absorption. Hepatic metabolism with hydroxylation and glucuronide conjugation. Excreted renally. High protein binding 99%	Nonselective COX-1 and COX-2 inhibition. Analgesic, Antipyretic and anti-inflammatory	Oral tablets IV/IM injectable	Limit use to ≤5 days due to GI toxicity risk. It is recommended to discontinue ketorolac at least 4 to 6 half-lives before major dental surgical procedures to minimize the risk of perioperative bleeding.
Flurbiprofen	Good oral absorption. Bioavailability %96. Primarily hepatic metabolism via CYP2C9. protein binding >99%. Renal excretion	Nonselective COX-1, COX-2 inhibitor. Analgesic, Antipyretic and anti-inflammatory	Oral tablets	Avoid in patient with GI bleeding. It may cause drowsiness and blurred vision; caution patients about activities requiring alertness.
Celecoxib	Solution well and rapidly absorbed while capsule absorption prolonged due to low solubility. Protein binding 97%. Metabolized via CYP2C9. Excreted in feces and urine.	Selective COX-2 inhibitor (dose-dependent selectivity). Does not inhibit COX-1 at therapeutic concentrations. Analgesic, Antipyretic and anti-inflammatory.	Oral capsules Oral solution	Medication overuse headache (>14 days per month). Caution with patients with sulfonamide allergy, aspirin sensitive asthma, bariartic surgery, hepatic and renal impairment.
Etoricoxib (Not Approved by FDA)	Strong oral bioavailability 100%. Metabolized by liver, excreted Renally. Long half-life permitting once-daily dosing	Highly selective COX-2 inhibitor. Analgesic, Antipyretic and anti-inflammatory.	Oral tablets	Cardiovascular risk increases with higher doses and in smokers; use caution in patients with cardiovascular risk factors.
Naproxen (>2 years)	Well GI absorption. Bioavailability 95%. Protein binding %99. Hepatically metabolized and renally excreted.	Nonselective COX-1 / COX-2 inhibitor. Analgesic, Antipyretic and anti-inflammatory.	Tablets/capsules/ suspension. Extended and delayed release forms	May cause drowsiness and blurred vision; periodic eye exams are recommended during long-term use. All NSAIDs increase the risk of hyperkalemia particularly in patients ≥ 65 years. Could increase the risk of aseptic meningitis in patients with SLE. Use with caution in patients with hepatic and renal impairment.

Table 1. (Continued)

Drug	Pharmacokinetics (PK)	Pharmacodynamics (PD)	Forms (Topical/Systemic)	Precautions
Diclofenac	Variable Bioavailability; protein binding >99%. High first-pass metabolism. Mixed hepatic Metabolism. Excretion via urine and bile.	Relatively COX-2 selective at low doses, nonselective at higher doses	Oral tablets Topical/gel/patch Injectable forms	GI risk, hepatic enzyme elevation possible. Also has some CV risks. Topical forms can be beneficial if local inflammation is superficial
Etodolac	Rapid Absorption. Hepatic metabolism (CYP2C9). Renal excretion	Preferential COX-2 inhibition at lower doses	Oral capsules/tablets	Take with food to reduce GI upset. Monitor renal function in at-risk patients.
Benzydamine	Minimal systemic absorption in rinse form. Local action primarily.	Topical anti-inflammatory effect. Local analgesic properties	Mouth rinse, spray, topical solution	Local irritation or Stinging. Generally low systemic risk. Used in inflammatory conditions (mouth ulcers, pharyngitis)

Table 2. Key NSAID parameters for dental pain: Dosage, duration, and indication (Motov et al., 2019; Laursen et al., 2025; Costa et al., 2017)

Drug	Adult Dose (Oral)	Pediatric Dose (Oral)	Duration of Action	Indication for Dental Pain
Paracetamol	325–650 mg every 4–6 hours or 1000 mg every 6 hours (max 4000mg/day).	10–15 mg/kg every 4–6 hours. (Max 75 mg/kg/day; do not exceed 4000 mg/day)	4–6 hours	Effective for mild to moderate pain; often combined with NSAIDs for synergistic effects. Safe for patients with GI risks.
Aspirin	325–1000 mg every 4–6 hours (not commonly used for dental pain). Max daily dose of 4 grams.	Avoid in children <18 years (risk of Reye's syndrome).	4–6 hours	Rarely used in dentistry due to bleeding risk. May be used for anti-inflammatory effects in specific cases.
Ibuprofen	200–400 mg every 4–6 hours (max 2400–3200 mg/day).	The dose for children ≥6 months and ≤11 years vary according to their weight and manufacturer recommendation. ≥12 years 200-400 mg every 4-6 hours less than 10 days.	4–6 hours	First-line NSAID for dental pain. Effective for post- surgical pain, inflammation, and swelling. Often combined with paracetamol for synergy.
Ketorolac	Oral: first dose 20 mg followed by 10 mg every 4–6 hours (max 40 mg/day; ≤5 days). The first dose of 20 mg was skipped for geriatric patients >65 years old.	Not recommended for children under 16 Years old as initial therapy. Limited data available	4–6 hours	Potent NSAID for severe dental pain (e.g., post-surgical). Short-term use only due to high GI and renal risks.
Flurbiprofen	50–100 mg every 6–8 hours	Not commonly used in children	4-6 hours	Flurbiprofen is notable in dentistry for its use as a topical oral rinse or lozenge, providing local pain and inflammation relief in the mouth and throat. Additionally, it has a superior role in managing periodontal inflammation and preventing bone destruction.

Table 1. Key properties and precautions of NSAIDs: Pharmacokinetics, pharmacodynamics, and dosage forms (Motov et al., 2019; Laursen et al., 2025; Costa et al., 2017)

Drug	Pharmacokinetics (PK)	Pharmacodynamics (PD)	Forms (Topical/Systemic)	Precautions
Paracetamol	Bioavailability is dose -dependent: it increases from 63% for 500 mg dose to 89% for 1000 mg dose, Hepatic metabolism (conjugation pathways), Renal excretion of metabolites	Inhibiting central prostaglandin synthesis, modulating serotonergic and endocannabinoid pathways, and has minimal peripheral anti-inflammatory effects. Analgesic/antipyretic, weak anti-inflammatory activity	Oral /Tablets/Liquid Rectal IV in some settings	Avoid exceeding 4 g/day in adults or 75 mg/kg/day in children to prevent hepatotoxicity. Check total dose for combination products
Aspirin	Rapid GI absorption. Aspirin is a prodrug, which is transformed into salicylate in the stomach, in the intestinal mucosa, in the blood and mainly in the liver. Salicylate metabolized by the liver. Renal excretion.	Irreversible COX-1 and COX-2 inhibitors. Inhibits formation of prostaglandin derivative Thromboxane A2 (Antiplatelet effect). Analgesic, Antipyretic and anti-inflammatory	Oral tablets (buffered, enteric-coated, chewable)/Capsule (extended release). Rectal	Avoid in children (Reye's syndrome risk). Risk of prolonged bleeding; caution in dental surgery. Avoid using in patients with dehydration, heavy ethanol use, gastrointestinal disease, severe hepatic failure.
Ibuprofen	Rapid GI absorption. Bioavailability %80 Hepatic metabolism into hydroxylated and carboxylated compounds. Renal excretion and 1% of the original drug is excreted unchanged	Nonselective COX-1 and COX-2 inhibition. Analgesic, Antipyretic and anti-inflammatory	Oral tablet/Chewable tablet/capsules/ liquids. IV	GI irritation, gastritis, ulcer risk. Caution with renal and hepatic impairment. Ibuprofen injections must be diluted prior to administration as hemolysis can occur. It is recommended to discontinue ibuprofen at least 4 to 6 half-lives before major dental surgical procedures to minimize the risk of perioperative bleeding.

Table 1. (Continued)

Drug	Pharmacokinetics (PK)	Pharmacodynamics (PD)	Forms (Topical/Systemic)	Precautions
Diclofenac	Variable Bioavailability; protein binding >99%. High first-pass metabolism. Mixed hepatic Metabolism. Excretion via urine and bile.	Relatively COX-2 selective at low doses, nonselective at higher doses	Oral tablets Topical/gel/patch Injectable forms	GI risk, hepatic enzyme elevation possible. Also has some CV risks. Topical forms can be beneficial if local inflammation is superficial
Etodolac	Rapid Absorption. Hepatic metabolism (CYP2C9). Renal excretion	Preferential COX-2 inhibition at lower doses	Oral capsules/tablets	Take with food to reduce GI upset. Monitor renal function in at-risk patients.
Benzydamine	Minimal systemic absorption in rinse form. Local action primarily.	Topical anti-inflammatory effect. Local analgesic properties	Mouth rinse, spray, topical solution	Local irritation or Stinging. Generally low systemic risk. Used in inflammatory conditions (mouth ulcers, pharyngitis)

Table 2. Key NSAID parameters for dental pain: Dosage, duration, and indication (Motov et al., 2019; Laursen et al., 2025; Costa et al., 2017)

Drug	Adult Dose (Oral)	Pediatric Dose (Oral)	Duration of Action	Indication for Dental Pain
Paracetamol	325–650 mg every 4–6 hours or 1000 mg every 6 hours (max 4000mg/day).	10–15 mg/kg every 4–6 hours. (Max 75 mg/kg/day; do not exceed 4000 mg/day)	4–6 hours	Effective for mild to moderate pain; often combined with NSAIDs for synergistic effects. Safe for patients with GI risks.
Aspirin	325–1000 mg every 4–6 hours (not commonly used for dental pain). Max daily dose of 4 grams.	Avoid in children <18 years (risk of Reye's syndrome).	4–6 hours	Rarely used in dentistry due to bleeding risk. May be used for anti-inflammatory effects in specific cases.
Ibuprofen	200–400 mg every 4–6 hours (max 2400–3200 mg/day).	The dose for children ≥6 months and ≤11 years vary according to their weight and manufacturer recommendation. ≥12 years 200-400 mg every 4-6 hours less than 10 days.	4–6 hours	First-line NSAID for dental pain. Effective for post- surgical pain, inflammation, and swelling. Often combined with paracetamol for synergy.
Ketorolac	Oral: first dose 20 mg followed by 10 mg every 4–6 hours (max 40 mg/day; ≤5 days). The first dose of 20 mg was skipped for geriatric patients >65 years old.	Not recommended for children under 16 Years old as initial therapy. Limited data available	4–6 hours	Potent NSAID for severe dental pain (e.g., post-surgical). Short-term use only due to high GI and renal risks.
Flurbiprofen	50–100 mg every 6–8 hours	Not commonly used in children	4-6 hours	Flurbiprofen is notable in dentistry for its use as a topical oral rinse or lozenge, providing local pain and inflammation relief in the mouth and throat. Additionally, it has a superior role in managing periodontal inflammation and preventing bone destruction.

Table 2. (Continued)

Drug	Adult Dose (Oral)	Pediatric Dose (Oral)	Duration of Action	Indication for Dental Pain
Celecoxib	For acute pain initial dose of 400 mg followed by 200 mg 12 hour later, if needed: thereafter at the second day 200 mg twice Daily. Maximum Daily dose 400 mg. For chronic pain 200 mg once Daily or 100 mg twice Daily.	50 mg twice daily for children ≥2 years and ≥10kg. >25 kg: 100 mg twice daily.	~8–12 hours (dose-dependent).	Useful for patients with GI risks who require NSAIDs. Limited use in dentistry due to cost and cardiovascular risks.
Etoricoxib	≥16 years and adults 30–120 mg once daily (not available in the US)	Not approved for pediatric use	~24 hours	May be used for moderate to severe dental pain in patients with GI risks. Long duration of action is advantageous for post-surgical pain.
Naproxen	For immediate release 500 mg once followed by 250–500 mg every 12 hours or 250 mg every 6-8 hours (max ~1250 mg/day and 1000 mg/day thereafter). Extended release: 1 g once daily increase to 1.5 g for acute pain, then reduce to 1 gram thereafter.	5–7 mg/kg every 8-12 hours (max 1000 mg/day).	8–12 hours	Effective for moderate to severe dental pain. Longer duration makes it useful for post-surgical pain management.
Diclofenac	50 mg every 8–12 hours (max ~150 mg/day depending on product).	Children ≥12 years and Adolescents: Immediate-release capsule 25 mg 4 times daily.	6–8 hours	Occasionally used for dental pain. Topical forms may be useful for localized inflammation (e.g., TMJ disorders).
Etodolac	200–400 mg every 6–8 hours (max ~1000 mg/day)	Not commonly used in children	6–8 hours	Rarely used in dentistry. May be considered for patients with moderate pain and GI risks.
Benzydamine	Mouth rinse: 0.15% solution, 15 mL q1.5–3 hours (topical)	Mouth rinse: 0.15% solution, 5–15 mL q1.5–3 hours (use smaller volume for younger children).	N/A (topical)	Topical NSAID for oral mucosal pain, ulcers, or post-surgical inflammation. Low systemic absorption makes it safe for most patients.

Table 3. NSAIDs in dental pain management: adverse effect, contraindication, drug interactions and patients education tips (Motov et al., 2019; Laursen et al., 2025; Costa et al., 2017)

Drug	Adverse Effects	Contraindication	Drug interactions	Patients education tips
Paracetamol	Hepatoxicity (overdose), nausea, vomiting, pruritus, insomnia, Constipation.	Severe liver impairment, or severe active liver disease. Hypersensitivity to paracetamol or any component of the formulation.	Alcohol (increased hepatotoxic effect). Paracetamol increases the adverse effect of atazanavir, belumosudil and increases the hepatotoxic effect of dasatinib, sorafenib. Increased the risk for methemoglobinemia with primaquine. Probencid increases serum concentration of paracetamol. Paracetamol decreases the therapeutic effect of vaccines.	Avoid exceeding 4g/day; check for paracetamol in combination products to avoid overdose. Administer without regard to food.
Aspirin	GI bleeding, tinnitus, Reye's syndrome (in children), hypersensitivity reactions include angioedema, urticaria, dyspnea, rhinorrhea, anaphylaxis, drug rashes.	Peptic ulcer, bleeding disorders, children with viral infections (Reye's syndrome). Patients with asthma, rhinitis, nasal polyps. Hypersensitivity to salicylates.	Aspirin have very serious drug interactions (Category X) with dexibuprofen, dexketoprofen, diclorphenamide, influenza vaccine, ketorolac, macimorelin, probencid, omecetaxine, sulfinpyrazine, varicella vaccine and concurrent use should be avoided. Increase anticoagulant effect of fondaparinux. increased GI bleeding and adverse effect of NSAIDs. Aspirin increase serum concentration of methotrexate, abrocitinib, Caplacizumab.	Take with food to reduce GI upset; avoid in children; inform about bleeding risk.
Ibuprofen	GI upset, peptic ulcers, kidney injury, cardiovascular risk. Prolonged bleeding time, hemolytic anemia. Hypersensitivity reaction, Stevens-Johnson syndrome.	Active GI bleeding, severe kidney impairment, heart failure and CABG. Hypersensitivity to ibuprofen or any component on the product. History of asthma, aspirin triad.	Ibuprofen has very serious drug interactions (Category X) with abrocitinib, tenoxicam, sulprostone, salicylates, ketorolac, and photosensitizing agents such as temoporfin and porfimer.	Use the lowest effective dose for the shortest duration; avoid alcohol to reduce GI risk. Take with food if there is a stomach upset.

Table 3. (Continued)

Drug	Adverse Effects	Contraindication	Drug interactions	Patients education tips
		Cerebrovascular bleeding or other bleeding disorders.	Increase serum concentration of methotrexate, pralatrexate, pemetrexed. Increase the anticoagulant effect of enoxaparin and fondaparinux. SSRIs increase the antiplatelet effect of ibuprofen.	
Ketorolac	Severe GI bleeding, kidney injury, cardiovascular events. Prolonged bleeding time, hemolytic anemia. Hypersensitivity reaction, Stevens-Johnson syndrome.	Same as Ibuprofen	Same as Ibuprofen Ketorolac nasal should be avoided when use systemic NSAIDs.	Limit use to 5 days; avoid in patients with kidney or GI issues.
Flurbiprofen	GI bleeding, cardiovascular risk, skin rashes, abdominal pain, constipation, diarrhea.	Same as ibuprofen	Same as ibuprofen	Take with food to reduce GI upset; avoid alcohol to reduce GI risk.
Celecoxib	Cardiovascular events (MI, stroke), GI upset (less than nonselective NSAIDs). Alopecia, rash, urticaria. Abdominal pain,	Hypersensitivity to sulfa drugs, celecoxib, aspirin. Perioperative pain in CABG surgery. Pregnancy and breastfeeding. Active cerebrovascular or gastrointestinal bleeding. Severe liver or renal impairment.	Celecoxib has interactions similar to ibuprofen, though the severity can vary among different NSAIDs.	Use the lowest effective dose for the shortest duration of time. Celecoxib may raise the cardiovascular risk. Take with food if it causes an upset stomach. The capsule is not chewable; its contents may be sprinkled on applesauce only and once mixed, kept refrigerated for no more than 6 hours.

Table 2. (Continued)

Drug	Adult Dose (Oral)	Pediatric Dose (Oral)	Duration of Action	Indication for Dental Pain
Celecoxib	For acute pain initial dose of 400 mg followed by 200 mg 12 hour later, if needed: thereafter at the second day 200 mg twice Daily. Maximum Daily dose 400 mg. For chronic pain 200 mg once Daily or 100 mg twice Daily.	50 mg twice daily for children ≥2 years and ≥10kg. >25 kg: 100 mg twice daily.	~8–12 hours (dose-dependent).	Useful for patients with GI risks who require NSAIDs. Limited use in dentistry due to cost and cardiovascular risks.
Etoricoxib	≥16 years and adults 30–120 mg once daily (not available in the US)	Not approved for pediatric use	~24 hours	May be used for moderate to severe dental pain in patients with GI risks. Long duration of action is advantageous for post-surgical pain.
Naproxen	For immediate release 500 mg once followed by 250–500 mg every 12 hours or 250 mg every 6-8 hours (max ~1250 mg/day and 1000 mg/day thereafter). Extended release: 1 g once daily increase to 1.5 g for acute pain, then reduce to 1 gram thereafter.	5–7 mg/kg every 8-12 hours (max 1000 mg/day).	8–12 hours	Effective for moderate to severe dental pain. Longer duration makes it useful for post-surgical pain management.
Diclofenac	50 mg every 8–12 hours (max ~150 mg/day depending on product).	Children ≥12 years and Adolescents: Immediate-release capsule 25 mg 4 times daily.	6–8 hours	Occasionally used for dental pain. Topical forms may be useful for localized inflammation (e.g., TMJ disorders).
Etodolac	200–400 mg every 6–8 hours (max ~1000 mg/day)	Not commonly used in children	6–8 hours	Rarely used in dentistry. May be considered for patients with moderate pain and GI risks.
Benzydamine	Mouth rinse: 0.15% solution, 15 mL q1.5–3 hours (topical)	Mouth rinse: 0.15% solution, 5–15 mL q1.5–3 hours (use smaller volume for younger children).	N/A (topical)	Topical NSAID for oral mucosal pain, ulcers, or post-surgical inflammation. Low systemic absorption makes it safe for most patients.

Table 3. NSAIDs in dental pain management: adverse effect, contraindication, drug interactions and patients education tips (Motov et al., 2019; Laursen et al., 2025; Costa et al., 2017)

Drug	Adverse Effects	Contraindication	Drug interactions	Patients education tips
Paracetamol	Hepatoxicity (overdose), nausea, vomiting, pruritus, insomnia, Constipation.	Severe liver impairment, or severe active liver disease. Hypersensitivity to paracetamol or any component of the formulation.	Alcohol (increased hepatotoxic effect). Paracetamol increases the adverse effect of atazanavir, belumosudil and increases the hepatotoxic effect of dasatinib, sorafenib. Increased the risk for methemoglobinemia with primaquine. Probencid increases serum concentration of paracetamol. Paracetamol decreases the therapeutic effect of vaccines.	Avoid exceeding 4g/day; check for paracetamol in combination products to avoid overdose. Administer without regard to food.
Aspirin	GI bleeding, tinnitus, Reye's syndrome (in children), hypersensitivity reactions include angioedema, urticaria, dyspnea, rhinorrhea, anaphylaxis, drug rashes.	Peptic ulcer, bleeding disorders, children with viral infections (Reye's syndrome). Patients with asthma, rhinitis, nasal polyps. Hypersensitivity to salicylates.	Aspirin have very serious drug interactions (Category X) with dexibuprofen, dexketoprofen, diclorphenamide, influenza vaccine, ketorolac, macimorelin, probencid, omecetaxine, sulfinpyrazine, varicella vaccine and concurrent use should be avoided. Increase anticoagulant effect of fondaparinux. increased GI bleeding and adverse effect of NSAIDs. Aspirin increase serum concentration of methotrexate, abrocitinib, Caplacizumab.	Take with food to reduce GI upset; avoid in children; inform about bleeding risk.
Ibuprofen	GI upset, peptic ulcers, kidney injury, cardiovascular risk. Prolonged bleeding time, hemolytic anemia. Hypersensitivity reaction, Stevens-Johnson syndrome.	Active GI bleeding, severe kidney impairment, heart failure and CABG. Hypersensitivity to ibuprofen or any component on the product. History of asthma, aspirin triad.	Ibuprofen has very serious drug interactions (Category X) with abrocitinib, tenoxicam, sulprostone, salicylates, ketorolac, and photosensitizing agents such as temoporfin and porfimer.	Use the lowest effective dose for the shortest duration; avoid alcohol to reduce GI risk. Take with food if there is a stomach upset.

Table 3. (Continued)

Drug	Adverse Effects	Contraindication	Drug interactions	Patients education tips
		Cerebrovascular bleeding or other bleeding disorders.	Increase serum concentration of methotrexate, pralatrexate, pemetrexed. Increase the anticoagulant effect of enoxaparin and fondaparinux. SSRIs increase the antiplatelet effect of ibuprofen.	
Ketorolac	Severe GI bleeding, kidney injury, cardiovascular events. Prolonged bleeding time, hemolytic anemia. Hypersensitivity reaction, Stevens-Johnson syndrome.	Same as Ibuprofen	Same as Ibuprofen Ketorolac nasal should be avoided when use systemic NSAIDs.	Limit use to 5 days; avoid in patients with kidney or GI issues.
Flurbiprofen	GI bleeding, cardiovascular risk, skin rashes, abdominal pain, constipation, diarrhea.	Same as ibuprofen	Same as ibuprofen	Take with food to reduce GI upset; avoid alcohol to reduce GI risk.
Celecoxib	Cardiovascular events (MI, stroke), GI upset (less than nonselective NSAIDs). Alopecia, rash, urticaria. Abdominal pain,	Hypersensitivity to sulfa drugs, celecoxib, aspirin. Perioperative pain in CABG surgery. Pregnancy and breastfeeding. Active cerebrovascular or gastrointestinal bleeding. Severe liver or renal impairment.	Celecoxib has interactions similar to ibuprofen, though the severity can vary among different NSAIDs.	Use the lowest effective dose for the shortest duration of time. Celecoxib may raise the cardiovascular risk. Take with food if it causes an upset stomach. The capsule is not chewable; its contents may be sprinkled on applesauce only and once mixed, kept refrigerated for no more than 6 hours.

Drug	Adverse Effects	Contraindication	Drug interactions	Patients education tips
Etoricoxib	Hypertension, cardiovascular events, GI upset	Severe hypertension, cardiovascular disease, severe kidney or liver impairment.	Anticoagulants (bleeding), antihypertensives (reduced efficacy), lithium (increased levels). Etoricoxib has interactions similar to ibuprofen, though the severity can vary among different NSAIDs.	Monitor blood pressure regularly; avoid in patients with cardiovascular risks. The medication should be stopped if a skin rash, mouth lesions, or any signs of an allergic appear.
Naproxen	GI side effects like dyspepsia, abdominal pain, constipation, diarrhea. Headache, dizziness, drowsiness, visual disturbance. Cardiovascular side effect <1%.	Hypersensitivity to naproxen, other NSAIDs, aspirin. Perioperative pain in CABG surgery Active GI and cerebrovascular bleeding. Severe kidney impairment, heart failure. Third trimester of pregnancy and breast feeding.	Anticoagulants (bleeding), antihypertensives (reduced efficacy), aspirin (interferes with cardioprotection). Itk has interactions similar to ibuprofen, though the severity can vary among different NSAIDs.	Take with food or antacids or milk to reduce GI upset; avoid alcohol to reduce GI risk. Extended- and delayed-release forms must be swallowed whole; do not break, crush, or chew.
Diclofenac	GI bleeding, hepatotoxicity, cardiovascular events	Active GI bleeding, severe liver or kidney impairment, heart failure	Anticoagulants (bleeding), antihypertensives (reduced efficacy), lithium (increased levels)	Avoid long-term use; monitor liver function; take with food to reduce GI upset.
Etodolac	GI upset, kidney injury, cardiovascular risk	Active GI bleeding, severe kidney impairment, heart failure	Anticoagulants (bleeding), antihypertensives (reduced efficacy), aspirin (interferes with cardioprotection)	Take with food to reduce GI upset; avoid alcohol to reduce GI risk.
Benzydamine	Local irritation (topical use), allergic reactions, dry mouth (oral rinse).	Hypersensitivity to benzydamine	Nonsignificant (topical use)	For topical use only; avoid swallowing oral rinse; discontinue if irritation occurs.

Table 4. Key parameters of opioid and combination products commonly used in dentistry (Becker, 2010)

Product / Opioid	Typical Dose (mg)	MME Conversion Factor	Onset (min)	Duration (hrs)	Key Pharmacokinetics	Notes
Morphine	30 (PO)	1	30–60	3–6	Hepatic metabolism; active metabolites	Standard reference; caution in renal impairment
Codeine	200 (PO)	0.1	30–60	4-6	Prodrug; CYP2D6 to morphine	Variable efficacy; avoid in children <12 and CYP2D6 ultra-rapid/poor metabolizers
Hydrocodone	5-10 (PO)	1	10–30	4–6	Hepatic metabolism (CYP3A4, CYP2D6)	Often combined with acetaminophen or ibuprofen; monitor for hepatotoxicity
Oxycodone	20 (PO)	1.5	10–15	3–6	Hepatic metabolism (CYP3A4, CYP2D6)	Higher potency; increased risk of misuse
Tramadol	100 (PO)	-	30–60	4–6	Prodrug; CYP2D6 to active metabolite	Seizure risk; serotonin syndrome; avoid in children <12
Hydromorphone	7.5 (PO)	4	15–30	3–4	Hepatic metabolism; no active metabolites	Potent; use with caution; not first-line in dentistry
Acetaminophen + Hydrocodone	325/5, 325/7.5, 325/10	1 (hydrocodone)	10–30	4–6	Hydrocodone: hepatic; acetaminophen: hepatic	Max acetaminophen 4g/day; monitor for hepatotoxicity; common first-line opioid combo
Ibuprofen + Hydrocodone	200/5	1 (hydrocodone)	10–30	4–6	Hydrocodone: hepatic; ibuprofen: renal	Avoid in renal impairment, GI risk with NSAID; max ibuprofen 3.2g/day
Acetaminophen + Oxycodone	325/5, 325/7.5, 325/10	1.5 (oxycodone)	10–30	3–6	Oxycodone: hepatic; acetaminophen: hepatic	Max acetaminophen 4g/day; higher misuse risk; potent analgesia
Acetaminophen + Tramadol	325/37.5	0.1 (tramadol)	30–60	4–6	Tramadol: prodrug, CYP2D6; acetaminophen: hepatic	Max acetaminophen 4g/day; seizure risk; serotonin syndrome; avoid in children <12

Table 5. Guidelines for drug prescription in dental pain management*

Pain Severity	Preferred NSAIDs	Indication in Dentistry	First-Line Recommendation	Comments
Mild	Ibuprofen, Naproxen.	Minor procedures (e.g., simple extraction, gingivitis, mild pulpitis)	NSAID (e.g., ibuprofen 400 mg q4–6h; Naproxen: 220–440 mg every 8–12 hours (max 1000 mg/day) or Acetaminophen. Use single agent; follow dosing instructions Opioid use is not Recommended.	Monitor for allergies, GI upset; acetaminophen if NSAIDs contraindicate.
Moderate	Ibuprofen, Naproxen	Moderate pain (e.g., surgical extraction, moderate pulpitis, periodontitis)	NSAID + Acetaminophen (alternating or combined). Combination more effective than opioids	Educate patient on alternating schedule; avoid exceeding max daily doses.
Severe	Ibuprofen, Naproxen	Severe pain (e.g., multiple extractions, extensive surgery, severe infection)	NSAID + Acetaminophen. As an alternative short course opioid (if non-opioids are inadequate). Only, if necessary, lowest effective dose, ≤3 days.	Assess risk, check Prescription Drug Monitoring Program, educate patient. Opioids only if absolutely necessary; document justification.
Special Populations	Adjusted per patient (e.g., avoid NSAIDs in pregnancy, GI disease, renal impairment)	As above, with caution	Adjust dose, consider acetaminophen if NSAIDs contraindicated. Avoid opioids if possible	Pediatric, elderly, pregnant, or medically complex patients require special consideration. Consider comorbidities and drug interactions.

*Extracted from American Dental Association practice guidelines.

Table 6. Corticosteroids in dentistry: Pharmacokinetics, pharmacodynamics, dosage forms, and precautions (Hodgens & Sharman, 2024; Satpathi et al., 2024; Kallali et al., 2011)

Drug	Pharmacokinetics	Pharmacodynamics	Dosage Forms	Precautions for Use
Hydrocortisone	Absorbed in the GI tract, metabolized in the liver, excreted in urine	Binds to glucocorticoid receptors to reduce inflammation	Tablets, injections, topical creams	Avoid in patients with systemic infections or severe hypertension.
Prednisolone	Rapid absorption, metabolized primarily in the liver, excreted primarily in urine	Suppresses immune response and reduces inflammation	Tablets, oral solution, injections	Use with caution in diabetic and hypertensive patients.
Dexamethasone	Highly bioavailable, metabolized in the liver, excreted in urine	Potent anti-inflammatory and immunosuppressive effects	Tablets, injections, topical solutions	Avoid long-term use to prevent adrenal suppression.
Triamcinolone	Absorbed systemically, metabolized in the liver, excreted in urine	Inhibits inflammatory mediators and immune response	Injections, suspensions, topical creams, dental pastes	Avoid in patients with fungal infections or peptic ulcers.
Methylprednisolone	Well absorbed orally, metabolized in the liver, excreted in urine	Reduces inflammation by inhibiting cytokine production	Tablets, injections	Monitor for osteoporosis and adrenal suppression in long-term use. High doses may induce toxic form of acute hepatitis.

Table 7. Commonly used corticosteroids in dentistry (Satpathi et al., 2024)

Drug	Adult Dose	Pediatric Dose	Duration of Action	Common Side Effects	Indication in Dentistry
Hydrocortisone	20-240 mg/day	2.5-10 mg/kg/day	8-12 hours	Nausea, headache, dizziness, adrenal suppression	Used for severe inflammation and adrenal insufficiency.
Prednisolone	10-60 mg/day	0.14-2 mg/kg/day	18-36 hours	Weight gain, mood changes, hyperglycemia	Used for oral lichen planus, pemphigus vulgaris, and erythema multiforme.
Dexamethasone	4-20 mg/day given in a single dose or 2 to 4 divided doses	0.02-0.3 mg/kg/day	36-54 hours	Insomnia, mood swings, increased infection risk	Used for postoperative swelling, Bell's palsy, and severe oral lesions.
Triamcinolone	4-32 mg/day	0.11-1.6 mg/kg/day	12-36 hours	Skin atrophy, oral thrush, delayed wound healing, joint swelling.	Used for central giant cell granuloma (intralesional) and oral submucous fibrosis.
Methylprednisolone	4-48 mg/day	Methylprednisolone sodium succinate 0.11-1.6 mg/kg/day in 3 to 4 divided doses IV/IM. Methylprednisolone acetate 0.11-1.6 mg/kg/day as one time dose or every 1 to 2 weeks (Depot).	Oral: 12–36 hours. 1 to 5 weeks (Depot)	Fluid retention, hypertension, osteoporosis	Used for severe inflammatory conditions and autoimmune diseases.

3.2. Local and General Anesthesia

3.2.1. Local Anesthesia

3.2.1.1. Mechanisms and Clinical Applications

Local anesthesia (LA) is one of the most important tools for providing painless treatment in dentistry. LA increases patient comfort and makes dental treatments more tolerable by blocking the transmission of pain to the brain. In this section, the pharmacological properties, mechanisms, clinical applications, and possible side effects of local anesthetics will be discussed in detail.

3.2.1.2. Pharmacodynamics of Local Anesthetics

The mechanism of action of LAs is determined by their ability to inhibit voltage-gated sodium channels in nerve cells. This process hinders nerve cell depolarization and, therefore, the transmission of pain signals. Thin-diameter and myelinated nerve fibers (such as those conducting pain and temperature) are the first to be blocked (Krogman et al., 2023). As a result, the sensation of pain fades before motor functions. These drugs have a higher affinity for open or inactivated sodium channels, making them more effective in situations involving significant neural activity, such as pain. The nerve-blocking effect of LAs is reversible; after the anesthetic wears off, normal nerve function is restored (Fozzard et al., 2005; Scholz, 2002).

The effect of LAs depends on the drug's pKa value and lipid solubility. The pKa value determines the ratio of the drug in its ionized (charged) or non-ionized (uncharged) form at physiological pH. The non-ionized form is necessary to cross the nerve membrane, while the ionized form exerts its effect by binding to the sodium channel. Therefore, both forms are important (Perrin et al., 2022). For instance, medications with a low pKa, like lidocaine, exhibit a rapid onset, while drugs with high lipid solubility, such as bupivacaine, have a prolonged effect. However, due to its higher pKa compared to lidocaine, bupivacaine has a slower onset time (Velioglu et al., 2020).

In infected or inflamed tissues, the low pH environment increases the proportion of LAs in their ionized form, making it more difficult for the drug to penetrate nerve membranes and reduces its effectiveness. Buffering LAs with sodium bicarbonate raises the pH, which helps more of the drug remain in its non-ionized, membrane-permeable form. This results in a faster onset of action, less injection pain, and more reliable anesthesia, ultimately making dental procedures more comfortable and effective in challenging cases (Tole & Neeli, 2024).

3.2.1.3. Pharmacokinetics of Local Anesthetics

A thorough understanding of the pharmacokinetics of LAs—including absorption, distribution, metabolism, and excretion—is essential, as these processes collectively determine both the efficacy and safety of these agents.

Absorption is primarily influenced by the blood supply at the injection site; regions with increased vascularity, such as the palate, facilitate more rapid absorption and elevate the risk of systemic toxicity. To mitigate this risk, vasoconstrictors (e.g., epinephrine) are often co-administered to decrease local blood flow, slow systemic absorption, prolong anesthetic action, and reduce toxicity (Michel, 2020).

Following absorption, local anesthetics are distributed preferentially to highly perfused organs, such as the brain, heart, and liver, which can further increase the potential for systemic toxicity. The extent of distribution, as well as the duration of action, is influenced by the physicochemical properties of the drug. Agents with greater lipid solubility, such as bupivacaine, have a larger volume of distribution and a prolonged effect. Other factors affecting systemic absorption and distribution include the administered dose, site of injection, presence of a vasoconstrictor, protein binding, and patient-specific variables such as age and hepatic or renal function, as well as the risk of accidental intravascular injection (Mazoit & Dalens, 2004).

Metabolism and excretion further impact the clinical profile of LAs. Amide-type agents (e.g., lidocaine, bupivacaine) are metabolized in the liver by cytochrome P450 enzymes, and impaired hepatic function can increase the risk of toxicity. In contrast, ester-type agents (e.g., procaine) are rapidly hydrolyzed in plasma by pseudocholinesterase, resulting in a shorter duration of action (Tucker & Mather, 1979). Metabolites are excreted via the kidneys, and elimination may be delayed in neonates, older adults, and individuals with renal or hepatic impairment (Arthur & Covino, 1971).

In summary, both drug-related properties (such as lipid solubility, protein binding, and vasodilator activity) and patient-specific factors (including age, clinical status, pregnancy, and concurrent medications) must be carefully considered to ensure the safe and effective use of LAs (Heavner, 2007).

3.2.1.4. Classification of Local Anesthetics

Local anesthetics are divided into two main groups based on their chemical structure: amide type and ester type. The most commonly used LAs in dentistry are amide-type agents, such as lidocaine, mepivacaine, bupivacaine, and articaine. Ester-type local anesthetics (e.g., benzocaine) are typically used for topical applications. Notably, some ester group anesthetics, such as benzocaine, have a higher potential to cause allergic reactions (Kramer et al., 2020).

In addition to chemical classification, LAs can also be categorized by their method of administration. Diffusive methods rely on the anesthetic diffusing through tissues to reach the nerves, as seen with topical applications, infiltration, and nerve blocks. Vascular-diffusive (spongy) methods utilize the vascular system within bone or ligaments to deliver the anesthetic directly to areas rich in nerves, offering effective and versatile anesthesia for a wide range of dental procedures (Petricas et al., 2016).

3.2.1.5. Clinical Uses of Local Anesthesia in Dentistry

Local anesthetics are utilized across a wide range of dental procedures to enhance patient comfort and procedural efficiency. In restorative and prosthetic dentistry, they facilitate painless tooth preparation and restoration for treatments such as fillings, crowns, and veneers. During oral surgery including extractions, biopsies, and minor surgical interventions, local anesthesia not only provides effective pain control but also promotes hemostasis, often reducing the need for general anesthesia. For periodontal procedures like scaling, root planing, and gum surgery, local anesthesia is essential for effective deep cleaning and surgical interventions. In endodontics, it controls pain during root canal therapy, particularly during pulp removal and canal shaping. Additionally, pediatric dentistry relies on special dosing and techniques to ensure safety and comfort for children undergoing dental procedures. During implant placement, LA minimizes discomfort of implant surgery. Finally, in emergency care, it allows for rapid pain relief and effective management of dental trauma or abscess drainage, supporting both patient comfort and infection control (Lottinger, 2019; Decloux & Ouanounou, 2020).

The choice of LA depends on the type of procedure, the patient's overall medical status, and the specific characteristics of the anesthetic agent. Short-acting local anesthetics, such as lidocaine and mepivacaine, are generally preferred for brief procedures due to their rapid onset. These agents are often combined with a vasoconstrictor, such as epinephrine, which prolongs the duration of action and reduces systemic absorption. In contrast, long-acting local anesthetics, such as bupivacaine, are selected when extended pain control is required. For instance, bupivacaine is often preferred to reduce postoperative pain following surgical tooth extractions. Studies have demonstrated that bupivacaine decreases analgesic consumption and provides a longer-lasting effect compared to lidocaine (Aguilera et al.,2024; Velioglu et al.,2020).

In addition to injectable agents, topical anesthetics, such as benzocaine, are commonly used prior to needle insertion or for short-term pain control. Benzocaine concentrations of 10% and 20% have been shown to be effective in reducing pain compared to placebo. Table 8 summarizes the different types of local anesthetics, their pharmacokinetic and pharmacodynamic profiles, and their uses in dentistry. The recommended dosages for these agents are provided in Table 9.

3.2.1.6. Dose Calculation for Local Anesthetics

A 6-year-old patient weighing 20 kg is scheduled to receive a mandibular block anaesthesia using 2% lidocaine with epinephrine (1:100,000). To determine the maximum safe dose, it is important to note that the maximum recommended dose of lidocaine for children is 4.5 mg/kg without epinephrine and 7 mg/kg with epinephrine (Deluke et al., 2018). Since epinephrine is being used in this case, the maximum dose is 7 mg/kg. For a 20 kg child, this equates to a maximum dose of:

$$20\ kg \times 7\ mg/kg = 140\ mg$$

Next, we need to establish the concentration of the solution. Lidocaine 2% contains 20 mg/mL (calculated as: % concentration × 10; thus, 2 × 10 = 20 mg/mL).

To determine the maximum volume that can be safely administered, divide the maximum dose by the concentration:

$$140mg/20mg/ml = 7\ ml$$

Therefore, the maximum volume of 2% lidocaine with epinephrine (1:100,000) that can be administered to this child is 7 ml. However, in dental practice, it is common to use a dose significantly lower than the maximum for children. Typically, 1.5–2 mL is sufficient for a mandibular block. Thus, administering 1.5–2 mL of lidocaine in this situation is both safe and effective.

3.2.1.7. Nerve Block vs. Infiltration: Choosing the Best Approach in Local Anesthesia

In dentistry, nerve blocks are frequently used to control pain during various surgical and restorative procedures. For interventions such as tooth extraction, root canal treatment, implant placement, periodontal surgery, and jaw surgery, sensation in the targeted area is temporarily blocked by injecting an anesthetic near the relevant nerves. This approach reduces pain for the patient during and after the procedure, allowing the dentist to work more comfortably and with greater control (Reuss-Lamky, 2007).

Infiltration anesthesia, on the other hand, involves injecting an anesthetic solution directly into the tissue at the site of treatment. It is commonly preferred for smaller and more superficial procedures, such as fillings, scaling, and the extraction of primary teeth. This method is particularly effective in the upper jaw, as it numbs the nerve endings in the immediate area, thereby preventing pain during the procedure (Pan et al., 2023).

Both techniques are effective in preventing pain, but they are applied in different clinical situations. Nerve blocks are more suitable for numbing larger areas, while infiltration is ideal for smaller, localized regions. The choice of technique depends on the specific procedure and the individual needs of the patient (Kende et al., 2021; Fernandez & Angeles, 2025).

The required amounts and concentrations of LA also differ between the two techniques. Nerve blocks typically use more concentrated anesthetic solutions in smaller volumes to achieve anesthesia over a larger area. In contrast, infiltration often involves lower concentrations in larger volumes to provide adequate coverage of the targeted site. In certain cases, combining both techniques can enhance the anesthetic effect and further reduce intraoperative pain and bleeding (Li et al., 2020; Geng et al., 2023).

3.2.1.8. Side Effects and Complications of Local Anesthesia

Local anesthetics are generally safe, but side effects and complications can occur. These may result from systemic toxicity, allergic reactions, or improper injection techniques. Ocular side effects reported in the literature include diplopia, partial loss of vision, strabismus, blurred vision, uniocular blindness, disturbances of the eye muscles, ptosis, and excessive pupil contraction. Neurological complications such as trigeminal nerve injury, facial nerve paralysis, facial numbness, hearing loss, facial palsy, and ipsilateral ataxia have also been documented. Additional risks include nerve damage, transient neurological symptoms, tissue damage, vasoconstrictor-induced ischemia, and mydriasis (Helander et al., 2019; Aquilanti et al., 2022).

Systemic toxicity may occur with high doses or intravascular injection of LAs, presenting with neurological symptoms such as dizziness, tinnitus, seizures, and loss of consciousness, as well as cardiac symptoms including arrhythmias and cardiac arrest. For example, high plasma concentrations of lidocaine can cause seizures and arrhythmias, while bupivacaine carries a particularly high risk of cardiotoxicity. Intravenous lipid emulsion therapy is effective in treating cardiotoxicity from lipophilic local anesthetics like bupivacaine by removing the drug from plasma (Antel & Ingelmo, 2022).

Ester-type LAs are more likely to cause allergic reactions, often due to para-aminobenzoic acid, a metabolite of benzocaine. In contrast, amide-type LAs have a much lower risk of allergies. Incorrect injection techniques can lead to complications such as hematoma or trismus (jaw muscle spasm), for which pressure and warm compresses are recommended. Although rare, cases of osteonecrosis following intraosseous anesthesia and skin necrosis after dental local LA have been reported. Some LAs, such as prilocaine and benzocaine, can cause methemoglobinemia, reducing hemoglobin's oxygen carrying capacity and leading to hypoxia; intravenous methylene blue is the treatment of choice. Other reported complications include persistent jaw stiffness and swelling, osteomyelitis following maxillary infiltration anesthesia, and needle fractures during administration (Ho et al., 2021; Ghafoor et al., 2023; Janev & Ouanounou, 2023).

3.2.1.9. Contraindications for Local Anesthesia

Contraindications for LA include a known allergy to LAs, particularly to amide or ester types. Severe cardiovascular disease, especially in patients receiving vasoconstrictors, and uncontrolled hypertension or arrhythmias are also important contraindications when vasoconstrictors are used. In patients with severe liver dysfunction, the use of amide-type anesthetics should be avoided. Prilocaine and benzocaine are contraindicated in individuals with methemoglobinemia. Additionally, the presence of an acute infection at the injection site is considered a relative contraindication. These considerations apply to pediatric, adult, and elderly patients undergoing procedures with local anesthesia (Janev & Ouanounou, 2023; Suri et al., 2022).

3.2.1.10. Local Anesthesia in Special Patient Groups

When administering LAs, the general health status of the patient should always be considered. Special precautions are necessary in cases such as diabetes, hypertension, heart disease, or pregnancy. Studies evaluating the impact of epinephrine in LA on diabetic patients have indicated that adrenaline does not significantly affect healthy or diabetic individuals. However, in patients with untreated diabetes, glucose levels tend to increase notably when LA containing adrenaline is administered. Therefore, dental local anesthetic solutions that contain epinephrine are considered safe for use in all healthy and diabetic patients, regardless of gender, except for those diabetics who have not taken their pre-operative hypoglycemic medication (Tily & Thomas, 2007; Santos-Paul et al., 2015).

Recent studies have shown that the use of epinephrine is not completely contraindicated in patients with heart disease and may even be beneficial in some cases. By prolonging the effect of LAs, epinephrine allows for lower doses, which can reduce the risk of systemic toxicity. Its vasoconstrictor effect also slows the absorption of anesthetics into the systemic circulation, potentially minimizing cardiac side effects. Low-dose epinephrine (such as 1:200,000 or 1:100,000) is generally considered safe for these patients, as studies have found no clinically significant increases in blood pressure or heart rate at these concentrations (Ismail, 2018).

Alternatively, LAs that do not contain epinephrine, such as mepivacaine, may be used for short-term procedures. However, because they lack the vasoconstrictive properties of epinephrine, their effects are often shorter in duration and may require higher doses, which increases the risk of systemic toxicity. Therefore, agents that contain epinephrine, such as lidocaine or articaine, are often more advantageous for patients with heart disease due to their longer-lasting effects and the potential for safer, lower dosing (Su et al., 2014).

A study comparing pregnant women who received LA with those who did not found that the rate of major anomalies in the experimental group was 4.8%, while the control group had a rate of 3.3% (Hagai et al., 2015). Importantly, no statistical differences were observed between the two groups, suggesting that local anesthesia does not increase the risk of major anomalies during pregnancy. Among LAs, lidocaine is classified as category B, indicating it is safe for use during pregnancy, with lower placental transfer and a shorter duration of action. In contrast, articaine, mepivacaine, and bupivacaine are classified as category C, and their use should be approached with greater caution (Fuchi & Noda, 2010).

Given these considerations, elective dental treatments should be avoided during the first trimester whenever possible. When LAs are required in pregnant women, it is essential to carefully consider the effects on both the mother and the fetus, and to determine the dosage with particular care (Zhou et al., 2023; Ming et al., 2021).

3.2.1.11. Innovative Approaches in Local Anesthesia

Several innovative approaches have been developed for the administration of LAs. Computer-controlled injection systems have been introduced to provide less painful and more effective anesthesia by precisely controlling injection pressure and speed. Ultrasound-guided nerve blocks utilize ultrasound technology to visualize nerve structures, thereby improving the accuracy of injections and reducing the risk of complications (Tan et al., 2022). The use of pH-buffered anesthetics, which involves increasing the pH of the anesthetic solution, results in a faster onset and a more effective nerve block, an approach particularly beneficial in infected tissues (Aulestia-Viera et al., 2018). Additionally, next-generation LAs that selectively target specific sodium channel subtypes are being developed, offering the potential for more effective pain control with fewer side effects (Sarı et al., 2021).

3.2.1.12. Practical Tips for Safe Administration

To ensure the safe and effective use of LAs in dentistry, clinicians should always aspirate before injection to avoid intravascular administration and reduce the risk of systemic toxicity. It is important to use the lowest effective dose, select the appropriate anesthetic agent and concentration for the procedure, and monitor the patient for early signs of adverse reactions such as dizziness, tinnitus, or changes in heart rate. Proper injection technique, slow administration, and careful observation during and after the procedure are essential for minimizing complications. Additionally, having emergency equipment and medications readily available is crucial for prompt management of rare but serious reactions (Decloux & Ouanounou, 2020; Bahar & Yoon, 2021).

3.2.1.13. Patient Communication

Clear communication with patients is vital for reducing anxiety and ensuring cooperation, especially in children and those with dental fear. Before administering LA, dentists should explain the procedure, what sensations to expect, and possible side effects in simple, reassuring language. Addressing patient concerns, answering questions, and providing aftercare instructions help build trust and improve the overall dental experience. In pediatric and anxious patients, using age-appropriate explanations and a calm, supportive approach can significantly enhance comfort and compliance during dental treatment (Sivrikaya et al., 2021).

Table 8. An overview of local anesthetics: Pharmacokinetics, pharmacodynamics, and dental applications(Decloux & Ouanounou, 2020)

Agent	Half-life (hour)	Pharmacokinetic properties	Pharmacodynamic properties	Dental Application
Lidocaine	1.6	Fast onset, medium duration of effect	Transient neurologic symptoms specially with spinal anesthesia	Standard agent, widely used for infiltration and nerve block
Articaine	0.5	Better tissue penetration, shorter half-life	Risk of paresthesia, neurotoxicity at high concentrations	Popular in dentistry, especially mandibular infiltrations
Mepivacaine	1.9	Vasoconstrictor effect, medium duration of action	Slow metabolism in the fetus, should be used with caution during pregnancy	Preferred in short procedures
Bupivacaine	3.5	Long-lasting effect, safe at low doses	High risk of cardiotoxicity	Used for long-term pain control
Prilocaine	1.5	Fast metabolism, low risk of toxicity	Risk of methemoglobinemia	Safe for short procedures
Ropivacaine	1.8-2	Less cardiotoxic, long-lasting effect	Lower potency, higher dose may be required	Preferred in high volume blocks
Procaine	0.1	Fast metabolism, low risk of toxicity	Short duration of effect, risk of allergic reactions	Rarely used in dentistry
Tetracaine	0.1	Long-lasting effect, effective in spinal anesthesia	High risk of toxicity, use with caution	Topical used in dentistry
Benzocaine	-	Effective for superficial anesthesia	Methemoglobinemia risk	Used for topical anesthesia
Cocaine	2	Vasoconstrictor effect, superficial anesthesia	Addiction potential, systemic toxicity	Not used in dentistry

Table 9. Tailoring local anesthetic doses for dental procedures (FDA)

Agent	Maximun dose mg/kg	With epinephrine maximum dose mg/kg	Adult maximum total dose mg	Maximum dose for children mg /kg	With epinephrine. Maximum dose for children mg /kg
Lidocaine*	4.5	7.0	300-500**	4.5	7.0
Articaine	NA	7.0	500	N/A	7.0(age>4)
Mepivacaine	6.6	6.6	400	6.6	6.6
Bupivacaine	2.0	2.5	90	NA	NA
Prilocaine	8.0	8.0	600	8.0	8.0
Ropivacaine	3.0	3.5	200	2.5	3.5
Procaine	7.0	10	600	7.0	10
Tetracaine	1.5	2.0	100	1.0	2.0

Note: MRDs vary by guideline; the AAPD specifically recommends a conservative limit of 4.4 mg/kg for lidocaine with epinephrine in pediatric patients.

Conclusion

LA is a cornerstone of modern dental practice, enabling safe, effective, and comfortable treatment for a wide range of procedures. Understanding the pharmacology, clinical applications, and potential complications of LAs is essential for optimizing patient care. With ongoing innovations and careful consideration of individual patient needs, LA continues to evolve, offering improved outcomes and enhanced safety in dental practice.

3.2.2. General Anesthesia

Today, the vast majority of dental procedures are performed under local anesthesia. However, in some cases, local anesthesia may be insufficient, and sedation or general anesthesia may be preferred. General anesthesia may be necessary, especially for uncooperative young children, individuals with mental disabilities, patients who are allergic to local anesthetics, or for procedures that are lengthy and cannot be tolerated by the patient. General anesthesia has both benefits and risks, so it should be administered only in a hospital setting by a skilled anesthesiologist. This chapter will explore the history of general anesthesia in dentistry, its indications, methods of administration, and important considerations for its use.

3.2.2.1. The History of General Anesthesia

General anesthesia in dentistry dates back to the mid-19th century. Nitrous oxide was first used by Horace Wells in 1844 to relax patients. Two years later, dentist William Morton applied the first ether anesthesia in Massachusetts. In 1846, British dentist James Robinson performed the first general anesthesia in dentistry. During this period, substances such as nitrous oxide, chloroform, and ether were widely used. However, a decline in the use of general anesthesia has been observed since the 1960s, mainly due to the widespread adoption of local anesthetics such as lidocaine (Matsuki & Zsigmond, 1973; Weaver, 2019; López-Valverde et al., 2011).

A report published in 1990 by Professor David Poswillo made major recommendations concerning the safety of general anesthesia, sedation, and resuscitation during dental practice. The recommendations from the Poswillo Report revolutionized the practice of dental anesthesia, with patient safety as the prime consideration. This was to be achieved by limiting the administration of general anesthesia to those trained as anesthetists in appropriately equipped facilities and dental teams trained to deal with emergencies. Following the report, there was a dramatic decline in the number of general anesthetics performed in dental offices, with most cases being referred for hospital treatment (Macpherson & Binnie, 1996; Smith & Alexander, 1992).

3.2.2.2. Evaluation for General Anesthesia

Before undergoing general anesthesia, patients must be evaluated by an anesthesiologist. This evaluation includes a thorough medical history, physical examination, and any necessary laboratory tests. Patients are assessed using the American Society of Anesthesiologists (ASA) classification system, which helps determine the risk of anesthesia based on the patient's overall health status. Other important preoperative considerations include the patient's age, general health, and the expected duration of the procedure. For pediatric patients, preoperative fasting times and fluid intake must be carefully managed, and psychological preparation, along with pharmaceutical premedication if needed, may be implemented (Valdez, 2020).

The ASA classification system categorizes patients as follows:

ASA I: A healthy individual with no systemic disease

ASA II: A patient with mild systemic disease

ASA III: A patient with severe systemic disease that is not immediately life-threatening

ASA IV: A patient with severe, life-threatening systemic disease

ASA V: A patient who is not expected to survive more than 24 hours without surgery

ASA VI: A patient who has been declared brain dead and is considered for organ donation (Hackett et al., 2015; Horváth et al., 2021).

3.2.2.3. Indications for General Anesthesia in Dentistry

General anesthesia is often the method of choice for complex and lengthy dental procedures. It ensures total unconsciousness, thereby eliminating pain and discomfort, minimizing tension and anxiety, and allowing multiple procedures to be performed in a single session. This approach is particularly beneficial for patients with a pronounced gag reflex, those requiring extensive treatment, and individuals whose motor control is affected by certain therapies or medications. General anesthesia also provides a safe treatment environment for young children and patients with special needs (Yeo et al., 2025; López-Velasco et al., 2021).

The main indications for general anesthesia in dentistry include:

- Patients who are uncooperative due to intellectual, physical, or behavioral disabilities
- Patients (children or adults) with severe dental anxiety or phobia that makes treatment impossible by other means
- Very young children, individuals unable to communicate, or those who cannot understand instructions
- Cases requiring extensive or complex dental treatment, such as multiple extractions, multiple restorations, or full-mouth rehabilitation
- Patients with contraindications to local anesthesia or sedation, such as allergies to anesthetics or sedatives, certain medical conditions, or unsuccessful attempts with other methods
- Special care dentistry cases, where adults or children with complex medical or social needs require multidisciplinary management

Despite its advantages, general anesthesia also has disadvantages. Possible side effects include stomach discomfort, nausea, sore throat, and fatigue. There is an increased risk of aspiration, and the procedure is more costly and requires a longer recovery time compared to local anesthesia. Additionally, general anesthesia introduces extra risks for patients with heart, lung, or systemic disorders (Doshi et al., 2024; McLennan & Ward, 2023).

3.2.2.4. Techniques of Anesthesia Delivery in Dentistry

General anesthesia delivery techniques in dentistry vary based on the patient's condition and the specific procedure. Mask anesthesia, which typically uses inhalation agents such as nitrous oxide or sevoflurane, is suitable for short-term procedures. For longer procedures or patients at risk of aspiration, intubation either nasotracheal or endotracheal is preferred. Intravenous anesthesia with agents like propofol or thiopental is favored for its rapid onset and short duration of action. Regardless of the technique, continuous monitoring of the patient's vital signs is essential to minimize the risk of complications (McLennan & Ward, 2023; Shehabi et al., 2025).

3.2.2.5. Characteristics of General Anesthesia Agents

The goal of optimal general anesthesia is to ensure loss of consciousness, pain relief (analgesia), muscle relaxation, and hemodynamic stability throughout the procedure. Additionally, rapid induction, ease of management, and prompt, smooth recovery after the procedure are essential criteria. An ideal anesthetic agent should have minimal side effects, not adversely affect organ function, and be non-toxic. However, it is generally not possible to achieve all these characteristics with a single agent. Therefore, modern anesthesia practice typically employs a "balanced anesthesia" technique, using a combination of agents. Intravenous drugs such as propofol are used for induction, while inhalational agents like sevoflurane are preferred for maintenance. Opioids are included for analgesia, and muscle relaxants are used to facilitate surgery. This combination allows for lower doses of each medication, reducing side effects and enhancing the safety of anesthesia management (Brown et al., 2018; Joshi, 2020).

3.2.2.6. Pharmacokinetics of General Anesthetic Agents

Intravenous anesthetics such as propofol and thiopentone have a rapid onset of action due to their high lipid solubility, which allows them to quickly cross the blood-brain barrier. Their short duration of action is primarily the result of rapid redistribution from the brain to other tissues, rather than immediate elimination. Inhalational agents like sevoflurane are absorbed through the lungs, and their low blood solubility enables both rapid induction and easy adjustment of anesthetic depth. Most intravenous agents are metabolized in the liver, with elimination half-lives typically ranging from 2 to 6 hours, although some agents are metabolized even more quickly. In contrast, inhalational agents are mainly eliminated unchanged via the lungs, with only minimal hepatic metabolism. Furthermore, muscle relaxants, which are hydrophilic, are primarily excreted by the kidneys, and their effects can be prolonged in patients with renal failure (Duvaldestin, 1981; Paulraj & Lakshmanan, 2021; De Lacerda et al., 2024).

3.2.2.7. Induction and Maintenance of General Anesthesia

The induction and maintenance of anesthesia are critical components of anesthetic management, particularly in oral and maxillofacial surgery. These phases involve the careful selection and administration of anesthetic agents to achieve a smooth transition to unconsciousness (induction) and to sustain the desired level of anesthesia throughout the procedure (maintenance) (Wiemer et al., 2020; Boubacar et al., 2025). Total Intravenous Anesthesia (TIVA) combines agents like propofol and remifentanil for maintenance without the use of inhalational agents. TIVA reduces the risk of postoperative nausea and vomiting (PONV) and malignant hyperthermia and provides precise control over anesthetic depth. Balanced anesthesia combines inhalational agents (e.g., sevoflurane) with intravenous agents (e.g., opioids, propofol) to achieve the desired effects while minimizing side effects (Lone et al., 2021).

3.2.2.8. Pharmacological Agents Used in General Anesthesia

3.2.2.8.1. Common Intravenous Agents Used in General Anesthesia

- Benzodiazepines

Benzodiazepines (such as midazolam, diazepam, and remimazolam) are commonly used during the induction phase of anesthesia, primarily to provide sedation and anxiolysis. They can be administered orally or intravenously to help patients relax and induce preoperative sedation. Benzodiazepines act as positive allosteric modulators of GABA-A receptors, enhancing the binding of GABA, which opens chloride ion channels and causes neuronal hyperpolarization. This results in central nervous system depression, anxiolysis, sedation, and amnesia (Kim et al., 2020).

Benzodiazepines are characterized by a wide therapeutic index, offering a notable safety advantage. When used alone, they do not significantly depress respiration. Their anxiolytic and sedative effects are particularly beneficial for patients with dental phobia, and their ability to cause anterograde amnesia increases patient comfort during surgical or invasive procedures. Additionally, their anticonvulsant properties make them useful in patients with epilepsy or an increased risk of seizures. The effects of benzodiazepines can be rapidly reversed with the antagonist flumazenil (Dundee et al., 2012).

Despite these advantages, benzodiazepines also carry potential risks. They may cause upper airway obstruction due to muscle relaxation. Long-acting benzodiazepines, such as diazepam, can lead to prolonged drowsiness or a "hangover effect" because of active metabolites. Paradoxical reactions, such as agitation and excitement, may occur, especially in sensitive populations like the elderly and children. Therefore, careful dose selection is essential, taking into account these potential risks (Schroeck et al., 2016).

Midazolam is often preferred for its rapid onset and short half-life, with its active metabolite being clinically insignificant. The typical intravenous dose is 1–2 mg, titrated to effect, while the oral dose for children is 0.5 mg/kg, up to a maximum of 20 mg. Diazepam has a longer duration of action and may cause hangover effects; its intravenous dose ranges from 2.5 to 5 mg by titration, and the oral dose is 2–10 mg. Remimazolam is an ultra-short-acting agent, metabolized by tissue esterases without producing active metabolites, allowing for rapid patient recovery. It is suitable for patients with liver or kidney impairment (Kim et al., 2020; Noor et al., 2021; Kim & Fechner, 2022).

- Propofol

Propofol is often the agent of choice for the induction of general anesthesia due to its rapid onset of action. It also plays a crucial role in the maintenance of anesthesia, particularly when used as a continuous infusion in TIVA techniques. Propofol acts as a positive allosteric modulator of GABA-A receptors, primarily enhancing the inhibitory action of the neurotransmitter gamma-aminobutyric acid (GABA). This increases chloride ion influx into neurons, leading to hyperpolarization and reduced neuronal excitability, which produces sedation and hypnosis (Trapani et al., 2000; Chidambaran et al., 2015).

Propofol is distinguished by its rapid onset, with effects typically seen within 30–60 seconds following intravenous administration. Its short duration of action allows for quick patient recovery, making it especially well-suited for ambulatory procedures. Its antiemetic properties significantly enhance patient comfort. Additionally, the ease of dose titration allows for precise adjustment of sedation levels, and the absence of active metabolites facilitates a rapid and uncomplicated recovery (Schraag et al., 2018; Trapani et al., 2000).

While propofol offers numerous benefits, it also has potential drawbacks. It can cause cardiovascular depression, leading to hypotension and bradycardia, which necessitates careful monitoring. Dose-dependent respiratory depression may also occur, resulting in decreased respiratory rate and tidal volume. Its narrow therapeutic index increases the risk of significant central nervous system depression in the event of an overdose. Furthermore, because propofol lacks analgesic properties, supplementary analgesics are required for effective pain management. These considerations require careful assessment and continuous monitoring during administration (Marik et al., 2004; Pigò et al., 2025).

Propofol dosing varies depending on its intended use. For induction, an intravenous bolus of 1.5–2.5 mg/kg is administered. Maintenance of deep sedation or general anesthesia typically involves a continuous infusion at a rate of 100–200 μg/kg/min, while moderate sedation requires a lower infusion rate of 25–50 μg/kg/min. For its antiemetic properties, propofol can be given as a continuous infusion at 15–20 μg/kg/min or as a bolus dose of 0.5–1 mg/kg at the end of the procedure (Sahinovic et al., 2018; Kim et al., 2019; Alshamoosi, 2021).

- Ketamine

Ketamine is frequently used as an induction agent, administered via intramuscular (IM) or intravenous (IV) routes, especially in children and uncooperative patients. Although less commonly used for this purpose, it can also provide analgesic support at low doses. Ketamine is a non-competitive antagonist of NMDA receptors, blocking excitatory signals by preventing glutamate binding. It also affects opioid receptors, monoamine reuptake, and voltage-gated ion channels. Its bronchodilator effects are particularly beneficial for asthmatics and individuals at risk of bronchospasm, promoting airway patency and easier breathing. Ketamine's cardiovascular stability is a significant advantage, as it can increase blood pressure and heart rate by stimulating sympathetic activity. It also provides pain relief due to its analgesic properties and preserves airway reflexes, reducing the risk of respiratory depression. The option for IM administration is useful when IV access is not available. However, side effects such as hallucinations and delirium (especially at higher doses or postoperatively), hypersalivation, increased cardiac workload, and postoperative nausea and vomiting can occur. Ketamine dosing depends on the clinical situation: for induction or procedural sedation, an IV bolus of 0.5–1.5 mg/kg or an IM bolus of 2–5 mg/kg is typical. For acute analgesic support, a lower, subanesthetic IV bolus of 0.25 mg/kg is used (Sun et al., 2020; Simonini et al., 2022; Zhou et al., 2023; Musale & Naveriya, 2024).

- Dexmedetomidine

Dexmedetomidine is used in anesthesia for its sedative, analgesic, and sympatholytic effects. The optimal dose depends on the route of administration, patient age, and clinical goal (e.g., sedation, emergence control, analgesia). It is typically administered as a continuous IV infusion for sedation and analgesia and may also be used for preoperative sedation to alleviate anxiety. Dexmedetomidine, an alpha-2 adrenergic agonist, provides sedation, analgesia, and anxiolysis by suppressing the sympathetic nervous system. It does not cause respiratory depression and preserves airway reflexes. Dexmedetomidine generally maintains hemodynamic stability, with significant adverse effects being rare except for possible moderate hypotension and bradycardia. It also reduces opioid requirements, has antisialagogues properties (reducing saliva production) and is useful for managing pre-procedure nervousness. Downsides include a delayed onset of sedation, higher cost compared to other agents, and dose-dependent hypotension and bradycardia. For procedural sedation, an IV loading dose of 0.5–1 μg/kg is administered slowly over 10 minutes, followed by an infusion at 0.2–1 μg/kg/hour (commonly 0.6 μg/kg/hour). For prevention of emergence delirium, dexmedetomidine can be given intranasally at 1 μg/kg or as an IV subanesthetic bolus of 0.25 μg/kg (Wang et al., 2019; Yu et al., 2023; Zheng et al., 2024; Li et al., 2024).

- Opioid Agonists (Fentanyl, Morphine, Hydromorphone)

Opioid agonists are typically used alongside other medications to provide analgesia during the maintenance phase of anesthesia, and less frequently for rapid analgesia during induction. Opioids block pain signals by activating mu, delta, and kappa opioid receptors, and enhance pain modulation in the medulla and spinal cord. They are effective for managing postoperative pain and may have sedative properties at higher doses. Cardiovascular stability is generally maintained, though dose-dependent hypotension can occur. Opioids decrease respiratory rate in a dose-dependent manner, and long-term use may lead to addiction, postoperative nausea and vomiting, and constipation. Fentanyl is favored for its rapid onset and high potency, especially in cardiac and high-risk surgeries, while morphine and hydromorphone are also used for intraoperative and postoperative pain control. Fentanyl is about 100 times more potent than morphine, with hydromorphone's potency between the two. Morphine is typically administered at a total dose of 10–20 mg per case (median 15 mg, or about 200 μg/kg), though this varies by patient and procedure. Fentanyl is usually given in amounts ranging from 500 to 2000 μg per case, with an average dose of approximately 1139 μg. Higher doses are often used in cardiac surgery, and dosing practices vary among providers (Hutchison et al., 2006; Trescot, 2008; Naik et al., 2021; Patočka et al., 2024).

- Inhalation Agents (Sevoflurane, Desflurane, Nitrous Oxide)

Inhalational anesthetics are dosed using minimum alveolar concentration (MAC) values, which vary by agent, patient age, and other factors. For adults, 1.0 MAC is considered a standard maintenance dose, but actual doses often range from 0.5 to 1.3 MAC depending on surgical needs and patient characteristics (Jedlička et al., 2021). Sevoflurane is frequently favored for mask induction, particularly in pediatric patients, and is also used for maintenance via continuous inhalation during general anesthesia (Lerman, 2022).

Sevoflurane is an inhalational anesthetic that acts on the central nervous system. While its mechanism of action is not fully understood, it is believed to enhance inhibitory signals by modulating GABA-A receptors in the brain, thereby reducing neuronal excitability. It also inhibits synaptic transmission by blocking voltage-dependent sodium channels and NMDA receptors, contributing to its overall anesthetic effect (Xu et al., 2019). Both sevoflurane and desflurane have rapid onset and recovery times, allowing for easy titration of anesthesia duration.

Nitrous oxide primarily functions as an NMDA receptor antagonist, with minimal to no effect on GABA-A receptors. It is also known for its stimulatory effects on dopamine, α1- and α2-adrenergic, and opioid receptors. Nitrous oxide provides analgesic benefits with few adverse effects (Alitalo et al., 2024; Maze & Fujinaga, 2000).

Despite these advantages, inhalational agents including nitrous oxide, sevoflurane, and desflurane also have potential drawbacks. Volatile agents can increase the risk of malignant hyperthermia and may cause dose-dependent respiratory resistance. Desflurane, in particular, may lead to airway irritation. Therefore, the choice of anesthetic agent should be based on patient characteristics, the duration of the surgical procedure, and the experience of the anesthesia provider (Lavelle & Kurra, 2018; Bogari et al., 2022; Zhou et al., 2023). A summary of the key features and differences among commonly used volatile anesthetic agents is provided in Table 10.

3.2.2.8.2. Reversal Agents and Antidotes in General Anesthesia

The use of reversal agents, or antidotes, is a crucial aspect of anesthesia management, especially in cases of overdose, prolonged sedation, or adverse reactions. Among the most commonly used antidotes in general anesthesia are naloxone and flumazenil. Naloxone, an opioid receptor antagonist, rapidly reverses the effects of opioid agonists such as fentanyl, morphine, and hydromorphone, while flumazenil is used to counteract benzodiazepine effects; both are routinely administered in overdose situations to quickly address life-threatening respiratory depression and other toxic effects (Wong, 2022). For neuromuscular blockade, sugammadex has become the preferred agent for reversing steroidal neuromuscular blockers like rocuronium and vecuronium, providing rapid and reliable recovery. In contrast, traditional anticholinesterases such as neostigmine, used for non-depolarizing agents, may cause cardiovascular side effects, making sugammadex a safer and more effective alternative (Greco et al., 2023; Wang et al., 2025). Additionally, intravenous lipid emulsion (ILE) is the first-line treatment for local anesthetic systemic toxicity, working through the "lipid sink" effect and other mechanisms (Jaffal et al., 2023). The choice and administration of these reversal agents should be tailored to the specific medication used, the clinical situation, and the patient's underlying health status. Careful monitoring is essential after administration, as re-sedation or recurrence of respiratory depression may occur, particularly with long-acting agents.

3.2.2.9. General Anesthesia Considerations for Special Populations

3.2.2.9.1. Pediatric Population

Children have increased sensitivity to anesthetic agents, higher metabolic rates, and immature organ systems (e.g., liver and kidneys). Psychologically, anxiety and fear are common, necessitating premedication or a calm environment. Additionally, the risk of airway obstruction is higher due to smaller airways and anatomical differences. In pediatric patients, specific agents and techniques are preferred to ensure safety and comfort. For premedication, midazolam is commonly used at a dose of 0.5 mg/kg orally (up to a maximum of 20 mg) to provide anxiolysis, while dexmedetomidine at 1 μg/kg intranasally is effective for sedation. Induction is often achieved with sevoflurane, favored for its non-irritating properties and rapid onset, or with ketamine at 2–5 mg/kg intramuscularly or 0.5 - 1.5 mg/kg intravenously, particularly in uncooperative children. Maintenance of anesthesia can be accomplished with sevoflurane or propofol, the latter administered at 100–200 μg/kg/min for TIVA. For intraoperative analgesia, fentanyl is typically given at 1–2 μg/kg intravenously. One of the main challenges in pediatric anesthesia is the occurrence of emergence delirium, especially with sevoflurane; this risk can be mitigated by administering low-dose dexmedetomidine (0.25 μg/kg IV) (Lerman & Jöhr, 2009; Kaye et al., 2020; Pieri et al., 2024).

3.2.2.9.2. Geriatric Patients

In geriatric patients, physiological changes such as decreased cardiac output and alterations in renal and hepatic function are common. The increased prevalence of cardiovascular, respiratory, and neurological diseases, along with prolonged drug metabolism and elimination, leads to heightened sensitivity to anesthetic agents. This may result in an extended duration of effects, requiring dose adjustments and careful monitoring. In elderly patients, certain agents and techniques are preferred to enhance safety and efficacy. For premedication, midazolam is administered intravenously at 1–2 mg, with careful titration to prevent oversedation. Induction is typically achieved with propofol at a reduced dose of 1-1.5 mg/kg IV, reflecting the increased sensitivity of older adults, or with etomidate at 0.2-0.3 mg/kg IV to maintain hemodynamic stability. Maintenance of anesthesia often involves sevoflurane or desflurane, both of which require lower MAC values in the elderly, or dexmedetomidine at 0.2–0.7 μg/kg/h for combined sedation and analgesia. For analgesia, fentanyl is used at 0.5–1 μg/kg IV for intraoperative pain control, while morphine at 0.05–0.1 mg/kg IV may be given postoperatively, though with caution due to slower drug clearance in this population. A significant challenge in elderly patients is the increased risk of postoperative cognitive dysfunction (POCD) and delirium, so it is advisable to avoid benzodiazepines and anticholinergics whenever possible (Wellner & Goettel, 2020; Rana et al., 2017; Shetti et al., 2025).

3.2.2.9.3. Patients with Systemic Diseases

When managing anesthesia in patients with systemic diseases, specific agents and techniques are chosen to address their unique needs. For patients with cardiovascular diseases, it is prudent to avoid drugs that may cause substantial hemodynamic alterations; for instance, ketamine is contraindicated in hypertensive patients. Etomidate at 0.2 - 0.3 mg/kg IV is preferred for induction due to its minimal impact on cardiovascular function, while dexmedetomidine at 0.2 - 0.7 μg/kg/h is used for sedation and analgesia.

In patients with respiratory disease, drugs with bronchodilator effects, such as sevoflurane, are preferred, while agents that may induce respiratory problems should be avoided. Sevoflurane is favored for both induction and maintenance because of its bronchodilatory properties, and ketamine at 0.5–1 mg/kg IV is particularly useful for induction in asthmatic individuals.

For those with renal disease, it is advisable to avoid drugs with active metabolites (e.g., morphine) and to adjust the dosages of drugs eliminated by the kidneys. Propofol at 1–2 mg/kg IV is selected for induction since it is metabolized in the liver, and remifentanil at 0.05–0.1 μg/kg/min is used for analgesia due to its metabolism by plasma esterases.

In cases of hepatic disease, drugs with extrahepatic metabolism (e.g., propofol, remifentanil) are preferred. Either etomidate or propofol can be used for induction, with remifentanil providing safe analgesia. Across all these conditions, careful monitoring of fluid balance and hemodynamics is crucial to ensure patient safety (Darwish et al., 2024).

3.2.2.9.4. Mentally Retarded Patients

Patients with intellectual disabilities often experience heightened anxiety, fear, and challenges with cooperation during medical procedures. They also have a higher incidence of epilepsy, cardiovascular abnormalities, and respiratory issues, and may struggle to communicate pain or discomfort effectively. For premedication, midazolam at 0.5 mg/kg can be given orally or intranasally for anxiolysis, while dexmedetomidine at 1 μg/kg intranasally is effective for sedation. Induction is commonly achieved with ketamine at 2–5 mg/kg intramuscularly for uncooperative patients, or with sevoflurane for inhalation induction. Maintenance of anesthesia may involve propofol at 100–200 μg/kg/min for TIVA or sevoflurane for inhalation maintenance. Fentanyl at 1–2 μg/kg IV is typically used for intraoperative pain control. These patients are at increased risk of airway obstruction due to hypotonia or anatomical abnormalities and may also experience postoperative agitation or confusion, which could necessitate additional sedation, such as dexmedetomidine (Chaudhary et al., 2017; Şitilci et al., 2017; Auerbacher et al., 2023).

3.2.2.10. Management of General Anesthesia Complications

3.2.2.10.1. Postoperative Care and Complications

The most common complications following general anesthesia are nausea, vomiting, and pain. To prevent and manage these issues, several precautions can be taken. Prophylactic antiemetic medications may be administered to reduce the risk of nausea and vomiting. Some studies report a modest reduction in mild pain when local anesthetics are used in conjunction with general anesthesia, but most do not find a significant impact on moderate or severe pain (Parekh et al., 2014; Ali & Hammuda, 2019; Lipp et al., 2021). Careful patient follow-up is essential, with patients kept under observation until they are fully awake and stable. Before discharge, it is important to ensure that the patient is alert and oriented; vital signs are stable, and both pain and nausea are well controlled. Additionally, patients should receive clear instructions regarding diet and medication use after the procedure (Brailo et al., 2019).

3.2.2.10.2. Respiratory Complications

Anesthetic medications, particularly benzodiazepines and propofol, can relax airway muscles, potentially resulting in upper airway obstruction—especially in patients with anatomical predispositions or excessive sedation. Hypoventilation often arises from the use of opioids, propofol, or benzodiazepines, with the risk increasing when these agents are used together. Bronchospasm may be triggered by airway irritation, allergic reactions, or preexisting conditions such as asthma. The risk of bronchospasm can be reduced by using drugs with bronchodilator properties, such as ketamine. Measures to reduce airway obstruction include repositioning the patient (e.g., head tilt-chin lift or jaw thrust), using airway adjuncts such as oropharyngeal or nasopharyngeal airways, administering 100% oxygen, and, if necessary, performing bag-mask ventilation. Additionally, behavioral support and nonpharmacological techniques can help reduce anxiety (Hillman et al., 2003; Qian et al., 2024; Frasca et al., 2025).

3.2.2.10.3. Hypoventilation

Management of hypoventilation includes reducing or discontinuing respiratory depressants and providing assisted ventilation or intubation if necessary (Visvanathan et al., 2005).

3.2.2.10.4. Bronchospasm

In cases of bronchospasm, administer bronchodilators (e.g., albuterol). Ketamine (0.5–1 mg/kg IV) may be used for its bronchodilatory effects. For severe cases, corticosteroids and epinephrine should be considered (Ali et al., 2018; Anderson et al., 2020).

3.2.2.10.5. Cardiovascular Complications

Hypotension may result from vasodilation induced by drugs such as propofol or volatile anesthetics, or from hypovolemia. In contrast, hypertension is frequently attributable to discomfort, inadequate anesthesia, or sympathetic activation. Bradycardia often occurs due to vagal stimulation or the administration of medications such as dexmedetomidine, while arrhythmias can be induced by electrolyte imbalances, hypoxia, or anesthetic agents. Management of intraoperative hemodynamic disturbances involves several strategies. For hypotension, intravenous fluids such as crystalloids or colloids are administered, and if fluid resuscitation is inadequate, vasopressors like phenylephrine or ephedrine may be used. In cases of hypertension, deepening the level of anesthesia or providing additional analgesia can help, and antihypertensive agents such as beta-blockers or calcium channel blockers may be administered if necessary. Bradycardia is typically managed with atropine or glycopyrrolate, with epinephrine reserved for more severe cases. For arrhythmias, it is important to identify and address underlying causes such as hypoxia or electrolyte imbalances, and antiarrhythmic medications like amiodarone or lidocaine can be used when indicated (Nateghi et al., 2021; Brzezinski-Sinai et al., 2021; Abebe et al., 2022).

3.2.2.10.6. Postoperative Nausea and Vomiting (PONV)

The use of volatile anesthetics, opioids, or nitrous oxide increases the risk of postoperative nausea and vomiting (PONV), with additional patient-specific risk factors including female gender, a history of motion sickness, and nonsmoking status. To prevent PONV, antiemetics such as ondansetron or dexamethasone can be given prophylactically, and utilizing TIVA with propofol may further reduce the risk. If PONV occurs, treatment involves administering rescue antiemetics like promethazine or metoclopramide and providing intravenous fluids to manage dehydration (Gan et al., 2020; Weibel et al., 2020; Yang et al., 2024).

3.2.2.10.7. Agitation and Delirium

Emergence delirium is especially common in children, often associated with the use of sevoflurane, while postoperative delirium tends to occur more frequently in elderly patients, typically due to lingering anesthetic effects, discomfort, or hypoxia. Management of emergence delirium includes administering low-dose dexmedetomidine (0.25 μg/kg IV) or midazolam, along with ensuring a calm and quiet recovery environment. For postoperative delirium, it is important to first rule out causes such as hypoxia, hypoglycemia, or electrolyte imbalances. In cases of severe agitation, medications like haloperidol or dexmedetomidine may be used. Continuous monitoring of vital signs including heart rate, blood pressure, and oxygen saturation is crucial for patient safety. The depth of anesthesia should be assessed using clinical indicators or devices such as bispectral index monitors, and anesthetic dosing should be adjusted according to the patient's response and the demands of the surgical procedure (Zhang et al., 2020; Chen et al., 2024; Dalamagka, 2024; Dragovic et al., 2023).

Table 10. Comparison of volatile anesthetic agents:
Key features and differences (Michenfelder et al., 1987; Houghton et al., 1993; Jedlicka et al., 2021)

Agent	Rapid Onset of Effect and Recovery	Ease of Titration	Cardiovascular Effects	Effects on Respiration	Potency (MAC)	Advantage	Special Disadvantages
Sevoflurane	Rapid	Easy	Stable, low effects	Respiratory depression	~2.0%	Non-irritating, good for induction	Risk of malignant hyperthermia, nephrotoxicity (low probability)
Desflurane	Very rapid	very easy	Mild tachycardia and hypertension	Respiratory depression, airway irritation	~6.0%	Fastest recovery	Airway irritation, high cost
Isoflurane	Moderate	Easy	Mild hypotension	Respiratory depression	~1.2%	Greater cerebral protection during periods of reduced blood flow	More pungent, less used for induction Slower recovery time
Halothane	Slow	Middle	Cardiac depression, arrhythmia	Respiratory depression	0.68–0.77%	Smoother, non-irritating properties and pleasant odor	Hepatotoxicity, risk of malignant hyperthermia
Nitrous Oxide	Very rapid	Easy	Minimum impact	Minimal depression	>100% does not provide sufficient deep anesthesia alone	strong analgesic	Weak anesthetic, risk of hypoxia

Conclusion

General anesthesia plays a vital role in modern dental practice, especially for patients and procedures where local anesthesia is insufficient. A thorough understanding of its indications, pharmacology, delivery methods, and potential complications is essential for safe and effective patient care. With careful patient selection, appropriate agent choice, and vigilant monitoring, general anesthesia can be administered safely, providing comfort and optimal outcomes for a diverse range of dental patients.

3.3. Sedation in Dentistry

Despite recent advancements in local anesthetic drugs, dental anxiety and fear remain common. While most people admit to some level of apprehension, many others avoid dental treatment altogether. Sedation in dentistry is a drug-based technique used to reduce patient anxiety, pain, and discomfort during dental procedures (Almenrader et al., 2007). Sedation enables patients to tolerate unpleasant or lengthy procedures while maintaining safety and cooperation. The depth of sedation can range from mild anxiolysis to deep sedation and general anesthesia, depending on the patient's needs, the complexity of the procedure, and the individual's medical status.

3.3.1. Goals and Objectives of Sedation

The primary goals of sedation in dentistry are to provide anxiolysis, analgesia, amnesia, and muscle relaxation while maintaining patient safety. Sedation should allow the patient to remain responsive to verbal commands, maintain protective airway reflexes, and preserve spontaneous ventilation and cardiovascular function. By improving patient cooperation and reducing stress for both the patient and the clinician, sedation facilitates the successful completion of dental procedures (Almenrader et al., 2007; Wilson et al., 2014).

3.3.2. Levels of Sedation

Sedation is commonly classified into four levels based on the patient's level of consciousness and response to stimuli: minimal sedation (anxiolysis), moderate sedation (conscious sedation), deep sedation, and general anesthesia (Hara et al., 2023). Minimal sedation involves a slight depression of consciousness, where patients can maintain their airway and respond normally. Moderate sedation is a drug-induced depression of consciousness in which patients respond purposefully to verbal commands, maintain their airway without intervention, and have adequate spontaneous ventilation. Deep sedation and general anesthesia involve progressively deeper levels of unconsciousness, with impaired airway and ventilation that may require assistance. The Ramsey scale is often used to assess sedation depth, with scores ranging from 1 (anxious, agitated) to 8 (no response to stimuli) (Van Der Jagt, 2018; Wang et al., 2012; Wong et al., 2021).

3.3.3. Sedation in Dentistry: Practices and Safety

Sedation in dentistry is widely used to manage anxiety and facilitate treatment, especially in patients who are unable to tolerate procedures with local anesthesia alone. For both adults and children, midazolam is the most commonly used and well-studied sedative, demonstrating effectiveness and a good safety profile when administered orally or via other routes, although some side effects can occur at higher doses or with alternative delivery methods (Corcuera-Flores et al., 2016; Ashley et al., 2018; Ashley et al., 2021). In pediatric dentistry, oral midazolam is recommended as the first-line agent for conscious sedation, with nitrous oxide/oxygen and other delivery methods as alternatives, though evidence for these is less robust (Gao & Wu, 2023). Non-pharmacological techniques, such as behavioral management, can complement sedation to reduce medication needs and adverse events, particularly in children. Other agents like ketamine, dexmedetomidine, propofol, and herbal medicines have shown promise but require further comparative studies to establish their relative safety and efficacy (et al., 2024).

In adults, benzodiazepines such as midazolam, diazepam, and alprazolam are effective for reducing anxiety, but more research is needed to confirm the safety and optimal dosing of oral sedation regimens. Safe sedation practice requires careful patient selection, including a comprehensive medical history and American Society of Anesthesiologists (ASA) classification, identification of contraindications such as allergies or severe systemic disease, and adherence to preoperative fasting guidelines. Continuous monitoring of vital signs including oxygen saturation, heart rate, respiratory rate, and blood pressure is essential, and emergency equipment along with trained personnel must be readily available. Overall, while sedation is a valuable tool in dental care, ongoing research and adherence to best practice guidelines are essential to ensure optimal outcomes and minimize risks (De Oliveira Araújo et al., 2021). The American Dental Association (ADA) guidelines emphasize that sedation drugs and techniques must have a wide margin of safety to avoid unintended loss of consciousness. Practitioners must be trained to manage emergencies and rescue patients if sedation deepens beyond the intended level (Goodchild & Donaldson, 2017). The ASA classification is summarized in Table 11.

3.3.4. Sedation Techniques and Their Efficacy

Oral midazolam is a commonly used sedative in pediatric dentistry, known for its consistent effectiveness and safety (Arezzo et al., 2022; Wulifan et al., 2016; Carta et al., 2021). When combined with other agents, such as intranasal dexmedetomidine, the sedation success rate significantly improves, although the onset time is longer (Bambini et al., 2003; Bambini et al., 2005; Strappa et al., 2022). Using drug combinations often results in better cooperation and behavior during dental treatments, which can have lasting positive effects especially for children receiving care for conditions like early childhood caries (Inchingolo et al., 2024).

Another frequently used method is the inhalation of nitrous oxide-oxygen (N_2O-O_2), which is appreciated for its high success rate and safety profile. It effectively reduces anxiety and promotes cooperation during procedures, with only minor and temporary side effects (Inchingolo et al., 2023; Inchingolo et al., 2024). Research highlights that factors such as the patient's age and the practitioner's experience play important roles in the success of nitrous oxide sedation (Bambini et al., 2005).

Regarding behavioral effects, studies show that pharmacological management of dental anxiety not only improves immediate treatment outcomes but also positively affects children's behavior in future visits. For example, children sedated moderately with midazolam or a midazolam/ketamine combination demonstrate better cooperation in subsequent dental sessions compared to those who were not sedated. These results emphasize the importance of sedation in preventing negative dental experiences that could otherwise traumatize young patients (Dipalma et al., 2023).

Comparative research has explored various drug combinations for conscious sedation. Pairing midazolam with chloral hydrate or promethazine enhances cooperation during dental procedures, with each combination offering unique benefits. The chloral hydrate/midazolam combination provides deeper and longer-lasting sedation, while promethazine-based regimens tend to cause fewer postoperative side effects such as nausea. These findings support customizing sedation strategies based on the patient's individual needs and the specific procedure (Mehran et al., 2018; Chen et al., 2019).

The method of drug administration also affects sedation outcomes. Intranasal midazolam is often favored due to its rapid onset and ease of administration, particularly in uncooperative children. It is more effective at reducing crying and anxiety than buccal administration, while maintaining comparable safety and efficacy (Ferrante et al., 2024). The commonly used drugs for sedation in dentistry, along with their advantages and disadvantages, are summarized in Table 12.

3.3.5. Indications

Indications for sedation in dentistry include patients with dental anxiety or phobia, those requiring complex or lengthy procedures, individuals with special needs or significant medical comorbidities, and cases where cooperation with local anesthesia alone is not possible. It is also considered for children with low coping skills or behavioral challenges, as well as for patients classified as ASA I or II (Cusenza et al., 2024; Inchingolo et al., 2024).

3.3.6. Contraindications

Contraindications include the presence of severe systemic disease (ASA III or IV), known allergies to sedative agents, inadequate fasting, or significant airway abnormalities. Sedation is also not recommended for children under one year of age or for individuals with documented allergies to sedative medications. Additional contraindications include pregnancy, certain drug interactions, severe psychiatric disorders, and lack of appropriate monitoring or trained personnel (Mason & Young, 1989; Santos et al., 2019; Aljohani et al., 2021).

3.3.7. Monitoring Protocols During Sedation

Effective monitoring during sedation is critical to ensure patient safety and timely detection of adverse events. Continuous monitoring should include pulse oximetry to assess oxygen saturation, electrocardiography (ECG) for cardiac rhythm, non-invasive blood pressure measurement, and capnography to monitor end-tidal CO_2, especially during moderate to deep sedation (American Society of Anesthesiologists, 2018). Vital signs should be recorded at baseline, every five minutes during sedation, and until full recovery. Proper documentation of these parameters is essential for quality assurance and medico-legal purposes (Malamed, 2017). The use of capnography has been shown to significantly reduce the incidence of hypoxemia during sedation (Cote et al., 2016).

3.3.8. Emergency Preparedness and Management of Sedation-Related Complications

All dental practitioners administering sedation must be prepared to manage potential emergencies such as airway obstruction, respiratory depression, hypotension, or allergic reactions. Emergency equipment including oxygen delivery systems, suction devices, airway adjuncts (e.g., oropharyngeal airways), and resuscitation drugs (e.g., epinephrine, naloxone) should be immediately accessible (ADA, 2016). Regular training in basic and advanced life support (BLS and ACLS) is mandatory to ensure prompt and effective response (Wilson et al., 2014). Protocols for escalation of care and transfer to hospital settings should be established. Studies emphasize that preparedness and simulation training improve outcomes in sedation-related emergencies (Nielsen et al., 2021).

3.3.9. Legal and Ethical Considerations in Sedation Practice

Sedation in dentistry carries significant legal and ethical responsibilities. Practitioners must obtain informed consent after explaining the risks, benefits, and alternatives to sedation in language understandable to the patient or guardian (ADA, 2016). Documentation of consent and sedation details is crucial. Adherence to local regulations and guidelines, such as those from the

ASA and the ADA, is mandatory to maintain licensure and avoid malpractice claims (Goodchild & Donaldson, 2017). Ethical practice also involves careful patient selection, avoiding sedation in high-risk individuals unless in appropriate settings, and ensuring sedation is used solely for patient benefit (Malamed, 2017).

3.3.10. Patient Consent and Communication Strategies

Effective communication before sedation is essential to reduce patient anxiety and improve cooperation. Practitioners should provide clear instructions regarding fasting, medication adjustments, and post-sedation care. Using visual aids or written materials can enhance understanding, especially in pediatric or special needs populations (Gao & Wu, 2023). Establishing trust through empathetic dialogue helps alleviate fears and sets realistic expectations. In pediatric dentistry, involving parents or guardians in the consent process and sedation planning is critical. Follow-up communication to assess patient recovery and satisfaction is also recommended (Ashley et al., 2021).

Table 11. ASA physical status classification for sedation assessment

ASA Class	Description	Sedation Considerations
ASA I	Normal healthy patient	Generally safe for all sedation levels; routine monitoring required
ASA II	Mild systemic disease (e.g., controlled hypertension, mild asthma)	Usually safe for sedation with standard monitoring; caution advised
ASA III	Severe systemic disease (e.g., poorly controlled diabetes, COPD)	Increased risk; sedation requires careful assessment and advanced monitoring
ASA IV	Severe systemic disease that is a constant threat to life (e.g., unstable angina, severe heart failure)	Sedation generally contraindicated or requires hospital setting with full resuscitation capabilities
ASA V	Moribund patient not expected to survive without the operation	Sedation contraindicated except in emergency situations
ASA VI	Brain-dead patient whose organs are being removed for donor purposes	Not applicable for sedation

Table 12. Common drugs used for sedation in dentistry (Malamed, 2017).

Drug	Route	Onset Time (min)	Duration (min)	Half-life (hours)	Pediatric Dose	Adult Dose	Advantages	Disadvantages
Midazolam	Oral/ IV/IM	5 (IV)	30	1.5-2.5	0.25-0.5 mg/kg oral	7.5-15 mg oral	Rapid onset and short duration; Provides anxiolysis, sedation, and amnesia	Risk of respiratory depression; Requires monitoring
Nitrous Oxide	Inhalation	2	5-10	NA	30-50% concentration inhaled	30-50% concentration inhaled	Rapid onset and recovery; Provides anxiolysis and mild analgesia; Safe with minimal side effects	Requires equipment; Not suitable for patients with respiratory issues
Diazepam	Oral/ IV/IM	15	60	20-50	0.1-0.3 mg/kg oral	5-10 mg oral	Provides anxiolysis, sedation, and amnesia; Oral administration available	Longer duration; Risk of accumulation
Hydroxyzine	Oral/IM	15-30	180	20-25	0.6-1 mg/kg oral	25-100 mg oral	Anxiolytic and sedative properties; Antihistamine	Sedation may be prolonged; Anticholinergic side effects
Chloral Hydrate	Oral	15-30	60-120	8	50-75 mg/kg oral	Not commonly used	Sedative and hypnotic; Used in pediatric sedation	Gastrointestinal irritation; Risk of overdose
Propofol	IV	1	5-10	1-3	1-2 mg/kg IV	1-2 mg/kg IV	Rapid onset and short duration; Used for deep sedation; Requires trained personnel	Requires monitoring; Risk of respiratory depression
Fentanyl	IV	1	30-60	2-4	1-2 mcg/kg IV	50-100 mcg IV	Potent analgesic; Rapid onset	Risk of respiratory depression; Requires monitoring
Dexme-detomidine	IV	10-15	30-60	2	0.5-1 mcg/kg IV	0.2-0.7 mcg/kg/hr IV infusion	Sedation and analgesia with minimal respiratory depression; Useful in patients with behavioral disorders	Bradycardia and hypotension potential
Ketamine	IV/IM	1-2	15-30	2-3	0.5-1 mg/kg IV	0.5-1 mg/kg IV	Provides sedation and analgesia; Maintains airway reflexes	Emergence reactions; Increased salivation

Conclusion

Sedation in dentistry is a valuable tool for managing patient anxiety, facilitating complex procedures, and improving overall treatment outcomes. By carefully selecting appropriate candidates, adhering to safety protocols, and maintaining clear communication, dental practitioners can provide effective and safe sedation. Ongoing research, practitioner training, and adherence to ethical and legal standards are essential to ensure optimal patient care and minimize risks associated with sedation.

3.4. Topical Agents for Oral Conditions

Topical agents play an important role in the treatment of various diseases affecting the oral mucosa and teeth. These are drugs applied directly to the oral mucosa or tooth surfaces, exerting a local effect. By acting directly on the diseased area, topical agents increase treatment success while avoiding systemic side effects. New delivery systems (e.g., mucoadhesive gels, patches, nanocarriers) improve drug retention and effectiveness in the oral cavity, even in moist environments. Most topical agents, including herbal and hyaluronic acid preparations, have good safety profiles with minimal adverse effects. The use of topical agents is particularly common in clinical practice for conditions such as periodontal disease, aphthous ulcers, fungal infections, and traumatic lesions (Mombelli & Samaranayake, 2004; Casale et al., 2016; Nakajima et al., 2021).

Antimicrobial agents are used to treat infections caused by bacteria, fungi, or viruses in the mouth. Chlorhexidine gluconate is the most commonly preferred topical antimicrobial agent for treating periodontal disease and reducing the risk of post-surgical infection. It is beneficial in the early healing phase after periodontal surgery and as an adjunct in the management of periodontal pockets and peri-implant mucositis (Graziani et al., 2024). Chlorhexidine is also effective in preventing gingivitis due to its plaque-inhibiting effect. However, long-term use can cause side effects such as tooth discoloration and taste changes (Deus & Ouanounou, 2022; Batista et al., 2021). Additionally, antimicrobial gels (e.g., IDEA ion gel), hyaluronic acid, and locally administered antibiotics accelerate healing, diminish infections, and inhibit disease development, particularly as adjuncts to mechanical therapy (Casale et al., 2016; Nakajima et al., 2021).

The most common fungal infection in the mouth is oral candidiasis, caused by Candida albicans. Topical antifungal agents such as nystatin suspension, miconazole gel, and clotrimazole lozenges are used to treat this infection. Nystatin acts by targeting the fungal cell wall and is considered safe due to its low systemic absorption. Miconazole, on the other hand, is effective against both fungi and some bacteria and is particularly recommended for elderly denture wearers. Advanced nanocarrier formulations of antifungal drugs (e.g., nystatin, miconazole) provide targeted action and minimize systemic toxicity (Garg et al., 2020).

Local analgesics and anesthetics are used for the symptomatic treatment of painful oral lesions, such as aphthous ulcers. Lidocaine gel or benzocaine-containing preparations provide short-term relief for patients (Lau & Smith, 2022). Topical anesthetics have been shown to be more effective than corticosteroids for quick pain relief in recurring aphthous ulcers, making them a preferable option for acute symptom control (Prathoshini et al., 2020). These agents are particularly preferred for reducing discomfort during eating and speaking. They are usually applied directly to the ulcer surface and provide short-term relief, enhancing dental function and patient comfort. However, caution should be exercised, as excessive and uncontrolled use can cause local side effects such as mucosal irritation, burning, or allergic reactions (Milia et al., 2022). Careful dosing and patient education are required to reduce these hazards. Prolonged or frequent use should be avoided, especially in children, to prevent toxicity.

Topical corticosteroids are frequently prescribed for inflammatory oral diseases, such as aphthous ulcers, oral lichen planus, and pemphigoids. Agents such as triamcinolone acetonide and betamethasone are effective in reducing inflammation and symptoms. These drugs are applied directly to the lesion, avoiding systemic side effects. However, the risk of local immunosuppression and secondary infection should be considered with long-term use (Sheshaprasad & Pai, 2020). Additionally, other topical agents such as anti-inflammatories (amlexanox, diclofenac), anesthetics (lidocaine), licorice extract, herbal agents, and mucoadhesive delivery systems can reduce pain, speed healing, and minimize recurrence of aphthous ulcers (Muthu et al., 2021). Topical treatments, including hyaluronic acid, corticosteroids, and protective mucoadhesive substances, can facilitate healing and alleviate discomfort in cases of traumatic lesions (Casale et al., 2016; Suharyani et al., 2021).

Fluoride-containing gels, varnishes, and mouthwashes play an important role in preventing tooth decay and reducing tooth sensitivity. Fluoride supports the remineralization of tooth enamel and increases its resistance to acids. Meta-analyses show that these agents can reduce caries incidence by 26–43% compared to no treatment, with fluoride varnishes showing particularly strong effects in both primary and permanent teeth. High-concentration fluoride varnishes applied by dentists significantly reduce the incidence of caries, especially in individuals at high risk (Munteanu et al., 2022; Marinho et al., 2013). All formulations (gels, varnishes, mouthwashes) are efficacious, exhibiting comparable effectiveness; however, varnishes may provide practical benefits for young children and individuals with limited cooperation (Marinho et al., 2004).

3.5. Prescription-Strength Oral Hygiene Products

Some oral hygiene products can only be obtained with a prescription because they contain high concentrations of active ingredients or have specialized formulations. However, the regulations and specific uses of these prescription products may differ from country to country. These products are generally used in patients who are unresponsive to standard oral care products or are at high risk and should be applied under the supervision of a dentist or doctor.

Chlorhexidine gluconate-containing mouthwashes are used by prescription for the treatment of gum disease and the prevention of post-surgical infections. Chlorhexidine is highly effective in controlling plaque and gingivitis. However, long-term use can cause tooth discoloration, taste changes, and, rarely, mucosal irritation. Therefore, the duration and frequency of use should be determined by a dentist (Deus & Ouanounou, 2022; Batista et al., 2021; Muhammad et al., 2025).

High-concentration fluoride gels and varnishes are also prescribed and applied by dentists to patients at high risk of tooth decay. Products such as 1.1% sodium fluoride gel or 5% sodium fluoride varnish are effective in strengthening tooth enamel and preventing caries. These products are particularly preferred for children, those undergoing orthodontic treatment, and elderly individuals at high risk of root surface caries (Mahalingam, 2025).

Some topical agents used to treat fungal or viral infections in the mouth are also available by prescription. Products such as miconazole oral gel and acyclovir cream are effective in reducing the spread of infection and the severity of symptoms. Additionally, topical corticosteroids, used to treat inflammatory diseases of the oral mucosa, are usually prescribed. These medications act locally, eliminating the need for systemic treatment, especially in severe and widespread lesions (Muhammad et al., 2025).

The use of prescription-strength oral hygiene products should be planned according to the patient's individual needs and risk factors. Because incorrect or unnecessary use of these products can increase the risk of side effects, they should always be administered under the supervision of a dentist or relevant specialist.

Conclusion

Topical agents are essential in managing oral diseases, offering effective local treatment with minimal systemic side effects. Their careful selection and use, especially for prescription products, ensure optimal outcomes and patient safety.

3.6. Antibiotics in Dentistry: Use, Challenges, and Stewardship

3.7.1. Introduction to Antibiotics in Dentistry

Antibiotics have revolutionized healthcare, playing a critical role in managing bacterial infections and saving lives. In dentistry, antibiotics are primarily used to treat odontogenic (tooth-related) and non-odontogenic infections, prevent surgical site infections, and provide prophylaxis for high-risk patients. However, their misuse and overuse have led to significant challenges, including antimicrobial resistance (AMR), adverse effects, and unnecessary healthcare costs. This chapter explores the appropriate use of antibiotics in dentistry, the challenges associated with their misuse, and strategies for effective stewardship.

3.7.2. Odontogenic Infections

Odontogenic infections are infections that originate within the tooth and its supporting structures, such as the periodontal tissues, and are among the most common types of orofacial infections. These infections can result from conditions such as dental caries, pulpal necrosis, dental trauma, and periodontal diseases. If left untreated, they can lead to severe consequences affecting both the soft and hard tissues of the oral cavity. Gram-positive cocci are responsible for approximately 65% of odontogenic infections, while Gram-negative bacilli are found in about 25% of cases (Kuriyama et al., 2002a; Kumar et al., 2022). These infections are most prevalent in individuals aged 21–40 and are not gender-specific. Common symptoms include pain and swelling in the oral region. If not treated promptly, odontogenic infections can lead to complications ranging from sinusitis and osteomyelitis to more serious conditions such as airway obstruction, septicemia, brain abscess, and, in rare cases, life-threatening outcomes like cavernous sinus thrombosis and loss of vision. The most frequent complication of odontogenic infections is the dentoalveolar abscess (Mariño et al., 2023). Treatment typically involves a combination of surgical interventions, such as debridement, incision and drainage, and endodontic therapy, along with the judicious use of antibiotics. Antibiotics should be prescribed only after the source of infection has been addressed, and their use should be limited to acute infections to help prevent the development of bacterial resistance. Comprehensive guidelines and ongoing education for dental practitioners are essential to ensure the effective management of odontogenic infections and to minimize the risks associated with unnecessary antibiotic use (Kudiyirickal & Hollinshead, 2012; Nadig & Taylor, 2018; González et al., 2012).

3.7.3. Indication of Antibiotics in Dentistry

Antibiotics are an essential component of dental practice, used both for prophylaxis and for the treatment of odontogenic and non-odontogenic (non-tooth-related) infections. However, their use must be carefully considered to avoid unnecessary prescriptions and the development of antibiotic resistance.

3.7.3.1. Prophylactic Use of Antibiotics

In dentistry, prophylactic antibiotics have been used for many years to prevent serious complications such as infective endocarditis and prosthetic joint infections. However, due to the risks associated with antibiotic resistance and unnecessary prescribing, significant changes have been made to the guidelines in recent years (Vidović et al., 2024). The new guidelines emphasize that antibiotic prophylaxis should be recommended only for certain high-risk patient groups. According to the American Heart Association (AHA) and the European Society of Cardiology (ESC), antibiotic prophylaxis before invasive dental procedures is recommended only for patients at high risk—specifically, those with a history of infective endocarditis, prosthetic heart valves, certain congenital heart diseases, or valve disease following heart transplantation. For patients considered to be at moderate or low risk, antibiotic prophylaxis is not recommended (Sperotto et al., 2024; Thornhill et al., 2024).

In these high-risk patients, certain dental procedures that increase the risk of infection require prophylaxis, such as dental extractions, surgical periodontal procedures, dental implant placement, endodontic procedures or surgeries, subgingival placement of antibiotic fibers or strips, and intraligamentary local anesthetic injections (Tong & Rothwell, 2000; Kumar et al., 2014; Dar-Odeh et al., 2010; Kussainova et al., 2025).

The majority of dentists administer antibiotic prophylaxis to high-risk patients, but full compliance with guidelines varies, and some patients may receive unnecessary or inadequate antibiotics (Dios et al., 2023; Havers-Borgersen et al., 2023). Therefore, it is important to accurately identify the patient's risk group and to act in accordance with current guidelines.

3.7.3.2. Therapeutic Use of Antibiotics

Antibiotics are indicated for the treatment of several acute dental infections. These include necrotizing ulcerative gingivitis, Stage III-grade C/incisor-molar pattern periodontitis (previously known as localized aggressive periodontitis), acute periapical abscess, cellulitis, and periodontal abscesses that show local or systemic spread of infection. Additionally, antibiotics are recommended for pericoronitis, peri-implantitis, and infections affecting the deep fascial layers of the head and neck. Finally, any cases presenting with fever and/or malaise also warrant antibiotic treatment (Bascones et al., 2010; Dar-Odeh et al., 2018). Antibiotics should be adjuncts to local treatment, not substitutes, and their use is justified only in cases with systemic involvement or risk of spread (Ahmadi et al., 2021; Cope et al., 2014).

3.7.4. Challenges in Antibiotic Use

Antibiotics are often overused and misused in dentistry, with patients frequently not adhering to prescriptions, and antimicrobial resistance (AMR) is on the rise due to improper use of antibiotics (Contaldo et al., 2023). Additionally, overuse leads to allergic reactions and other side effects. Only about 12% of dentists prescribe antibiotics correctly, highlighting the need for better guidelines (Ahmadi et al., 2021; Elhassy et al., 2024). In India, significant misuse of antibiotics for dental diseases is observed, including inappropriate use, unrecommended combinations, and self-medication by the general population (Bhuvaraghan et al., 2021). The misuse of antibiotics contributes to the global problem of AMR (Stein et al., 2018). Interventions in dentistry can reduce antibiotic prescriptions and increase prescription accuracy (Löffler & Böhmer, 2017). These interventions include the development of antibiotic stewardship programs, which aim to optimize antibiotic use, minimize resistance, and improve patient outcomes. Key principles of stewardship in dentistry include evidence-based prescribing, appropriate drug selection, correct dosage and duration, patient education, monitoring and feedback, and the use of alternatives such as nutraceuticals when available (Teoh et al., 2025). The future of antibiotics in dentistry should focus on minimizing use through accurate diagnosis, local application, and adherence to guidelines to prevent AMR and ensure effective treatment.

3.7.5. Commonly Used Antibiotics in Dentistry

Dentists rely on a limited range of antibiotics, selected according to the specific pathogens involved in oral infections. The most commonly prescribed antibiotics include beta-lactam antibiotics, macrolides, nitroimidazoles, and lincosamides.

3.7.5.1. Beta Lactam Antibiotics

Beta-lactam antibiotics are among the most widely used classes of antibiotics in medicine and dentistry. They are characterized by the presence of a beta-lactam ring in their chemical structure, which is essential for their bactericidal activity (Balsalobre et al., 2019). These antibiotics work by inhibiting bacterial cell wall synthesis, leading to cell lysis and death. Beta-lactam antibiotics include penicillins, cephalosporins, carbapenems, and monobactams, with penicillins being the most commonly used in dental practice.

3.7.5.1.1. Mechanism of Action

Beta-lactam antibiotics target penicillin-binding proteins (PBPs), which are enzymes involved in the synthesis of peptidoglycan, a critical component of the bacterial cell wall. By binding to PBPs, beta-lactams inhibit the cross-linking of peptidoglycan chains, weakening the cell wall and causing bacterial death, particularly in actively dividing cells (Waxman & Strominger, 1983; Balsalobre et al., 2019; Zabiszak et al., 2023).

3.7.5.1.2. Beta-Lactam Antibiotics in Dentistry

In dentistry, beta-lactam antibiotics—particularly penicillins—are the first-line treatment for odontogenic infections due to their efficacy, safety, and narrow spectrum of activity against oral pathogens. These infections are often polymicrobial, involving both aerobic and anaerobic bacteria, such as *Streptococcus mutans*, *Peptostreptococcus*, *Prevotella*, and *Fusobacterium* species (Kuriyama et al., 2002b; Davis, 2010).

3.7.5.1.3. Penicillins

- Mechanism of Action

Penicillin antibiotics are beta-lactam antibiotics that inhibit bacterial cell wall synthesis, making them bactericidal. They are widely used in dentistry due to their effectiveness against many oral pathogens, including *Streptococcus* species and anaerobic bacteria (Balsalobre et al., 2019).

- Penicillin Use in Dentistry

Penicillin is primarily used in dentistry to treat bacterial infections. Common applications include the treatment of dental abscesses, management of periodontal infections, prophylaxis for bacterial endocarditis in high-risk patients undergoing dental procedures, and post-operative infection prevention following dental surgeries (Barone et al., 2025).

- Pharmacokinetics of Penicillin Antibiotics

The most commonly used penicillin antibiotics in dentistry are penicillin V, amoxicillin, amoxicillin-clavulanate, and ampicillin. They are generally water-soluble, have moderate to low protein binding, are primarily eliminated by the kidneys, and their effectiveness depends on maintaining drug concentrations above the minimum inhibitory concentration (MIC) for a sufficient portion of the dosing interval. The most important pharmacokinetic features of penicillins are rapid absorption (for oral forms), short half-lives, and renal elimination, which require frequent dosing to maintain therapeutic levels. The pharmacokinetic properties of these antibiotics are presented in Table 13.

Table 13. Pharmacokinetic profiles of common β-lactam antibiotics in dental practice (Aksoy, 2022a; Aksoy, 2022b)

Antibiotics	Route of administration /Absorption	Distribution	Metabolism	Excretion
Penicillin V	Oral -Bioavailability 60-73%	Highly protein binding 80% widespread distribution	Hepatic 55%	Parent drug and metabolites are excreted in the urine.
Amoxicillin	Orally, IV and IM. -Bioavailability 75% -Does not affect absorption when taken with food.	Low protein binding (17%) -Widespread distribution -Crosses only inflamed meninges.	Hepatic 10%	Excreted unchanged in the urine.
ampicillin	Oral, IV and IM. -Bioavailability 40% -Absorption decreases when taken with food.	Low protein binding 17% Widespread distribution Crosses only inflamed meninges.	Hepatic 10%	Excreted unchanged in the urine.
Amoxicillin-Clavulanate	Amoxicillin absorption is not affected by food but clavulanate potassium absorption improves when taken with meals	Clavulanic acid is about 25% bound.	Clavulanate is metabolized considerably	25% and 40% of the Clavulanate is excreted unchanged in the urine. The half-life is 1.3 hours for amoxicillin and 1 hour for clavulanic acid.
Cephalexin	Oral	Distributes well into body tissues and fluids	Not metabolized.	Half-life:0.9–1.5 hours Excreted unchanged in urine.
Cefazolin	IV, IM	It enters most tissues well; does not pass into the Cerebrospinal fluid.	Not metabolized.	Half-life :1.4–2 hours. Excreted unchanged in urine.
Cefadroxil	Rapid and well absorbed from GI tract.	Protein binding: 20%.	Not metabolized.	1 to 2 hours; 20 to 24 hours in renal failure. Urine (>90% as unchanged drug within 24 hours
Cefuroxime	PO, IM, IV	Pass well into Cerebrospinal fluid	Not metabolized.	Half-life: 1.2–1.9 hours. Excreted unchanged in urine.
Ceftriaxone	IM ve IV	Widespread distribution Can pass into cerebrospinal fluid.	Not metabolized	It is excreted unchanged in feces and urine.

Table 14. β-lactam antibiotic dosing across special populations (Aksoy, 2022a; Aksoy, 2022b)

Antibiotics	Indication	Children dose	Adult dose	Kidney impairment Dose	Liver impairment dose	Pregnancy and breastfeeding consideration
Penicillin V	Dental Abscess	25 to 50 mg/kg/day in divided doses every 6 hours; maximum daily dose: 2,000mg/day	500 mg every 6 to 8 hours*. For 5-7 days	No dose adjustment	No dose adjustment	compatible for use during pregnancy and breastfeeding
Amoxicillin	First choice in dental infection	Oral: 40 to 45 mg/kg/day in divided doses every 8 hours; maximum dose: 500 mg/dose. 3-7 days	500 mg every 8 hours or **875** -1000 mg every 12 hours. 3-7 days	GFR 10 to 29 mL/minute/1.73 m2: The dose given every 12 hours. GFR <10mL/minute/1.73 m2: The dose given every 12-24 hours	No dose adjustment	Compatible for use during pregnancy and breastfeeding when given within the recommended doses
ampicillin	Unable to take oral medication	IV, IM: 50 to 200 mg/kg/day divided every 6 hours; maximum daily dose: 8 g/day	1 to 2 g every 6 hours	GFR 10 to 29 mL/minute/1.73 m2: the dose given every 8-12 hours. GFR <10mL/minute/1.73 m2: The dose given every 12 hours	No dose adjustment	Compatible for use during pregnancy and breastfeeding when given within the recommended doses
Amoxicillin-Clavulanate	Failure of first choice antibiotic	20–40 mg/kg/day divided every 8 hours or 25–45 mg/kg/day divided every 12 hours, based on infection severity. Maximum dose 1000–2800 mg amoxicillin/143–400 mg clavulanic acid	Oral: 875 mg every 12 hours; continue until clinical resolution, typically for 7 to 14 days. 14 days for Periodontitis, severe, plaque-associated	Avoid IR 875 mg tablet or ER tablets in patients with CrCl <30 mL/minute.	No dose adjustment. Contraindicated in patients with a history of amoxicillin-clavulanate-associated liver dysfunction	Compatible for use during pregnancy but should be avoided in patients at risk for preterm delivery.

Antibiotics	Indication	Children dose	Adult dose	Kidney impairment Dose	Liver impairment dose	Pregnancy and breastfeeding consideration
Cefazolin	Alternative to penicillin. . IM, IV	25 to 100 mg/kg/day divided every 8 hours	1 to 2 g every 8 hours	CrCl 30 to <50 mL/minute: the dose every 8-12 hours CrCl >10 to <30 mL/minute: the dose every 12 hours CrCl ≤10 mL/minute: the dose every 24 hours.	No dose adjustment.	Compatible for use during pregnancy. Caution be exercised when administering cefazolin to breastfeeding women.
Cephalexin	Alternative to penicillin. . Oral	25–100 mg/kg/day, divided 6_8 hours	250 mg to 1 g every 6 hours or 500 mg every 12 hours (maximum: 4 g/day).	CrCl 15 to <30 minute: the dose every 8-12 hours CrCl ≤15 mL/minute: the dose every12- 24 hours.	no dose adjustments	
Cefadroxil	Alternative to penicillin. . Oral	Oral: 30 mg/kg/day divided every 12 hours; maximum daily dose: 2,000 mg/day	1 g every 24 hours or 500 mg every 12 hours. In sever cases 1 g every 12 hours	20 to <40 mL/minute: the dose every 12-24 hours. <20 mL/minute: the dose every 48 hours	no dose adjustments	Outcome information specific to maternal use of cefadroxil during pregnancy is limitEd, caution Caution should be exercised when administering cefadroxil to breastfeeding patients.

Table 14. (Continued)

Antibiotics	Indication	Children dose	Adult dose	Kidney impairment Dose	Liver impairment dose	Pregnancy and breastfeeding consideration
Cefuroxime	Necessity of broad-spectrum action.	IV, IM: 100 to 150 mg/kg/day in divided doses every 8 hours; maximum daily dose: 6,000 mg/day. 20 to 30 mg/kg/day in divided doses every 12 hours; maximum daily dose: 1,000 mg/day	500 mg twice daily in combination with metronidazole for 7 to 14 days	10 to 29 mL/minute/1.73 m2: The IV dose every 12 hours but the oral dose 250 mg every 12 hours. <10 mL/minute/1.73 m2: the doses for IV and oral every 24 hours	no dose adjustments	The risk and benefit should be evaluated for breastfeeding. However cephalosporins consider safe during pregnancy and breastfeeding.
Ceftriaxone	Odontogenic soft tissue infection.	IM, IV: 50 to 75 mg/kg/day in divided doses every 12 to 24 hours; maximum daily dose: 2,000 mg/day	Odontogenic soft tissue infection :2 g once daily in combination with metronidazole; following clinical improvement, transition to oral step-down therapy and continue antibiotics until resolution, typically for a total of 7 to 14 days	a maximum daily dose $\leq$2,000 mg/day is suggested.	no dose adjustments	The risk and benefit should be evaluated for breastfeeding. However cephalosporins consider safe during pregnancy and breastfeeding.

*Generally combined with metronidazole for dental abscess for 5 to 7 days.

- Dosage and Administration

Administration of penicillin antibiotics is typically oral, but intravenous or enteral routes may be used in hospital settings or for severe infections (Hanberg et al., 2024). For dental procedures with a risk of bacteremia (such as extractions), penicillin has been used prophylactically, often started 24 hours before the procedure and continued afterward, especially in patients at risk for endocarditis (Glaser et al., 1948). The doses of penicillin antibiotics for various populations, according to their clinical application in dentistry, are listed in Table 14.

- Adverse Drug Reaction

Penicillin is a widely used antibiotic, but it can cause side effects ranging from mild to life-threatening. The most important and common side effects are allergic reactions (Udhnawala et al., 2024). Penicillins can cause IgE-mediated (Type 1) allergic reactions, such as pruritus, erythema, urticaria, angioedema, wheezing, hypotension, laryngeal edema, and anaphylaxis. Delayed reactions, such as serum sickness, may occur and present with fever, rash (often urticarial), lymphadenopathy, arthritis, and glomerulonephritis. Severe cutaneous reactions—including erythema multiforme, exfoliative dermatitis, toxic epidermal necrolysis, and photosensitivity—are rare but serious.

Neurological side effects, such as encephalopathy, altered consciousness, hyperreflexia, myoclonus, and seizures, can occur with high doses, particularly in patients with renal failure. Gastrointestinal side effects, including diarrhea, are common, especially with amoxicillin-clavulanate and ampicillin. Prolonged use (e.g., ampicillin for more than two months) increases the risk of *Clostridioides difficile*-associated diarrhea (CDAD) and superinfections, such as fungal (e.g., vaginal candidiasis) or bacterial infections (Bhattacharya et al., 2010; Udhnawala et al., 2024). Amoxicillin-clavulanate is also associated with rare cases of hepatitis and cholestatic jaundice (Larrey et al., 1992; Vaishnani et al., 2019).

Renal effects, such as allergic interstitial nephritis (e.g., with methicillin or ampicillin) and glomerulonephritis, may occur, along with hematological effects like eosinophilia, neutropenia, thrombocytopenia, and thrombopathy (e.g., with ticarcillin) (Galpin et al., 1978; Woodroffe et al., 1975). Cross-reactivity with other beta-lactams (e.g., cephalosporins, carbapenems) is possible, and patients with a history of allergic diseases (e.g., asthma, allergic conjunctivitis) are at higher risk of penicillin allergy (Romano et al., 2016).

The cross-reactivity between cephalosporins and penicillins varies depending on the cephalosporin generation and the similarity of their side chains. For first- and second-generation cephalosporins, the risk of cross-reactivity is less than 10%, while for third- and fourth-generation cephalosporins, it is less than 5%. However, when cephalosporins share identical side chains with penicillins, the risk of cross-reactivity increases significantly, exceeding 30% (Chaudhry et al., 2019; Romano et al., 2016).

- Warning

Penicillins are primarily excreted by the kidneys, so dose adjustments are required for certain medications (Kumar et al., 2016). Hemodialysis removes ampicillin, requiring additional doses post-dialysis, while peritoneal dialysis does not affect penicillin levels. Penicillins containing sodium (e.g., carbenicillin, ticarcillin) should be used cautiously in patients with hypertension or heart failure. Probenecid increases penicillin serum levels by inhibiting renal excretion. Penicillins may reduce the efficacy of live vaccines (e.g., Bacillus Calmette-Guérin [BCG], typhoid, cholera) and sodium picosulfate for bowel cleansing (Jauro et al., 2020). Chloroquine and lanthanum reduce ampicillin levels, so ampicillin should be taken two hours later. Neomycin reduces penicillin V absorption by 50%, and amoxicillin or ampicillin may cause oral contraceptive failure, requiring additional contraception. Long-term use requires monitoring of renal, hepatic, and hematological functions. Penicillin V and ampicillin should be taken on an empty stomach. Patients allergic to one penicillin are at higher risk of reacting to other beta-lactams. Blood pressure monitoring is advised for patients with hypertension due to sodium or potassium content. Patients should complete prescribed doses and be monitored for anaphylaxis during initial use (Aksoy, 2022a).

- Mechanism of Resistance

Bacteria have various mechanisms by which they may resist penicillin action. They may produce beta-lactamase enzymes, which inactivate penicillin by breaking the beta-lactam ring, or decrease the number of porin channels in the outer membrane, thereby restricting the entry of penicillin. Additionally, bacteria may alter the structure of their PBPs so that they have a lower affinity for penicillin. This is the mechanism by which *MRSA* and *Streptococcus pneumoniae* develop resistance. Some bacteria have efflux pumps that expel penicillin from the cell, and efflux may provide synergy with other resistance mechanisms. The combination of these mechanisms can make bacteria highly resistant to penicillin.

3.7.5.1.4. Cephalosporins

- Overview of Cephalosporins

Cephalosporins are a class of beta-lactam antibiotics derived from *Acremonium* (formerly known as *Cephalosporium*). They are structurally and functionally related to penicillins but have a broader spectrum of activity and greater resistance to beta-lactamases (Williams et al., 2001). Cephalosporins are classified into five generations based on their antimicrobial spectrum and clinical applications (Sturaro et al., 2025). Each generation has unique characteristics that make it suitable for specific types of infections.

- Mechanism of Action

Cephalosporins exert their bactericidal effect by inhibiting bacterial cell wall synthesis. They bind to penicillin-binding proteins (PBPs), which are essential for the cross-linking of peptidoglycan chains in the bacterial cell wall (Curtis et al., 1979; Chase et al., 1981). This disruption weakens the cell wall, leading to bacterial lysis and death. Cephalosporins are effective against a wide range of Gram-positive and Gram-negative bacteria, although their spectrum varies by generation.

- The Role of Cephalosporins in Dental Infections

Dental infections are typically polymicrobial, involving both aerobic and anaerobic bacteria. Common pathogens include *Streptococcus* species (e.g., *Streptococcus mutans*, *Streptococcus viridans*), *Peptostreptococcus* species, *Prevotella* species, *Fusobacterium* species, and *Porphyromonas* species (Larsen & Fiehn, 2017). Cephalosporins are particularly useful in treating dental infections due to their efficacy against many of these organisms (Manoharan & Rajesh, 2019).

- Indications for Cephalosporin Use in Dentistry

Cephalosporins are generally not considered first-line antibiotics for dental infections, as penicillins such as amoxicillin are typically preferred (Sato et al., 2022). However, cephalosporins may be indicated in certain scenarios, including patients with mild hypersensitivity to penicillins (excluding those with a history of anaphylaxis or severe allergic reactions), infections caused by beta-lactamase-producing bacteria that are resistant to penicillins, and severe or spreading infections such as cellulitis or Ludwig's angina, where broad-spectrum antibiotic coverage is necessary (Campagna et al., 2012). Additionally, cephalosporins can be used for prophylaxis in dental procedures for patients at high risk of infective endocarditis or those with prosthetic joint replacements, particularly when penicillins are contraindicated.

- Commonly Used Cephalosporins in Dental Practice

First-generation cephalosporins, such as cephalexin and cefadroxil, are effective against Gram-positive cocci, including *Streptococcus* species, and are commonly used for mild to moderate dental infections. Second-generation cephalosporins, such as cefuroxime and cefaclor, have broader activity against Gram-negative bacteria and are occasionally used for more complex infections. Ceftriaxone and cefotaxime are examples of third-generation cephalosporins that are reserved for severe infections, such as deep neck infections or odontogenic infections with systemic involvement. Fourth- and fifth-generation cephalosporins are rarely used in dental practice due to their advanced spectrum and are typically reserved for hospital settings or multidrug-resistant infections (Guo et al., 2024; Ishikane et al., 2019).

- Pharmacokinetics of Cephalosporins

Cephalosporins are well absorbed orally (for oral formulations) and distributed widely in body tissues and fluids. They achieve therapeutic concentrations in bone and soft tissues, making them effective for dental infections (Kanan et al., 2023). Most cephalosporins are excreted renally, and dose adjustments may be necessary in patients with renal impairment (Pais et al., 2022). The pharmacokinetic properties of the most commonly used cephalosporins are presented in Table 13.

- Advantages of Cephalosporins in Dental Infections

Cephalosporins have broad-spectrum activity against both aerobic and anaerobic bacteria, a good safety profile with relatively low rates of adverse effects, and stability against beta-lactamase enzymes produced by some oral pathogens (Thornsberry et al., 1985). In addition, their availability in both oral and parenteral formulations allows flexibility in treatment.

- Limitations and Considerations

Cephalosporins are not effective against methicillin-resistant *Staphylococcus aureus* (MRSA) or certain anaerobes, such as *Bacteroides fragilis* (Kesado et al., 1984; Tally et al., 1975). Cross-reactivity with penicillins can occur in patients with a history of beta-lactam allergy, although the risk is low (approximately 1–10%). Overuse or inappropriate use of cephalosporins can contribute to antibiotic resistance.

- Clinical Scenarios and Recommendations

For localized dental abscesses, first-generation cephalosporins such as cephalexin can be used when penicillins are contraindicated, although drainage of the abscess remains the primary treatment approach. In cases of periapical or periodontal infections, cephalosporins may serve as adjuncts to mechanical debridement and root canal therapy, particularly in severe infections. For more serious conditions like cellulitis or Ludwig's angina, third-generation cephalosporins such as ceftriaxone, often combined with metronidazole, are utilized to provide broad-spectrum coverage, especially in infections that require hospitalization. Additionally, cephalexin is commonly prescribed for prophylaxis in dental procedures for patients with prosthetic joints or other high-risk conditions when penicillins cannot be used (Sato et al., 2022; Hirayama et al., 2025). The doses for the most commonly used cephalosporins are listed in Table 14.

- Adverse Effects

Cephalosporins are generally well-tolerated but can cause various adverse effects, including allergic reactions such as anaphylaxis, particularly in patients with a history of penicillin allergy. The risk of cross-reactivity is about

10% with first-generation cephalosporins and 2–3% with second- and third-generation drugs, with lower risks reported for cefuroxime, ceftriaxone, and ceftazidime (Chaudhry et al., 2019; Romano et al., 2016). Common side effects include fever, skin rash, nephritis, granulocytopenia, and hemolytic anemia (Mathew et al., 2024; Harrison & Bratcher, 2008). Intravenous administration may lead to local irritation or thrombophlebitis, while intramuscular injections of certain cephalosporins (e.g., ceftaroline) can cause severe pain (Prince & Villar, 1983).

Cephalosporins with a methylthiotetrazole side chain (e.g., cefotetan, cefoperazone) may disrupt vitamin K metabolism, increasing bleeding risk, and can cause disulfiram-like reactions when combined with alcohol. Close monitoring and appropriate management are essential in such cases (Harrison & Bratcher, 2008).

- Warning

Patients are encouraged to complete the full course of cephalosporins prescribed to them, as doing so helps prevent the development of resistance. Long-term use of cephalosporins can lead to the development of superinfections, such as *C. difficile* infection and candidiasis. Cephalosporins with a methylthiotetrazole side chain (e.g., cefazolin) can increase bleeding risk, especially in patients who are malnourished or have liver or kidney disease; therefore, blood tests to monitor bleeding—such as prothrombin time (PT) and international normalized ratio (INR)—should be carried out. Cefuroxime should not be taken with proton pump inhibitors (PPIs), as they interfere with its absorption, and antihistamines should be taken two hours before or after cefuroxime. Live vaccines (such as BCG and typhoid vaccine) may not work as well; therefore, immunization should be delayed until at least three days after cefuroxime therapy is completed. Ceftriaxone may cause biliary sludge or gallstones and should not be given to newborns with jaundice; it should also not be mixed with calcium-containing intravenous solutions. Patients should be monitored for anaphylaxis after the first dose and for kidney, liver, and blood disorders if cephalosporins are used long-term. Most cephalosporins should be taken on an empty stomach (with the exception of cefuroxime). Alcohol should not be consumed with cephalosporins that contain a methylthiotetrazole side chain, as this can lead to a disulfiram-like reaction (Dancer, 2001; Aksoy, 2022b).

3.7.5.1.5. Nitroimidazole Antibiotics

Dental abscesses are localized infections that occur within the teeth, gums, or surrounding tissues, often resulting from bacterial invasion due to untreated dental caries, periodontal disease, or trauma (Bertossi et al., 2017). These infections are typically polymicrobial in nature, involving both aerobic and anaerobic bacteria. Effective management of dental abscesses requires a combination of mechanical intervention, such as drainage or tooth extraction, and appropriate antibiotic therapy to control the spread of infection (Dedha et al., 2024; Herrera et al., 2000). Among the antibiotics used, nitroimidazole derivatives—particularly metronidazole—play a significant role due to their potent activity against anaerobic bacteria, which are commonly implicated in dental abscesses (Herrera et al., 2000).

- Mechanism of Action of Nitroimidazole Antibiotics

Nitroimidazole antibiotics, such as metronidazole, are synthetic antimicrobial agents that exhibit bactericidal activity primarily against anaerobic bacteria and certain protozoa. Their mechanism of action involves the reduction of the nitro group within the bacterial cell by anaerobic metabolic pathways. This reduction generates reactive intermediates that interact with bacterial DNA, leading to strand breakage, inhibition of nucleic acid synthesis, and ultimately, bacterial cell death (Li et al., 2019). This selective mechanism makes nitroimidazoles highly effective against obligate anaerobes, which are prevalent in dental abscesses (Müller, 1983).

- Pharmacokinetics of Metronidazole

Metronidazole is nearly entirely absorbed when taken orally, exhibiting a bioavailability close to 100%. Its absorption is not substantially influenced by food consumption. It is widely distributed throughout the body, including the central nervous system, and tissue levels frequently approximate serum levels. Metronidazole is extensively metabolized in the liver to create two principal oxidative metabolites: hydroxyl and acetic acid. The drug and its metabolites are mostly eliminated in the urine, with less than 20% of the administered dose excreted as an unmodified drug (Tabari et al., 2021; Ralph et al., 1974).

- Microbial Profile of Dental Abscesses

Dental abscesses are typically caused by a mixed population of bacteria, with anaerobes such as *Prevotella*, *Porphyromonas*, *Fusobacterium*, and *Peptostreptococcus* species being the predominant pathogens. Facultative anaerobes, including *Streptococcus* species, may also be present (Siqueira et al., 2013). The anaerobic environment within the abscess cavity provides an ideal niche for these bacteria to thrive, making nitroimidazole antibiotics particularly suitable for targeting the causative organisms.

- Clinical Use of Nitroimidazole Antibiotics in Dental practice

Metronidazole antibiotics are indicated in several dental scenarios, including the management of acute dental abscesses where anaerobic bacteria are the primary pathogens, and in cases of refractory or recurrent infections when initial antibiotic therapy fails, as metronidazole can help target resistant anaerobic organisms. It is often prescribed in combination with other antibiotics, such as amoxicillin, to provide broader coverage against both aerobic and anaerobic bacteria. This combination therapy is particularly useful in severe or spreading infections where mixed bacterial populations are suspected (McGowan et al., 2018). Additionally, when a dental abscess leads to systemic complications such as cellulitis or sepsis, metronidazole is often included in the treatment regimen. However, a systematic review by Cooper et al., (2022) concluded that metronidazole does not provide superior clinical outcomes, either alone or in combination with a beta-lactam, compared to beta-lactam antibiotics alone for the treatment of non-periodontal dental infections in general dental practice (Cooper et al., 2022).

- Dosage and Administration

For acute plaque-mediated gingivitis, metronidazole is administered orally at a dose of 500 mg every 8 hours alongside penicillin V for 5 to 7 days, with systemic use reserved for severe, rapidly progressive cases or immunocompromised patients. In cases of severe plaque-mediated periodontitis, the recommended regimen is 500 mg orally every 8 hours with amoxicillin for 14 days or until clinical improvement, combined with periodontal debridement. For pyogenic odontogenic infections, metronidazole can be given intravenously at 500 mg every 8 hours as part of a combination regimen for 7 to 14 days, in conjunction with appropriate surgical intervention such as drainage or extraction; alternatively, it may be administered orally at the same dose and interval for 7 to 14 days (Chow, 2025).

Pediatric oral dosing ranges from 15 to 50 mg/kg/day in divided doses every 8 hours, with a maximum daily dose of 2,250 mg, while intravenous dosing is 22.5 to 40 mg/kg/day in divided doses every 6 or 8 hours, with a maximum daily dose of 4,000 mg. In patients with renal failure (CrCl <10 mL/minute), the dosing interval may be extended to every 12 hours, and for children with GFR <10 mL/minute/1.73 m^2, a dose of 4 mg/kg every 6 hours is recommended. In cases of severe liver impairment, the dose should be reduced by 50%, and based on adult experience, the dosage interval may be extended while maintaining the usual individual dose, such as administering the regular dose every 12 hours instead of every 6 hours (Lau et al., 1987).

- Adverse Effect of Metronidazole

Metronidazole side effects include nausea, vomiting, diarrhea, metallic taste in the mouth, and peripheral neuropathy. The most common adverse events are headache, vaginitis, and nausea (each occurring in more than 10% of patients). Rarely, transient leukopenia, neutropenia, or severe neurological disturbances may occur with prolonged therapy (McKendrick & Geddes, 1979). Metronidazole carries a black box warning due to the potential for carcinogenicity observed in animal studies; however, the risk in humans is considered minimal. Additional warnings and precautions for metronidazole exist. Prolonged courses can cause severe neurological disturbances due to the risk of cumulative neurotoxicity. Furthermore, long-term use may result in superinfections, including Clostridioides difficile-associated diarrhea (CDAD) (Saginur et al., 1980; Hernández et al., 2019).

- Contraindication to Metronidazole

Metronidazole is contraindicated in patients with a previous history of sensitivity to metronidazole; and within 2 weeks of disulfiram use. Alcohol consumption during metronidazole therapy and for at least 3 days after completion of treatment should be avoided due to the risk of disulfiram-like reactions (Finegold, 1980). CBC and neurologic symptoms should be monitored with prolonged use, in elderly patients or in those with severe hepatic or renal impairment.

- Drug Interaction

Metronidazole has a large number of interactions with other drugs, and combinations to avoid include alcohol, disulfiram, and propylene glycol (Risk X). Use is also contraindicated with *Bacillus clausii*, BCG (intravesical), cholera vaccine, fecal microbiota (live), mebendazole, and ritonavir (Risk X). Caution is advised with busulfan, sodium picosulfate, and vitamin K antagonists (Risk D) (Dighriri et al., 2021; Gussow, 2023).

- Pregnancy and Lactation

Metronidazole penetrates the placenta, resulting in fetal exposure, which has raised concerns about its use in the first trimester of pregnancy. However, numerous studies have found no increased risk of birth defects or adverse effects. Certain authorities recommend that the drug should be avoided in the first trimester unless absolutely necessary. Nevertheless, it is widely used in the treatment of bacterial vaginosis and trichomoniasis, both of which can have adverse effects if left untreated during pregnancy (CDC, 2021). Therefore, the risks and benefits should be carefully considered when prescribing metronidazole.

Metronidazole is excreted into breast milk at concentrations similar to those found in maternal plasma. Thus, breastfeeding may be withheld for 12–24 hours following a single 2 g dose. The mother can express and discard milk for 48 hours after the last dose and feed the infant stored human milk or formula (CDC, 2021; Workowski et al., 2021; WHO, 2002).

3.7.5.1.6. Macrolides

Macrolides are a class of antibiotics that are widely used in the treatment of bacterial infections. They are characterized by a macrocyclic lactone ring and are primarily derived from *Streptomyces* species (Dinos, 2017). Macrolides are known for their broad-spectrum activity, particularly against Gram-positive bacteria, some Gram-negative bacteria, and atypical pathogens (Cunha, 2006). In dentistry, macrolides are often used as an alternative to penicillins, especially in patients with penicillin allergies (Sefton, 1999).

- Mechanism of Action

Macrolides work by inhibiting bacterial protein synthesis. They bind reversibly to the 50S ribosomal subunit of bacterial ribosomes, blocking the translocation step during protein elongation. This prevents the synthesis of essential proteins, leading to a bacteriostatic effect (Sturgill & Rapp, 1992).

- Therapeutic Uses of Macrolides in Dentistry

Macrolide antibiotics are an alternative to penicillins and are indicated when there is an allergy to penicillins. The newer macrolides have many advantages over erythromycin, including a longer duration of action, greater acid stability, better tissue penetration, and reduced gut-related adverse effects. They are effective in the treatment of oral and dental infections. Additionally, macrolides are utilized in the management of periodontal disease due to their efficacy in reducing key pathogenic organisms, including black-pigmented anaerobes and spirochetes, thereby contributing to improved clinical outcomes.

Table 15. Pharmacokinetic profiles and recommended dosing of common macrolides in dental practice (Amsden, 1996; Contaldo et al., 2023)

Macrolide	Pharmacokinetics	Adult Dose	Children Dose
Erythromycin	Absorbed in the small intestine; metabolized in the liver; half-life ~1.5 hours. Excretion: Primarily feces; urine (2% to 15% as unchanged drug).	250-500 mg every 6 hours	30-50 mg/kg/day in divided doses every 6-8 hours
Clarithromycin	Well absorbed; metabolized in the liver; half-life ~3-4 hours. Urine (20% to 40% as unchanged drug; additional 10% to 15% as metabolite); feces (29% to 40% mostly as metabolites.	250-500 mg every 12 hours	7.5 mg/kg every 12 hours (max 500 mg/dose)
Azithromycin	Rapidly absorbed; long half-life (~68 hours); excreted in bile	500 mg on day 1, then 250 mg once daily for 4 days	5 to 12 mg/kg/dose; typically administered as 10 to 12 mg/kg/dose on day 1 (usual maximum dose: 500 mg/dose) followed by 5 to 6 mg/kg once daily (usual maximum dose: 250 mg/dose) for remainder of treatment duration.

Another indication for macrolides is the prevention of bacterial endocarditis in high-risk patients undergoing dental procedures. Macrolides are also used in children; therefore, they are included in antibiotic prophylaxis (preventive) regimens for local and systemic infections caused by dental treatments in pediatric patients (Moore, 1999; Sefton, 1999; Piekoszewska, 2022).

- Considerations for Macrolide Use in Dental Practice

The use of macrolides in dental practice can lead to an increase in antibiotic-resistant oral streptococci; however, this resistance is typically transient and does not result in significant clinical problems. Despite their effectiveness and benefits, the high cost of newer macrolides compared to erythromycin often limits their routine use in dental settings. As a result, while macrolides remain a valuable option for managing certain infections, their use must be carefully considered to balance cost, resistance concerns, and clinical outcomes (Sefton, 1999; Moore, 1999). Table 15 explains the use of macrolides in dental practice.

- Azithromycin and Clarithromycin Differences

Azithromycin has a broader spectrum of activity and fewer drug interactions, while clarithromycin is more potent against certain pathogens but has stronger CYP3A4 inhibition, leading to more drug interactions. Both drugs can cause gastrointestinal side effects, QT prolongation, and rare cardiovascular risks, with clarithromycin generally being less well tolerated. Azithromycin is commonly used in pregnancy, though its safety in the first trimester is unclear, while clarithromycin is avoided unless no alternatives exist. Resistance to both drugs is increasing, primarily due to ribosomal methylation and efflux pumps (Amsden, 1996; King et al., 2002; Schildkraut et al., 2019).

3.7.5.1.7. Tetracyclines Antibiotics

Tetracyclines are predominantly bacteriostatic drugs effective against numerous Gram-negative bacteria, including potential periodontopathogens like *Aggregatibacter actinomycetemcomitans* (previously known as *Actinobacillus actinomycetemcomitans*) (Slots et al., 1986). The effectiveness of this class of medications in treating periodontal disorders may be attributed not solely to their antibacterial capabilities, but also to several recently recognized additional attributes. These include collagenase inhibition, anti-inflammatory effects, suppression of bone resorption, and facilitation of fibroblast attachment to root surfaces (Kounatidis et al., 2024).

- Pharmacodynamics of Tetracyclines

  - Mechanism of Action

Tetracyclines penetrate the bacterial cell wall via two mechanisms: passive diffusion and an energy-dependent active transport pathway, likely regulated by changes in pH. Upon entering the cell, tetracyclines reversibly attach to the 30S ribosomal subunit at a location that obstructs the binding of aminoacyl-tRNA to the acceptor site on the mRNA–ribosome complex. Protein synthesis is ultimately suppressed, resulting in a bacteriostatic effect (Kounatidis et al., 2024; Nguyen et al., 2014).

  - Mechanism of Resistance

Resistance occurs through failure of uptake or active efflux from the cell, and resistance to one tetracycline confers resistance to all. However, tigecycline kills many bacteria that are normally resistant to tetracyclines because it is able to overcome certain resistance mechanisms. In *Proteus* bacteria, tigecycline resistance is due to overexpression of an efflux pump, thus limiting the effectiveness of tigecycline in these bacteria (Zhanel et al., 2004; Schnappinger & Hillen, 1996).

- Pharmacokinetics and Doses of Common Tetracyclines that Used in Dentistry

The levels of tetracyclines are found to be higher in the gingiva and gingival crevicular fluid than in the serum. In a study that measured the concentration of tetracycline in gingival fluid following the oral administration of single doses of 250 or 500 mg to seven volunteers, it was shown that tetracycline concentrations in gingival fluid are typically 2–10 times higher than blood levels after a single dose, with peak levels at 3.5–7 hours and persisting for at least 19 hours (Gordon et al., 1981). The pharmacokinetic properties of the most commonly used tetracyclines are listed in Table 16.

Table 16. Pharmacokinetic characteristics and recommended dosing of tetracyclines commonly used in dental practice (Aksoy, 2022c)

Tetracyclines	Pharmacokinetics	Clinical Use in Dentistry and adult Dose	Dose Modification in renal and hepatic failure
Tetracycline Oral and topical	Bioavailability decreases by 50% when taken with food. It is well distributed in tissues and body fluids. It passes through the placenta and breast milk. Protein binding: 55-64%. Minimal hepatic metabolism 5% metabolized to a less active metabolite. Half-life 6-11 hours. It is excreted in urine and 20-60% in feces.	Acute infection: 250 to 500 mg 4 times daily or 500 mg twice daily.	**Avoided** in renal failure. **Hepatic:** Use with caution.
Doxycycline Oral and Topical	Bioavailability >80% (with or without food). It is well distributed in tissues and body fluids. It passes into the placenta and breast milk. It is partially inactivated by chelate formation in the gastrointestinal system. 18-22 hours 30% of the dose is excreted in the feces. 40% of the dose is excreted in the urine.	Acute infection dose 100 mg once or twice daily. For periodontal therapy: 20 mg twice daily for up to 3-9 months.	No dose adjustment in renal failure. **Hepatic:** Use with caution.
Minocycline Oral	Bioavailability 95% (with food or on an empty stomach) It is well distributed in tissues and body fluids. It passes through the placenta and breast milk.. It is metabolized by the liver to at least six inactive metabolites. 4-9% is excreted in urine and 34% in feces within 16 hours	Acute infection :50-100 mg twice daily. periodontal pockets: A 1 mg dose of minocycline microspheres is applied directly into the periodontal pocket, where it provides sustained release over several days	No dose adjustment **Hepatic:** Use with caution.

*As safer alternatives are present, tetracyclines are rarely used for acute infection in dentistry.

- Clinical Use of Tetracyclines in Dentistry

Doxycycline is widely used in dentistry, particularly for its antimicrobial and anti-inflammatory properties. It is commonly employed in the treatment of periodontal diseases, such as chronic periodontitis, where it can be administered systemically or locally. Subantimicrobial doses of doxycycline (20 mg twice daily) have been shown to inhibit matrix metalloproteinases (MMPs), enzymes that contribute to tissue destruction in periodontal disease, without significantly affecting bacterial resistance (Preshaw et al., 2004; Lee et al., 2004). Studies have demonstrated that adjunctive use of doxycycline with scaling and root planing (SRP) improves clinical outcomes, such as reducing gingival inflammation, bleeding, and pocket depth (Machion et al., 2006; Sgolastra et al., 2011). Additionally, slow-release doxycycline gels applied subgingivally have been effective in targeting periodontal pockets (Gorle & Khairnar, 2018). Its use is also considered in cases of systemic involvement or when local treatments alone are insufficient (Slots et al., 1983). However, its application should be guided by clinical judgment and patient-specific factors to optimize outcomes and minimize risks.

Chemically modified tetracyclines (CMTs) are derivatives of tetracyclines that have been structurally altered to eliminate their antimicrobial properties while retaining their ability to modulate the host response (Golub et al., 1992). In dentistry, CMTs are primarily used as host-modulating agents in the management of periodontal diseases, such as chronic periodontitis. These compounds inhibit MMPs, which are enzymes responsible for the breakdown of connective tissue and bone in periodontal disease. By suppressing MMP activity, CMTs help reduce tissue destruction and promote healing without contributing to antibiotic resistance, a common concern with traditional tetracyclines (Gu et al., 2012; Swamy et al., 2015; Agnihotri & Gaur, 2012).

CMTs also exhibit anti-inflammatory properties by reducing the production of pro-inflammatory cytokines such as interleukin-1 (IL-1) and tumor necrosis factor-alpha (TNF-α), as well as by inhibiting bone resorption. For example, CMT-3 and CMT-8 have shown promise in reducing osteoclastic activity and promoting bone formation, making them valuable in periodontal therapy. Additionally, their ability to enhance fibroblast attachment and connective tissue repair further supports their role in periodontal regeneration (Swamy et al., 2015; Gu et al., 2012).

These properties make CMTs a novel adjunctive treatment option in periodontal therapy, particularly for patients with severe or refractory periodontitis. Their non-antimicrobial nature also allows for long-term use without the risk of developing antibiotic resistance or the gastrointestinal side effects commonly associated with traditional tetracyclines (Swamy et al., 2015).

- Adverse Effects of Tetracyclines

The use of oral tetracycline and intravenous tigecycline can lead to gastrointestinal side effects that vary with the dosage. These effects include abdominal discomfort, epigastric pain, nausea, vomiting (most frequently observed with tigecycline), and a decrease in appetite (Angelette et al., 2023). Esophageal ulcers and esophageal strictures usually develop from tetracycline use. To avoid this, the medication should be taken with plenty of water and should not be used prior to bedtime. Changes in intestinal flora may lead to diarrhea, while alterations in vaginal flora can result in vaginal candidiasis, including *Clostridioides difficile* infections. Allergic reactions and other hypersensitivity responses are uncommon with tetracyclines. The onset of an allergic reaction to one tetracycline suggests that an allergy to all tetracyclines could potentially arise, so caution is advised (Maciag et al., 2020; Aksoy, 2022c).

- Warning and Consideration for Tetracyclines

Tetracycline antibiotics carry significant warnings related to their effects on dental health, particularly in children and during pregnancy. These antibiotics bind to calcium in developing bone and tooth tissues, leading to permanent discoloration of teeth, enamel hypoplasia, and structural deformities. When used during pregnancy, tetracyclines can cause developmental abnormalities in the teeth and bones of the fetus, including dentin hypoplasia and permanent tooth damage. For this reason, tetracyclines are contraindicated in pregnant women and children under the age of 8, as they can result in brown staining and weakened enamel in both primary and permanent teeth (Yordanova et al., 2018). Additionally, their use in children under 8 should only occur under strict medical supervision when no safer alternatives are available. Patients should be informed of these risks, and dental professionals should be cautious when treating individuals with a history of tetracycline use, as it may affect the appearance and integrity of their teeth (Yordanova et al., 2018; Aksoy, 2022c).

Furthermore, tetracyclines can cause cutaneous reactions, including erythema, dermatitis, and photosensitivity. Patients should avoid prolonged exposure to sunlight and use sun protection measures such as sunscreen, sunglasses, and protective clothing. Tetracyclines can also cause hepatotoxicity, which is more common with high dosages or in patients with poor liver function; liver damage can be fatal during pregnancy. Tetracyclines are known to be nephrotoxic and are primarily eliminated by the kidneys. In individuals with renal dysfunction, tetracycline antibiotics can cause acidosis and other reversible conditions; therefore, they require careful consideration. Doxycycline and tigecycline are exceptions because they are eliminated through the feces rather than the kidneys. They are less nephrotoxic and do not require dose adjustment in renal insufficiency, making them safer options for patients with kidney problems (LaPlante et al., 2022). Tetracyclines are also known to cause hematotoxicity, including thrombocytopenia, leukopenia, and hemolytic anemia, which is most likely to occur in patients with liver or kidney disease and with long-term use (Sainz et al., 2021). Neurotoxicity is another side effect of tetracyclines, and it is predominantly associated with minocycline, which is more lipophilic than other tetracyclines (Ahuja et al., 2008).

Tetracyclines undergo extensive interactions with drugs and various minerals, leading to significant changes in their efficacy. They form chelates with calcium, magnesium, and iron, which prevents their absorption (Wiesner et al., 2024). Tetracyclines should not be used with penicillins because they can make penicillins less effective by antagonizing their antibacterial activity. Carbamazepine, phenytoin, and barbiturates increase the rate of metabolism of doxycycline in the liver, leading to earlier elimination and lower plasma concentrations. The dose of doxycycline may need to be adjusted if the patient is also taking any of these drugs (Zaccara & Franco, 2022). Tetracyclines enhance the effects of retinoic acid derivatives, neuromuscular blockers, and nephrotoxic drugs (e.g., methoxyflurane); therefore, concomitant administration should be avoided if possible. Chronic alcohol consumption decreases the plasma concentration of doxycycline (Angelette et al., 2023; Warner et al., 2022).

3.7.5.1.8. Lincosamide Antibiotics

Lincosamide antibiotics, particularly clindamycin, are effective alternatives for dental infections, especially in patients with penicillin allergies; however, their increased use raises concerns about antibiotic overuse and resistance. Studies have shown that clindamycin is a promising antibiotic for periodontal treatment due to its bacteriostatic effect, inhibition of bacterial protein synthesis, and synergistic stimulation of the immune system (Mahmoud et al., 2023; Addy & Martin, 2005; Luchian et al., 2021).

- Clindamycin: Mechanism of Action

It reversibly binds to the 50S ribosomal subunit, preventing peptide bond formation and thereby inhibiting bacterial protein synthesis. Its effect can be either bacteriostatic or bactericidal, depending on factors such as drug concentration, infection site, and the organism involved (Spížek & Řezanka, 2017).

- Pharmacokinetics of Clindamycin

Clindamycin is quickly absorbed when taken orally, with approximately 90% bioavailability, and is extensively distributed throughout body fluids and tissues; however, it does not reach significant concentrations in the cerebrospinal fluid. It is significantly bound to proteins (94%) and is mainly metabolized by CYP3A4 into both active and inactive metabolites. The half-life varies with age, ranging from 2 to 6 hours in neonates and infants, 2 to 3.5 hours in children and adolescents, and approximately 3 hours in adults (up to 4 hours in the elderly). Peak serum levels are attained within 60 minutes when taken orally or within 1 to 3 hours when administered intramuscularly. Clindamycin is eliminated through urine (approximately 10%) and feces (around 3.6%) in the form of active drug and its metabolites. Effectiveness is linked to AUC24/MIC (target ≥27), and steady-state drug exposure differs by age and dosage, with higher levels observed in children than in adults (Levison & Levison, 2009; Muller et al., 2010; Gonzalez et al., 2016).

- Clinical Use and Doses of Clindamycin

Clindamycin is commonly used in dental practice to treat bacterial infections such as dental abscesses, periodontitis, and jawbone infections (osteomyelitis), especially when first-line antibiotics like amoxicillin or metronidazole are ineffective or when patients are allergic to penicillin. It is also used as prophylaxis for infective endocarditis in high-risk patients undergoing dental procedures. The usual prophylactic dose is 600 mg orally before the procedure or 600 mg intravenously in both penicillin-allergic patients and those who cannot take medication by mouth (Thornhill et al., 2015). Additionally, clindamycin is used for preventing post-surgical infections and as an adjunct in periodontal therapy. Its excellent penetration into bone and soft tissues makes it particularly useful in severe or recurrent infections (Thabit et al., 2019).

For adults, the typical oral dosage is 300–450 mg every 6 hours, with a duration of 7–10 days depending on the severity. For children, the oral dosage is weight-based, typically 10–30 mg/kg/day divided into 3 or 4 doses (Luchian, 2021; Gordon, 1985; Segura-Egea et al., 2017). No dose adjustment is required in renal or liver failure. Clindamycin mucoadhesive films were used to treat periodontal diseases like gingivitis and periodontitis, with maximum drug release at 98.16% (Pulate et al., 2021). Furthermore, some studies have shown that clindamycin might reduce the risk of dry socket after extraction (Peedikayil, 2016).

- Adverse Effects of Clindamycin

Clindamycin, an antibiotic frequently employed to address bacterial infections, may lead to various adverse effects, which can range in severity from mild to serious. One of the major risks associated with clindamycin is Clostridioides difficile-associated diarrhea (CDAD), which has the potential to result in severe colitis and, in rare cases, life-threatening complications. Common gastrointestinal side effects include nausea, vomiting, abdominal pain, and diarrhea. Allergic reactions can manifest as rash, itching, and, in rare instances, anaphylaxis. Prolonged use of clindamycin may disrupt the natural equilibrium of gut flora, increasing the likelihood of secondary infections such as oral or vaginal yeast infections (Lusk et al., 1977). Furthermore, certain individuals may experience liver dysfunction, indicated by increased liver enzymes, or blood disorders, including neutropenia. While clindamycin is effective in treating infections, its potential for serious side effects requires careful monitoring and it should be used under medical supervision (Jeffres et al., 2022; Duffy et al., 2019). Clindamycin is contraindicated in patients with cirrhosis and in those with a history of ulcerative or pseudomembranous colitis (Tedesco, 2020).

- Pregnancy and Lactation Consideration

Clindamycin is generally considered safe during pregnancy and is classified as FDA Category B, with studies showing no increased risk of birth defects or complications, especially when used in the second and third trimesters to treat infections such as bacterial vaginosis (Subtil et al., 2018). However, some literature has noted a small increase in specific birth defects with first-trimester use (Muanda et al., 2017). During lactation, clindamycin is excreted in small amounts into breast milk and is usually safe for breastfeeding infants, though rare side effects such as diarrhea or thrush may occur. Monitoring the infant for adverse effects is recommended, and its use should always be guided by a healthcare provider (Wan-Jun, 2008; Bookstaver et al., 2005).

3.7.5.1.9. Fluoroquinolones Antibiotics

Fluoroquinolones are broad-spectrum bactericidal antibiotics that primarily target Gram-negative bacilli, Gram-positive aerobic cocci, and anaerobic organisms by inhibiting DNA synthesis (Hooper, 2001). These agents demonstrate greater tissue penetration compared to other antibiotics frequently prescribed in dental practice (Guentsch et al., 2008).

- Pharmacodynamic and Mechanism of Action of Fluoroquinolones

Fluoroquinolones are antibiotics that have a concentration-dependent effect, functioning by inhibiting bacterial DNA gyrase, which results in bacterial cell death. Their pharmacodynamic efficacy is most accurately predicted by the AUC/MIC ratio. These antibiotics are effective against a wide variety of pathogens, though there is a possibility of developing resistance (Turnidge, 2012).

- Pharmacokinetic Properties of Fluoroquinolones

Fluoroquinolones demonstrate remarkable absorption in the gastrointestinal tract, with bioavailability differing among the various agents. Levofloxacin and gatifloxacin, which are newer fluoroquinolones, exhibit bioavailability rates exceeding 95%, whereas sparfloxacin and moxifloxacin show slightly lower rates. These drugs effectively distribute into tissues, reaching elevated concentrations in respiratory tissues, kidneys, and bile, yet demonstrate restricted penetration into cerebrospinal fluid. Protein binding varies significantly, with some agents such as levofloxacin exhibiting low binding (20–40%), while others like rufloxacin demonstrate high binding (60–80%), which influences the availability of free drugs. Elimination occurs through both renal and nonrenal pathways, with renal clearance being the primary method for levofloxacin and gatifloxacin, whereas moxifloxacin and sparfloxacin depend more on hepatic metabolism and biliary excretion. The half-life of ciprofloxacin ranges from 3 to 5 hours, while sparfloxacin has a half-life of 15 to 24 hours, which supports different dosing regimens (Aminimanizani et al., 2001).

- Clinical Application of Fluoroquinolones in Dentistry

Fluoroquinolones, especially ciprofloxacin and moxifloxacin, are important antibiotics in dentistry for the treatment of odontogenic and periodontal infections, owing to their broad effectiveness against both Gram-positive and Gram-negative bacteria. Ciprofloxacin, a second-generation fluoroquinolone, is frequently prescribed at a dosage of 500 mg every 12 hours for odontogenic infections. It demonstrates strong antibacterial efficacy with relatively few side effects, the most common being gastrointestinal issues such as nausea, vomiting, and diarrhea. Dental practitioners should carefully review patients' medical histories, particularly regarding the concurrent use of theophylline, as drug interactions may result in significant theophylline toxicity, which can manifest as symptoms such as nausea and vomiting (Zhang et al., 2018; Dar-Odeh et al., 2010; Bem & Mann, 1988). Moxifloxacin, a fourth-generation fluoroquinolone, demonstrates high efficacy against aerobic and anaerobic bacteria, as well as Gram-positive and Gram-negative strains, and exhibits excellent penetration into periodontal and bone tissues. It is often used as a preventive measure in patients with beta-lactam allergies to prevent bacteremia or as an alternative treatment when first-line antibiotics and surgical options are unsuccessful. Moxifloxacin, administered at a dose of 400 mg once daily, is especially effective for treating chronic infections; however, it is avoided in pregnant and adolescent patients because of its potential impact on cartilage maturation. Although effective, its high cost limits its use as a primary treatment in dental practice (Diz Dios et al., 2006; Loyola-Rodriguez et al., 2019).

- Adverse Effects and Contraindication

Fluoroquinolones can cause various adverse effects, including central nervous system toxicity, gastrointestinal problems, tendon disorders, cardiovascular events, and disturbances in glucose metabolism. They are contraindicated in patients with seizure disorders, cardiovascular conditions, and those at risk for QTc (corrected QT interval) prolongation or tendinopathy (Mathews et al., 2019; Wierzbiński et al., 2023).

- Special Consideration and Warning

Fluoroquinolones are generally avoided during pregnancy and lactation due to concerns about potential cartilage damage and arthropathy in the developing fetus or infant, as observed in animal studies. During lactation, fluoroquinolones such as ciprofloxacin are excreted in breast milk in small amounts, with a low risk to infants, though concerns about cartilage development remain. Their use is typically reserved for severe infections when no safer alternatives are available (Wolfson & Hooper, 1991; Maggiolo et al., 1990).

Fluoroquinolone use in children should be limited to situations where there is no safe and effective alternative to treat multidrug-resistant bacteria, or for cases where oral treatment is needed, parenteral therapy cannot be used, and no other effective oral agent is available (Powell et al., 2006; Jackson et al., 2016).

- Drug Interactions

Fluoroquinolones interact with multivalent cations, leading to reduced absorption, and can inhibit the metabolism of methylxanthines and other drugs, potentially causing significant drug interactions (Pitman et al., 2019). Fluoroquinolones can also prolong the QT interval, increasing the risk of arrhythmias. Caution is advised when they are co-administered with other QT-prolonging drugs (e.g., amiodarone, macrolides, antipsychotics) (Falagas et al., 2007; Owens & Ambrose, 2002). Quinolone antibiotics can reduce the clearance of co-administered drugs such as theophylline, requiring caution when these drugs are used together (Edwards et al., 1988). Co-administration with NSAIDs may increase the risk of central nervous system (CNS) side effects, such as seizures.

Conclusion

Antibiotics are a vital tool in dentistry, but their misuse poses significant risks to both individual and public health. Dentists must adopt evidence-based practices, embrace antibiotic stewardship, and explore alternative therapies to ensure the continued efficacy of these life-saving drugs. By doing so, the dental profession can play a crucial role in combating the global antimicrobial resistance (AMR) crisis and safeguarding the health of future generations.

3.8. Antiviral Drugs Used in Dentistry

3.8.1. Introduction

Viral infections are a significant concern in dentistry due to their potential to cause oral lesions, systemic complications, and occupational hazards for dental professionals. These infections, caused by a variety of viruses such as herpes simplex virus (HSV), Epstein-Barr virus (EBV), human papillomavirus (HPV), varicella-zoster virus (VZV), Coxsackie virus, and others, often present with distinct oral manifestations. Early diagnosis and appropriate treatment are critical for managing these conditions and preventing their spread. This chapter explores therapeutic strategies for common viral infections encountered in dental practice (McCullough & Savage, 2005).

3.8.2. Common Viral Infections in Dentistry

Herpes Simplex Virus (HSV): HSV-1 and HSV-2 are DNA viruses that target epithelial cells and establish latency in sensory ganglia. Reactivation may occur as a result of stress, immunosuppression, or trauma. HSV infections typically present as primary herpetic gingivostomatitis, particularly in children. Symptoms include fever, lymphadenopathy, and painful vesicles on the oral mucosa, gingiva, and tongue. These vesicles rupture to form ulcers characterized by a yellowish base and red edges. Other clinical manifestations of HSV include recurrent herpes labialis, which presents as vesicles on the lips or perioral skin that rupture and crust over, healing within 7–10 days. Another manifestation is herpetic whitlow, a painful finger infection commonly seen in dental professionals due to contact with infected oral secretions (Arduino & Porter, 2006; McCullough & Savage, 2005).

HSV infection is generally diagnosed by clinical examination, cytological smears, and polymerase chain reaction (PCR) for viral DNA. For treatment in the acute phase, oral antiviral agents such as acyclovir, valacyclovir, or famciclovir can be administered. Topical acyclovir is effective if applied during the prodromal phase. However, the use of personal protective equipment (PPE) and adherence to infection control protocols are necessary to prevent HSV infection (McCullough & Savage, 2005). The pharmacokinetic and pharmacodynamic properties of these drugs are emphasized in Table 17.

Epstein-Barr Virus (EBV) and Associated Conditions: EBV is associated with conditions such as infectious mononucleosis, which is characterized by pharyngitis, lymphadenopathy, and fatigue. Oral manifestations include petechiae on the palate and oral hairy leukoplakia (OHL)—white, corrugated lesions on the lateral tongue, often seen in immunocompromised patients (Slots et al., 2006). EBV-related conditions are generally diagnosed by serological tests and histopathological examination (Abusalah et al., 2020). Antiviral therapy is generally not required for OHL, but management of underlying immunosuppression is crucial.

Varicella-Zoster Virus (VZV): Infection with VZV can present as a primary infection (chickenpox), with a vesicular rash on the skin and oral mucosa, which is usually self-limiting in children. Reactivation (shingles) presents with unilateral vesicles and ulcers along the distribution of the trigeminal nerve (Kolokotronis et al., 2001). Ramsay Hunt syndrome involves facial palsy and vesicles in the ear and oral cavity (Sweeney & Gilden, 2001). Treatment generally involves high-dose acyclovir or valacyclovir for acute episodes, in addition to pain management for postherpetic neuralgia (Kern, 2023; Kim et al., 2017).

Human Papillomavirus (HPV): The oral manifestations of HPV include squamous cell papilloma (benign, cauliflower-like growths on the oral mucosa), condyloma acuminatum (sexually transmitted warts that can appear in the oral cavity), and focal epithelial hyperplasia (FEH), which presents as multiple nodular lesions, often asymptomatic (Betz, 2019). These conditions are generally diagnosed by histopathological examination and HPV typing. Treatment involves surgical excision of lesions, and vaccination against high-risk HPV types is recommended for prevention (Mo et al., 2022).

Coxsackie virus: Coxsackie virus infection can present as herpangina, with vesicles on the soft palate and tonsillar pillars, or as hand, foot, and mouth disease, which is characterized by fever, sore throat, and vesicular lesions on the hands, feet, and oral cavity, primarily affecting children (Fujimoto et al., 2012). Supportive care, hydration, and pain relief are necessary for treatment (Saguil et al., 2019).

Table 17. Pharmacokinetic properties and doses of antiviral drugs (Gao et al., 2024)

Antiviral Drug	Pharmacokinetics	Use	Adult Dose	Pediatric Dose
Acyclovir	Poorly absorbed, widely distributed. Metabolized to the active form triphosphate by cellular enzymes. Excreted in urine (62% to 91% as unchanged drug and metabolite).	Orolabial HSV	Initiate therapy at earliest symptom. Orally:400 mg 3 times daily for 5 to 10 days and until complete lesion resolution in patients who are immunocompromised or IV dose 5 mg/kg/dose every 8 hours in sever cases. Suppressive therapy (eg, for severe and/or frequent recurrences) lesion resolution in patients who are immunocompromised. Oral: 400 mg twice daily.	Oral :20 mg/kg/dose 4 times daily for 5 to 7 days; usual maximum dose: 800 mg/dose.
Valacyclovir	Rapid absorption and widley distributed. Hepatic metabolism to acyclovir. Excreted primarily in urine, primarily as acyclovir (89%);	Orolabial HSV gingivostomatitis cold sores Suppressive therapy (eg, for severe and/or frequent recurrences) In immunocompromised patient initial or recurrent infection Suppressive therapy	Oral: 1 g twice daily for 7 to 10 days Oral: 2 g twice daily for 1 day Oral: 500 mg or 1 g once daily Oral: 1 g twice daily for 5 to 10 days and until complete lesion resolution Oral: 500 mg twice daily	Children ≥12 years and Adolescents: Oral: 2,000 mg every 12 hours for 1 day (2 doses)
Famciclovir	Absorption delayed with food, protein binding <20%. Famciclovir is rapidly deacetylated and oxidized to penciclovir. Urine (73% primarily as penciclovir); feces (27%).	Orolabial HSV Immunocompetent patients: initial infection (eg, gingivostomatitis) Recurrent infection (eg, cold sores) Immunocompromised patients Initial or recurrent infection Suppressive therapy	Oral: 250 mg 3 times daily or 500 mg twice daily for 7 to 10 days Oral: 1.5 g as a single dose. Oral: 500 mg twice daily for 5 to 10 days; extend treatment duration if lesions have not healed completely after 10 days Oral: 500 mg twice daily	Adolescents: Oral: 1,500 mg as a single dose

Table 17. (Continued)

Antiviral Drug	Pharmacokinetics	Use	Adult Dose	Pediatric Dose
Ganciclovir	Widely distributed to all tissues. Protein binding: 1% to 2%. Excreted in urine (80% to 99% as unchanged drug)	CMV mild to moderate disease treatment.	IV :5 mg/kg every 12 hours at least until cytomegalovirus viral load is undetectable for 1 or 2 consecutive weeks and symptoms are resolved (minimum treatment course: 2 weeks)	Limited data available: Infants: IV: 6 mg/kg/dose every 12 hours; transition to oral valganciclovir (when able) to complete total treatment duration of 6 months.

Human Immunodeficiency Virus (HIV): HIV causes oral problems due to immunosuppression. These include oral candidiasis (white plaques on the mucosa that are easily scraped off), Kaposi's sarcoma (purple-red lesions on the palate and gingiva), and oral hairy leukoplakia (OHL, associated with EBV, resulting in white lesions on the tongue). Treatment of these conditions requires antiretroviral therapy (ART) for HIV to control manifestations (Bukhnikashvili et al., 2021).

3.8.3. Therapeutic Strategies for Viral Infections

Preventive measures, such as vaccination with the HPV vaccine, are crucial. HPV vaccines lead to a substantial 88% reduction in oral or oropharyngeal HPV infections and stimulate the production of IgG antibodies in oral fluid following vaccination, which may contribute to a decrease in HPV-related oropharyngeal cancers (Nielsen et al., 2021; Zhang et al., 2021). Immunization against hepatitis B and HPV is also recommended (Pattyn et al., 2021). It is essential to strictly adhere to infection control protocols in dental settings, utilizing personal protective equipment such as gloves, masks, and eye protection. Consistent hand hygiene and the sterilization of instruments are also critical (Aderonke, 2025).

The implementation of teledentistry to reduce direct contact during pandemics represents a successful strategy to minimize occupational hazards and prevent the spread of viral infections (Wallace et al., 2021).

Supportive care, such as pain management with topical anesthetics or systemic analgesics, along with maintenance of hydration, nutrition, and oral hygiene, is important in the treatment of oral ulcers associated with herpes zoster (Matsuda et al., 2022).

Pharmacological intervention to treat viral infections in dentistry often involves antiviral agents such as acyclovir, valacyclovir, and famciclovir, which are most commonly used for treating HSV and VZV infections. Additionally, ganciclovir is used specifically for managing CMV infections.

3.8.4. Pharmacodynamics and Pharmacokinetics of Antiviral Agents

Antivirals act by inhibiting viral DNA synthesis and replication through selective interference with viral enzymes. Acyclovir is phosphorylated to the monophosphate form by virus-specific thymidine kinase and then to the triphosphate form by cellular enzymes. Acyclovir triphosphate competes with deoxyguanosine triphosphate for viral DNA polymerase and is incorporated into viral DNA, thereby inhibiting viral DNA synthesis and replication (Elion, 1982). Valacyclovir is a prodrug that is rapidly metabolized by intestinal and hepatic enzymes to acyclovir, and its mechanism of action is the same (Klysik et al., 2018). Famciclovir is a prodrug that is converted to the active drug penciclovir.

Penciclovir is phosphorylated in infected cells by viral thymidine kinase to the triphosphate form, which competes with deoxyguanosine triphosphate for HSV-2 polymerase, thereby selectively inhibiting herpes viral DNA synthesis (Hodge, 1993). Ganciclovir is phosphorylated by viral and cellular kinases to the triphosphate form, which competitively inhibits the binding of deoxyguanosine triphosphate to DNA polymerase, thereby suppressing DNA synthesis (Matthews & Boehme, 1988). Therefore, these agents exploit the unique enzymatic pathways of viruses to provide selective inhibition of viral replication with minimal effects on host cells.

The pharmacokinetics of antiviral drugs influence dosing, efficacy, and safety in dental practice. Many classic antivirals have low oral bioavailability, leading to the development of prodrugs (e.g., valacyclovir, famciclovir) and novel formulations to enhance absorption. These prodrugs are converted to their active forms in the liver or intestinal wall, improving systemic exposure. These drugs are generally well distributed in body fluids and tissues, including the oral mucosa, which is important for treating oral infections. Most antiviral drugs are eliminated via the kidneys, so dose adjustments may be needed in cases of renal impairment (Chen et al., 2021; Painter et al., 2012). The pharmacokinetic properties and dosing of common antiviral drugs used in dentistry are listed in Table 17.

3.8.5. Adverse Reactions and Contraindication of Antiviral Drugs

The prevalent side effects of this medication, especially with the intravenous form of acyclovir, include a reduction in absolute neutrophil count and diminished hemoglobin levels in newborns, while malaise may occur with oral doses (Klysik et al., 2018). Gastrointestinal side effects such as abdominal pain, nausea, and headache are common with valacyclovir, famciclovir, and ganciclovir. Other adverse effects include pruritus, skin rash, urticaria, diarrhea, thrombocytopenia, elevated serum bilirubin and transaminases, injection site inflammation and phlebitis, headache, increased blood urea nitrogen and serum creatinine levels (Gao et al., 2024). Contraindications for antiviral drugs include hypersensitivity to ganciclovir, valganciclovir, acyclovir, or any component of the formulation.

3.8.6. Dose Adjustment in Renal and Hepatic Failure

Dose adjustment is required when CrCl is less than 70 mL/minute for ganciclovir and less than 60 mL/minute for famciclovir. For valacyclovir and acyclovir, dose adjustment is necessary when CrCl is less than 50 mL/minute. No dosage adjustments are required in cases of liver impairment (Deray et al., 2015).

Conclusion

Viral infections present unique challenges in dental practice due to their diverse oral manifestations, potential systemic complications, and occupational risks. Early diagnosis, preventive measures such as vaccination and strict infection control, and appropriate use of antiviral agents are essential for effective management. Understanding the pharmacological properties, dosing, and potential adverse effects of antiviral drugs ensures safe and effective treatment. By staying informed and adhering to evidence-based protocols, dental professionals can minimize risks and improve outcomes for patients affected by viral infections.

3.9. Antifungal in Dentistry

Fungal infections in the oral cavity are a common concern in dental practice. These infections can cause discomfort, affect oral health, and complicate dental treatments. Antifungal drugs play a crucial role in managing these opportunistic infections. Understanding the types of fungal infections and the antifungal agents available is essential for effective management.

3.9.1. Types of Fungal Infections Affecting the Oral Cavity

The most prevalent fungal infection in the oral cavity is oral candidiasis, commonly caused by the *Candida* species, particularly *Candida albicans*, and is influenced by factors such as immune system status, oral microbiota balance, and predisposing conditions (Akpan & Morgan, 2002; Patel, 2022).

3.9.2. Various Forms and Diagnosis of Oral Candidiasis

A significant number of patients with oropharyngeal candidiasis exhibit no symptoms. When symptoms do manifest, patients frequently report a cotton-like sensation in the mouth, diminished taste perception, and, in certain instances, discomfort while eating and swallowing. Individuals with denture stomatitis typically experience pain. Immunocompromised patients with oropharyngeal candidiasis may also develop associated Candida esophagitis or, less commonly, laryngeal candidiasis. Laryngeal candidiasis should be considered in patients exhibiting signs of oropharyngeal infection accompanied by hoarseness.

There are five clinical forms of oropharyngeal candidiasis, each with distinct clinical features. The most common is pseudomembranous (exudative) candidiasis, which predominantly manifests as white plaques on the buccal mucosa, palate, tongue, and/or oropharynx. Depending on the extent of the lesions, disease severity can be classified as mild (scattered, nonconfluent lesions >2 mm in size), moderate (multiple lesions >2 mm in size), or severe (extensive, confluent lesions) (De Oliveira et al., 2024).

Another form is chronic atrophic stomatitis (denture stomatitis), typically observed in elderly individuals who use upper dentures. This type is located beneath the upper dentures and is distinguished by erythema without plaques (Budtz, 1981).

Angular cheilitis is also a recognized form, presenting as bilateral, vivid red erythematous fissures at the corners of the mouth (Sharon & Fazel, 2010). Chronic hyperplastic candidiasis (Candida leukoplakia), predominantly observed in males and closely linked to smoking, manifests as distinct, elevated whitish patches on the mucosal surfaces of the cheeks (Hussain & Al-Drobie, 2022).

Finally, median rhomboid glossitis (acute atrophic stomatitis) presents as symmetrical erythematous lesions at the center of the tongue accompanied by papillary atrophy (Li et al., 2021).

The diagnosis of oropharyngeal candidiasis is predominantly clinical, relying on the identification of distinctive symptoms in individuals with established risk factors. These risk factors include the use of dentures, recent antibiotic use, or inhaled corticosteroid therapy in immunocompetent patients. Immunocompromised individuals, such as those with AIDS, hematologic malignancies, or those receiving chemotherapy or radiation therapy, are at even greater risk.

While clinical assessment is usually sufficient, additional testing may be warranted if there is uncertainty about whether the findings are consistent with thrush, or if the patient lacks classic risk factors. In such cases, the presence of thrush should raise suspicion of HIV infection and prompt HIV testing. Diagnostic procedures may involve scraping lesions for a Gram stain or potassium hydroxide preparation to reveal yeasts or swabbing for culture. However, it is important to note that the clinical picture must align with thrush, since 20 to 55 percent of people are colonized by *Candida* species.

Given the overlap in clinical presentation, it is also essential to consider and exclude other conditions in the differential diagnosis. These include oral hairy leukoplakia, lichen planus, herpes simplex virus infection, squamous cell carcinoma (SCC), frictional keratosis, burning mouth syndrome, and coated or hairy tongue (Torres & Jewtuchowicz, 2025).

3.9.3. Treatment

3.9.3.1. Oropharyngeal Candidiasis

There are several topical and local treatment options available for mild cases (Shay et al., 1997; Darouiche, 1998), including clotrimazole troches (10 mg orally five times daily), miconazole mucoadhesive buccal tablets (50 mg once daily applied to the mucosal surface over the canine fossa), and nystatin suspension or pastilles (400,000 to 600,000 units orally four times daily). For moderate to severe cases, or those unresponsive to topical treatments, fluconazole (200 mg orally on day 1, then 100 to 200 mg daily) is recommended. In cases of refractory oropharyngeal candidiasis, the fluconazole dose can be doubled (up to 400 mg daily), or alternative treatments such as itraconazole oral solution (200 mg daily), posaconazole oral suspension (400 mg twice daily for 3 days, then 400 mg once daily), voriconazole (200 mg orally twice daily), or amphotericin B deoxycholate oral suspension may be used. Although echinocandins or IV amphotericin B can be considered for refractory disease, they are rarely indicated (Fichtenbaum et al., 2000). The initial treatment duration is 14 to 21 days, extended to 28 days for refractory cases (Laudenbach & Epstein, 2009; Qadir & Ahmad, 2023; Rajadurai et al., 2021).

3.9.3.2. Pharmacological Properties of Frequently Used Antifungal Agents in Dentistry

Antifungal agents work by targeting specific components of fungal cells. Polyenes (e.g., nystatin, amphotericin B) bind to ergosterol, forming pores in the cell membrane and leading to leakage of cell contents. However, some newly discovered polyenes (e.g., mandimycin) can also target phospholipids in the fungal membrane, broadening their antifungal spectrum and helping evade resistance (Deng et al., 2025). Recent research suggests that amphotericin B may also kill fungi by extracting ergosterol from the membrane, not just by forming pores (Maji et al., 2023). Azoles (e.g., clotrimazole, fluconazole) inhibit ergosterol synthesis by blocking the enzyme lanosterol 14-α-demethylase (CYP51/ERG11), thereby disrupting cell membrane integrity. Most azoles are fungistatic (inhibit growth rather than kill), though some, like posaconazole, can be fungicidal against certain fungi (Hof, 2006). The allylamines (e.g., naftifine and terbinafine) inhibit squalene epoxidase and prevent ergosterol synthesis (Ahmed et al., 2021a). The echinocandins, such as caspofungin, inhibit the enzyme β-(1,3)-D-glucan synthase, which is crucial for the synthesis of β-(1,3)-D-glucan, a major structural component of the fungal cell wall (Vanreppelen et al., 2023).

Understanding the pharmacology of antifungal agents is essential in dental practice, as their pharmacokinetic properties directly influence drug selection, route of administration, and monitoring strategies. For example, topical agents like nystatin are preferred for local infections because of their limited systemic absorption. In contrast, systemic azoles are reserved for more severe or refractory cases, where factors such as absorption, tissue penetration, and potential drug interactions must be carefully considered. A summary of the pharmacokinetic properties, adverse effects, and warnings for common antifungal drugs is provided in Table 18.

3.9.3.3. Mechanisms of Antifungal Drug Resistance

Prolonged use of azoles can lead to resistance, particularly in immunocompromised patients. Resistance mechanisms include mutations in the ERG11 gene, which alter the structure of 14-α-demethylase, thereby reducing azole binding and decreasing drug efficacy. Overexpression of ERG11 can also increase the amount of target enzyme, requiring higher drug concentrations for inhibition. Additionally, fungi can upregulate genes encoding efflux pumps (e.g., CDR1, CDR2, MDR1, SNQ2), which actively export azole drugs out of the cell, lowering intracellular drug concentrations (Pintye et al., 2024). Resistance to nystatin and amphotericin B is relatively rare but can occur through alterations in the ergosterol content of the fungal cell membrane, reducing the binding affinity of these drugs. Some resistant strains overproduce total sterols or specific sterol types (e.g., stigmasterol), diluting the effect of polyenes by reducing the proportion of ergosterol available for binding. In some cases, resistance especially to amphotericin B may involve changes in the cell wall that affect drug access or binding, independent of ergosterol alterations. Additionally, upregulation of drug transporters and stress response proteins can contribute to modest resistance by affecting ergosterol trafficking or cellular adaptation to drug exposure (Chiu et al., 2006; Hapala et al., 2005; Zhang et al., 2002).

3.9.3.4. Antifungal Drug Interactions

Antifungal agents, particularly azoles, are known for their significant drug interactions due to their effects on hepatic cytochrome P450 enzymes. Azoles such as fluconazole, itraconazole, voriconazole, and posaconazole act as inhibitors of various CYP enzymes, including CYP3A4, CYP2C9, and CYP2C19. This inhibition can lead to elevated plasma levels of co-administered drugs that are metabolized by these enzymes, potentially causing toxicity. For instance, drugs like alprazolam, ergot alkaloids, and lovastatin can have increased concentrations when taken with azoles. Conversely, certain agents such as rifampin and carbamazepine can decrease the plasma concentrations of azoles, reducing their efficacy. Additionally, some drug combinations with azoles are contraindicated due to severe interaction risks, such as with cisapride and certain statins. These interactions necessitate careful monitoring and dose adjustments to avoid adverse effects and ensure therapeutic efficacy (Sahadevan, 2021).

Table 18. Antifungal agents in dentistry: Pharmacokinetics, risks, and clinical cautions (Ahmed et al., 2021a)

Drug	Pharmacokinetics	Adverse Effects	Warnings
Nystatin	Not absorbed from the GI tract, skin, or vagina. Used for cutaneous, vaginal, or oral candidiasis.	Bitter taste, occasional nausea. Rarely causes adverse effects.	Not effective for infections of nails or hyperkeratinized skin lesions.
Amphotericin B	Poor GI absorption; administered IV. More than 90% are bound to plasma proteins. Limited penetration into CSF.	Fever, chills, nephrotoxicity, anemia, headache, nausea, vomiting, and phlebitis. Lipid formulations reduce nephrotoxicity.	Infusion-related reactions; caution in patients with renal impairment.
Miconazole	Readily penetrates the stratum corneum; less than 1% absorbed into the blood.	Burning, itching, irritation, pelvic cramps, headache, hives, or skin rash.	Considered safe during pregnancy, but some recommend avoiding use during the first trimester.
Itraconazole	Absorbed better in the fed state (capsule) or fasting state (solution). Metabolized in the liver; highly protein-bound. Does not appear in urine or CSF.	Hepatotoxicity, congestive heart failure, nausea, vomiting, hypertriglyceridemia, hypokalemia, rash.	Contraindicated in patients with ventricular dysfunction or heart failure. Avoid pregnancy for onychomycosis treatment.
Fluconazole, Voriconazole, Posaconazole	Includes fluconazole, voriconazole, posaconazole. Generally well absorbed orally. Fluconazole has good CSF penetration. Voriconazole has high oral bioavailability. Posaconazole absorption is enhanced by food.	Hepatotoxicity, QT prolongation, visual disturbances (voriconazole), nausea, vomiting, diarrhea, headache.	Voriconazole is contraindicated in pregnancy. Monitor liver function. Drug interactions due to CYP inhibition.

Conclusion

Fungal infections of the oral cavity, particularly those caused by Candida species, present significant challenges in dental practice. Effective management relies on accurate diagnosis, appropriate selection of antifungal agents, and an understanding of their pharmacological properties, resistance mechanisms, and potential drug interactions. By staying informed about these aspects, dental professionals can optimize treatment outcomes, minimize adverse effects, and help prevent the development of antifungal resistance.

3.10. Antiseptic in Dentistry

Antiseptics, disinfectants, and sterilant substances serve to inhibit the spread of microorganisms. Disinfection and sterilization methods are utilized to eliminate germs from both biotic and abiotic surfaces. Sterilization denotes the process of eradicating all living and active forms of germs from a material (Chauhan & Jindal, 2020). In other words, any approach that can deactivate both vegetative and spore forms is considered sterilization. Disinfection is the process of inactivating, destroying, or significantly reducing the concentration of pathogens (such as bacteria, viruses, and fungi) on hard surfaces. Processes designed to disinfect live organisms are termed antiseptics (Rutala & Weber, 2016).

The decision between disinfection and sterilization is contingent upon the medical procedure being performed and the materials involved. Medical instruments designed for use in sterile body areas, including cardiac or urinary catheters, must be devoid of any microorganisms. Therefore, the most appropriate approach for these instruments is sterilization. Disinfectants are adequate for items that come into contact with mucous membranes or potentially compromised skin.

Dental treatment surfaces can be contaminated by saliva, blood, and other infectious materials, which may include staphylococci, streptococci, Mycobacterium tuberculosis, cytomegalovirus (CMV), herpes simplex virus (HSV), hepatitis B virus (HBV), hepatitis C virus (HCV), human immunodeficiency virus (HIV), and upper respiratory tract viruses such as influenza and rhinoviruses (Abusalim, 2020). As it is impractical to sterilize all contaminated items or surfaces, the use of chemical disinfectants and disposable supplies is essential.

Disinfectants must eliminate a broad range of pathogenic organisms, encompassing their vegetative forms, and offer the widest antimicrobial spectrum. The chemical agent must maintain its activity in biological materials such as blood, saliva, and sputum. An ideal product is inexpensive, odourless, stable at room temperature, noncorrosive, nonstaining, nontoxic, and suitable for short exposure. Chemical disinfectants effectively reduce the number of viable pathogenic organisms on surfaces to levels that enable a healthy person's natural defences to ward off illness (Onemu et al., 2023).

On the other hand, the primary importance of antiseptics lies in their selective toxicity to microorganisms while sparing human cells. The selectivity of antiseptic agents can differ based on the tissues they encounter (Böhle et al., 2021). An antiseptic designed for handwashing may exhibit less selectivity compared to one formulated for oral rinsing, as the skin's highly keratinised epithelium provides a higher level of protection against the antiseptic than the oral epithelium does (Harnoss et al., 2018).

Antiseptics and disinfectants can be categorised based on their mechanism of action: those that denature proteins, those that induce osmotic disruption of the cell, and those that disrupt specific metabolic processes (McDonnell & Russell, 2001).

3.10.1. Alcohol and Aldehyde

Alcohol (70%), isopropanol (isopropyl alcohol; 70–90%), and n-propanol are the most commonly used antiseptics effective on the skin. Alcohols quickly target vegetative bacteria (including mycobacteria), pathogens, lipophilic viruses, and fungi. Alcohol irreversibly halts spore development; however, it does not possess sporicidal properties. Alcohol serves as an effective agent for surface disinfection and acts as a skin antiseptic, particularly in promoting hand hygiene. Both isopropyl and ethyl alcohol are rapidly bactericidal against vegetative bacteria, including common pathogens like *Staphylococcus aureus* and *Escherichia coli*, at concentrations of 60–90% (Al-Ogaili et al., 2024). Certain chemicals, such as chlorhexidine, can be combined with these agents to enhance their disinfectant properties (Sánchez-Guzmán et al., 2023). The mechanism of action of alcohol antiseptics involves damaging the microbial membrane and swiftly denaturing proteins, which is subsequently followed by metabolism disruption and cell lysis.

The saturated dialdehyde derivative glutaraldehyde solution (≥2%) is used for high-level disinfection of endoscopic and surgical tools (Bsg, 1988). Even though its chemical stability is good at low pH, its microbicidal efficacy is poor. The solution may kill spores in alkaline pH 7.5–8.5 settings. It also fixes tissue in electron microscopy (Russell & W, 1990). Due to its strong interaction with outer cell layers, glutaraldehyde inhibits spore germination at low concentrations and kills spores at high concentrations. Glutaraldehyde affects *Escherichia coli*, *Staphylococcus aureus*, protozoa, fungi, and viruses (Ashnagar et al., 2016). Its primary antibacterial mechanism involves cross-linking proteins and other cellular components, leading to rapid cell death (Navarro & Monsan, 1976).

Formaldehyde is a colorless, potent monoaldehyde, available in concentrations up to 35%. It is high level disinfectant, killing bacteria, spores, and viruses, although this effect is slower than that of glutaraldehyde. Its act by inhibiting DNA synthesis and forming protein-DNA cross-links. However, routine clinical use has declined due to its toxic, mutagenic, and carcinogenic effects. Because side effects such as respiratory, skin, and eye irritation can occur, it is primarily used for instrument sterilization or tissue preservation. Tissue samples should be stored in airtight containers at low temperatures and in well-ventilated areas (Gidley & Sanders, 1983; Subasi, 2020; La Torre et al., 2023).

Ortho-phthalaldehyde (OPA) is a high-level disinfectant alternative to glutaraldehyde, recommended at a concentration of 0.55%. It remains stable over a wide pH range, has a pleasant odor, requires no activation, and is non-irritating to the eyes and nose. It has high material compatibility. However, because it can stain proteins gray and cause skin discoloration, it should be used with gloves, goggles, and a liquid-impermeable apron. Equipment should be thoroughly rinsed after use. Caution should be exercised, especially in patients with bladder cancer, as OPA residue can cause serious reactions, and it should not be used for cystoscope disinfection (Iwasawa et al., 2011).

3.10.2. Halogens and Halogen-Releasing Compounds

Some of the most efficient disinfectants and antiseptic agents are halogens and halogen-releasing chemicals. Their main effect appears to be the free halogen interacting covalently with important microbial enzyme systems.

Hypochlorite salts, known as chloride lime, have been used for disinfection and antiseptic purposes since the 1800s. Sodium hypochlorite is particularly preferred in surface disinfectants due to its strong antimicrobial properties, despite its irritating effects. When dissolved in water, it rapidly transforms into hypochlorous acid, exhibiting a strong antimicrobial effect.. In hospitals, a 1:10 dilution of bleach is standard for destroying robust viruses like HBV. However, sodium hypochlorite corrodes metals, produces a foul odor, and must be diluted. Tuberculosis bacilli are more resistant to hypochlorite which require higher concentrations and extended contact times (Fiorillo et al., 2024).

Iodine is one of the oldest topical antiseptics. Iodine tincture, containing 2% iodine and 2.4% sodium iodide, and Lugol's solution are well-known forms. Iodine, with its antibacterial, antiviral, antiprotozoal, and antifungal properties, is used in the disinfection of medical equipment and in drinking water treatment. It is also effective as a pre-surgical skin antiseptic. However, iodine has some disadvantages, such as its corrosive nature, difficulty dissolving in water, and the potential to cause skin reactions like staining, rash, itching, redness, and swelling. The effectiveness (mechanism of action) of iodine is based on its ability to penetrate microorganisms and cause oxidative destruction of their cellular components (Rahman et al., 2019).

Iodophors are iodine combined with high-molecular-weight carriers (e.g., polyvinylpyrrolidone). They provide long-lasting, effective antimicrobial activity lasting 4–6 hours due to their gradual release of iodine. They are clinically preferred because their irritating and allergic effects are less than those of classic iodine. Iodophors are available in various forms, including solutions, ointments, foams, cleansing agents, gauze, and vaginal pessaries. They are used in surgical antisepsis, disinfection of blood cells, hydrotherapy tanks, thermometers, and endoscopes. Their effectiveness depends on pH, temperature, contact time, and storage conditions (Qiao-Ling, 2007).

In dentistry, hypochlorite salts—particularly sodium hypochlorite—are highly effective against a broad range of microorganisms, including bacteria and viruses, and are commonly used for root canal irrigation, surface cleaning, and decontamination of medical instruments (Qiu et al., 2023). Sodium hypochlorite, thanks to its ability to dissolve organic tissue and its broad antibacterial spectrum, is an indispensable disinfectant in dentistry. However, due to its corrosive effect on metals and its potential for irritation, it should be used with caution and diluted appropriately. Iodine and iodophors are preferred for surgical field antisepsis and the disinfection of sensitive surfaces. Both agents are important for infection control in dentistry, but the risks of allergic reactions and irritation should be considered during use, and appropriate concentration and contact time should be observed (Li & Wang, 2021).

3.10.3. Oxidizing Agents

Hydrogen peroxide (H_2O_2) serves as a mild antiseptic and oxidizing agent. H_2O_2 is a versatile agent in dentistry, primarily used for tooth whitening, oral disinfection, and biofilm control. Its applications range from professional in-office procedures to at-home oral care products, with varying concentrations and protocols tailored to specific dental needs (Altınışık & Nezir, 2025). Low concentrations (≤3%) of H_2O_2 are generally safe for daily use, with minimal risk of tissue damage. However, higher concentrations, as used in bleaching, can cause transient tooth sensitivity, soft tissue irritation, and, at very high levels, pulp damage or necrosis. Additionally, neutral pH formulations of H_2O_2 minimize enamel damage, while acidic solutions can increase surface alterations (Sun et al., 2011).

Peracetic acid (PAA) exhibits greater biocidal strength compared to hydrogen peroxide. It demonstrates sporicidal, bactericidal, virucidal, and fungicidal effects even at low concentrations. Furthermore, PAA shows strong antibacterial and antibiofilm effects, particularly against *Enterococcus faecalis*, a common endodontic pathogen. Its biofilm reduction is superior to EDTA and comparable to sodium hypochlorite. PAA is utilized in dentistry for instrument and equipment sterilization, disinfection of extracted teeth, dental impression disinfection, and endodontic irrigation. The products of its decomposition are safe and maintain their effectiveness even in the presence of organic loads. PAA does not corrode dental instruments or significantly alter the dimensions of dental impressions, making it suitable for routine use, but some formulations may have higher cytotoxicity, so selection and concentration should be carefully considered (Viola et al., 2022; Ali et al., 2021).

Potassium permanganate, in a 0.01% diluted solution, serves as a skin antiseptic in baths and wet bandages for treating eczema; however, it has the potential to stain skin and clothing. It is widely used for removing organic contaminants, bacteria, and algae from water (Wang et al., 2022).

Phenols, including both simple phenol (carbolic acid) and a range of natural and synthetic phenolic compounds, have a long history of use in dentistry. Their primary functions include serving as disinfectants, sedatives, and components in dental materials. Phenol has historically been used for cavity sterilization and desensitization, although its use and acceptance differ among practitioners. Several phenolic compounds—such as phenol, eugenol, thymol, and guaiacol—are utilized both as pulp sedatives and as disinfectants in the management of caries and root canal treatments. However, phenolic compounds show concentration-dependent cytotoxicity to human dental pulp fibroblasts but do not cause DNA damage (nongenotoxic); thus, care is needed to avoid pulpal or periapical irritation from overuse or accidental extrusion (Thomas, 1941; Chang et al., 2000). Furthermore, plant-derived polyphenols are increasingly incorporated into dental materials to enhance adhesion to enamel and dentin while also imparting antimicrobial properties. These modifications can improve the biological performance and durability of dental restorations. Additionally, certain phenolic lipids inhibit oral bacteria and bacterial collagenases, which may help reduce collagen breakdown in caries and promote tissue regeneration (Damé-Teixeira et al., 2022; Kharouf et al., 2020).

3.10.4. Heavy Metal and Quaternary Ammonium Compounds

Heavy metals and quaternary ammonium compounds are widely used for disinfection and preservation purposes because of their antimicrobial properties. Metals such as mercury and silver precipitate proteins and inactivate microbial enzymes, while quaternary ammonium compounds are effective disinfectants against both Gram-positive and Gram-negative bacteria(Aksoy & Dumlu, 2022). Although compounds such as benzalkonium chloride are used to clean surgical instruments and surfaces, the CDC does not recommend the use of such compounds as primary antiseptics.

3.10.5. Ultraviolet Irradiation

Ultraviolet germicidal irradiation (UVGI) serves as an electromagnetic radiation disinfection method aimed at curbing the transmission of specific infectious diseases. It offers decontamination of bacteria in approximately 25 minutes. Up to one hour should be allocated for decontamination of *Clostridioides difficile*. UVGI finds applications in diverse areas such as food, air, and water treatment (Aksoy & Dumlu, 2022).

3.10.6. Oral Antiseptics

When assessing different oral antiseptics, it is crucial to examine several fundamental factors, including their classification, mechanism of action, range of activity, and possible adverse effects.

Chlorhexidine (CHX) is a cationic surfactant regarded as the gold standard in oral antiseptics. Its significant substantivity and effectiveness against a broad spectrum of microorganisms, particularly Gram-positive bacteria, enhance its respected reputation. CHX operates by binding to negatively charged bacterial membranes, increasing their permeability and leading to cell death. As CHX binds to oral tissues and releases slowly, it provides prolonged antimicrobial effects. These properties, along with its effectiveness in reducing dental plaque and gingival inflammation, contribute to its widespread use as an antiseptic in dentistry. It is available in various formulations, including mouthwashes, gels, varnishes, and chips, and is used both professionally and for home care (Deus & Ouanounou, 2022; Thangavelu et al., 2020). CHX mouthwash is most effective for short-term use in situations where mechanical cleaning is limited, such as following surgery or in patients with physical or mental impairments. In periodontics and surgery, it is used to prevent complications like alveolar osteitis and bacteremia after tooth extraction and also serves as an adjunct in periodontal and implant procedures. In orthodontics, CHX mouthwash helps improve gingival health and plaque control during fixed appliance treatment. Additionally, mouthwash is employed in endodontics, caries prevention, and the management of oral infections (Pillai et al., 2023; Verma et al., 2023; Hussain et al., 2022). The most common side effect of CHX is tooth staining, particularly with prolonged use. Taste disturbance and irritation of the oral mucosa have also been reported in several studies. Although allergic reactions are possible, true allergies are very uncommon. Additionally, there is a potential concern for antimicrobial resistance with long-term use (Brookes et al., 2020; James et al., 2017).

Povidone-Iodine (PVP-I): PVP-I, an iodophor, exhibits a broad antibacterial spectrum and is efficacious against bacteria, fungi, and viruses. The process involves the oxidation of microbial proteins and nucleic acids, leading to cell death. PVP-I oral rinses at concentrations as low as 0.5% can completely inactivate viruses like SARS-CoV-2 within 15–60 seconds, outperforming some other antiseptics such as ethanol in speed and efficacy (Bakshi & Bakshi, 2021; Alqhtani et al., 2024). PVP-I is typically well-tolerated, with mild irritation or allergic reactions being rare side effects. However, prolonged or excessive use may impact thyroid function, necessitating caution in patients with pre-existing thyroid disorders or during pregnancy (Ibrahim, 2023).

Triclosan (TRC) is a nonionic phenolic compound that obstructs the formation of bacterial fatty acids, a crucial mechanism for preserving cell membrane integrity. TRC has shown efficacy against both Gram-positive and Gram-negative bacteria; nonetheless, questions exist regarding its potential contribution to antibiotic resistance and endocrine disruption. TRC is widely incorporated into dental products, especially toothpastes, to help control plaque, gingivitis, and oral bacteria (Monteiro et al., 2020; Stewart et al., 2020). Triclosan/copolymer toothpaste improves plaque control and gingival health around dental implants and in children at higher risk for aggressive periodontitis (Monteiro et al., 2020). Triclosan is generally well tolerated in oral care, with no serious adverse effects reported in studies lasting up to three years. Despite its established safety for dental applications, triclosan has been restricted or banned from certain consumer products due to environmental concerns and potential broader health implications. Nevertheless, it remains approved for use in toothpaste in many countries (Sinicropi et al., 2022).

Cetylpyridinium chloride (CPC) is a quaternary ammonium compound that operates by compromising bacterial cell membranes, leading to the efflux of cellular constituents. It has a broad antibacterial range and is less likely to cause stains than chlorhexidine (CHX), making it a more suitable option for patients with orthodontic devices. CPC is an active ingredient in mouthwashes and toothpastes. Its main roles are to reduce dental plaque, gingival inflammation, and oral microbial load, making it a valuable adjunct in oral hygiene and dental procedures (Setiawatie et al., 2023; Shijith, 2021). CPC is generally well tolerated and considered safe, with fewer side effects such as staining and taste alteration compared to chlorhexidine. However, certain CPC mouthwashes may impact the strength of orthodontic elastomeric chains, making careful product selection important. Additionally, overuse of CPC could contribute to antiseptic resistance, underscoring the need for prudent use (Mao et al., 2020; Castelló et al., 2024; Oo & Saddki, 2022).

Essential oils (EOs) are complex mixtures derived from plants, exhibiting antibacterial properties via denaturing proteins and compromising cell membranes. Essential oils have shown effectiveness against germs linked to caries and are considered harmless, with fewer unwanted effects than synthetic agents. However, efficacy may vary significantly based on the specific formulation and concentration utilized. EOs such as eugenol (clove), peppermint, tea tree, thyme, cinnamon, and others show significant inhibitory effects against common oral pathogens, including *Streptococcus mutans*,

Staphylococcus aureus, *Enterococcus faecalis*, *Escherichia coli*, and *Candida albicans* (Thosar et al., 2013; Fine et al., 2000). EOs are recommended for reducing bacterial load in dental aerosols, thereby contributing to infection control in dental settings. Additionally, EOs are being explored for special uses such as incorporation into dental materials, toothbrush sanitizers, and as agents for managing halitosis and oral candidiasis (Weber et al., 2023; Aires et al., 2020). Essential oil (EO) mouthwashes generally exhibit a favorable safety profile, presenting fewer side effects such as staining and taste alteration compared to chlorhexidine. While some individuals may experience mild burning sensations or taste changes, these occurrences are less frequent and severe than with other antiseptics. Despite their promise, further clinical trials are necessary to fully establish the safety and efficacy of EOs across diverse populations and formulations (Navabi et al., 2021; De Carvalho et al., 2024; Radu et al., 2023).

Octenidine (OCT) is a cationic bispyridinamine that demonstrates bactericidal properties similar to chlorhexidine (CHX), but with lower cytotoxicity. OCT binds to microbial cell membranes, resulting in cell lysis and subsequent cell death. It is recognized for its reduced unwanted effects, such as less staining and irritation, making it a viable option for oral care. OCT is considered a potential alternative to chlorhexidine, the current gold standard, due to its strong antimicrobial properties and favorable safety profile. OCT mouthwashes exhibit antimicrobial activity against key oral pathogens (e.g., *Streptococcus mutans*, *Candida albicans*, *Fusobacterium nucleatum*) that is comparable to, or even better than, chlorhexidine, especially at lower concentrations (Amrita et al., 2024).

OCT is effective in preventing biofilm formation and disrupting mature dental biofilms, leading to reduced bacterial viability and decreased biofilm thickness in situ. It demonstrates broad-spectrum activity against various bacteria and fungi, including those associated with periodontal disease and oral candidiasis (Dudek et al., 2023; Reda et al., 2021). OCT mouthwashes are highly effective in controlling plaque, gingival inflammation, and bleeding, showing significant benefits in both healthy individuals and those with gingivitis or periodontitis, often matching or surpassing the efficacy of chlorhexidine. In orthodontic patients with fixed appliances, OCT helps prevent gingival inflammation and limits the growth of periodontopathogens. Additionally, when used as an adjunct to scaling and root planing, OCT enhances clinical outcomes in periodontal therapy (Amrita et al., 2024; Vidovic et al., 2019).

OCT is generally well tolerated, with mild side effects such as slight tooth or tongue staining and taste disturbances, which are less pronounced than those seen with chlorhexidine. Additionally, OCT helps reduce pathogenic microorganisms while supporting the restoration of normal oral flora after use (Sabanceva et al., 2021; Sadanandan et al., 2021).

Conclusion

Effective infection control in dentistry relies on a comprehensive understanding of antiseptics, disinfectants, and sterilization methods. While chlorhexidine remains the benchmark for oral antiseptics, a range of alternative agents including povidone-iodine, triclosan, cetylpyridinium chloride, essential oils, and octenidine offer diverse mechanisms of action, antimicrobial spectra, and safety profiles. The selection of appropriate agents and methods should be guided by the clinical context, the nature of the surfaces or tissues involved, and individual patient needs. Ongoing research and prudent use of these agents are essential to maximize efficacy, minimize adverse effects, and prevent the development of resistance, ultimately ensuring optimal patient care and safety in dental practice.

Chapter 4

Special Considerations for Prescribing Medications in Dentistry

Abstract

When prescribing medications in dental practice, it is crucial to account for individual patient characteristics such as age, physiological status, and underlying health conditions. High-risk groups including pediatric and geriatric patients, pregnant and lactating women, and individuals with systemic diseases require special consideration due to their altered drug metabolism and heightened risk of adverse effects. For children, accurate dosing and awareness of developmental pharmacokinetics are essential. In the elderly, polypharmacy and age-related organ changes can increase drug sensitivity and interactions. Pregnant and breastfeeding women need medications with established safety profiles to avoid harm to the fetus or infant. Patients with systemic diseases, such as renal or hepatic impairment, may need dose adjustments or alternative therapies. This chapter provides an overview of key considerations and current approaches for safe and effective medication prescribing in special populations, including practical recommendations, risk mitigation strategies, and guidance on patient education to ensure optimal dental care outcomes.

Keywords: high-risk groups, drug metabolism, pediatric, geriatric, systemic diseases

4.1. Pediatric Dentistry

Pediatric dentistry requires a multidisciplinary approach that encompasses not only the prevention and treatment of dental and oral health issues but also addresses the overall health of children. In this context, prescribing medications for pediatric patients involves many specific considerations that differ from those for adults. Children's physiological, pharmacological, and psychosocial characteristics are key determinants in the selection and administration of medications.

4.1.1. Pharmacokinetic and Pharmacodynamic Differences in Children

Children should not be regarded as merely smaller versions of adults. Ongoing development and maturation of their organ systems result in substantial differences in the pharmacokinetics and pharmacodynamics of medications. These developmental variations significantly influence how pediatric patients absorb, distribute, metabolize, and excrete drugs, as well as how they respond to pharmacological interventions. As a result, drug dosing and monitoring in pediatric patients must be carefully tailored to account for these unique pharmacokinetic and pharmacodynamic characteristics (Lim & Pettit, 2019).

Pharmacokinetic changes in pediatric patients include several important differences compared to adults. In neonates, gastric pH is higher, gastric emptying is slower, and intestinal transit time can vary, all of which impact the absorption of orally administered drugs. Drug distribution is also affected, as infants have a higher total body water content and lower fat stores, along with reduced plasma protein binding, which increases the proportion of free drug in circulation. Additionally, the liver enzyme systems responsible for drug metabolism (both phase I and II) are immature at birth, resulting in slower metabolism and prolonged half-lives for many medications. Finally, renal function including glomerular filtration, tubular secretion, and reabsorption is not fully developed in neonates, leading to decreased drug clearance (Jovanović & Vučićević, 2022; Lu & Rosenbaum, 2014).

The pharmacodynamics of drugs also vary in children, especially in neonates, because both the number and function of drug receptors can differ from those in adults. These differences in receptor sensitivity can impact how children respond to medications and the likelihood of experiencing side effects. The most significant differences in pharmacokinetics and pharmacodynamics are observed during the first two years of life, as organ systems and receptor functions gradually mature toward adult levels. Additionally, there is considerable variability in how children respond to medications, which can be attributed to differences in developmental stages, genetic factors, and underlying health conditions (Watanabe et al., 2023; Meesters et al., 2024; Bardol et al., 2023).

4.1.2. Nonpharmacological Interventions in Pediatric Dentistry

Nonpharmacological interventions are frequently used in pediatric dentistry to reduce children's anxiety and fears, increase cooperation, and enhance the treatment process. Basic techniques such as tell-show-do, positive reinforcement, modeling, and distraction help make the child's experience with the dentist safer and more comfortable. Additionally, distraction methods such as storytelling, gamification, animations, and virtual reality can further facilitate children's compliance with treatment. Advanced approaches include cognitive behavioral therapy, relaxation exercises, sensory-adapted dental environments, and animal-assisted therapy. Applying these techniques in combination and tailoring them to the individual needs of each child can significantly reduce anxiety and increase treatment outcomes (Dhar et al., 2023; Alonazi et al., 2023).

4.1.3. Pharmacological Agents Commonly Used in Dentistry

The most frequently used drug groups in pediatric dentistry include analgesics, antibiotics, local anesthetics, and antifungal agents. Safe analgesics such as paracetamol and ibuprofen are generally preferred for pain management in children, while aspirin is not recommended due to the risk of Reye's syndrome (Harding, 1994). Amoxicillin is the first choice for the treatment of dental infections; however, clindamycin or macrolide antibiotics can be used as alternatives in children with a penicillin allergy. Prescribing antibiotics only when bacterial infections are confirmed and for appropriate indications is crucial to prevent the development of resistance (Marek & Timmons, 2019).

For procedures requiring local anesthesia, agents such as lidocaine, articaine, and mepivacaine are frequently used, with dosages carefully adjusted according to the child's age and weight (Klingberg et al., 2017). Prilocaine, however, should be used sparingly in children due to the risk of methemoglobinemia. When sedation is needed to manage dental anxiety, nitrous oxide is the most widely used agent, followed by oral benzodiazepines such as midazolam. In some cases, antihistamines may also be employed for mild sedation, offering the additional benefits of antiemetic and antisialagogue effects (Dowdy et al., 2023).

Topical antifungal agents such as nystatin and miconazole are preferred for the treatment of oral fungal infections. The selection and use of these drug groups should be meticulously planned to ensure the safety of pediatric patients and the success of treatment. Fluoride varnishes, silver diamine fluoride (SDF), and other silver compounds are also widely used in pediatric dentistry for the prevention and arrest of dental caries (Gao et al., 2016).

4.1.4. Drug Formulations and Administration Routes

Pediatric dental drug delivery relies on child-friendly formulations such as syrups, drops, chewables, orally disintegrating tablets (ODTs), and mini-tablets. Studies have shown that liquid forms can lead to dosing errors, while ODTs improve dose precision. Noninvasive methods like topical, sublingual, and intranasal administration are typically well accepted by children. Tablets or capsules are generally not suitable for young children. Furthermore, the taste and smell of medications can significantly affect children's compliance (Rautamo et al., 2020; Shaat et al., 2021; Frank et al., 2023). Numerous novel formulations, such as lozenges and jellies, can mask the unpleasant taste of prescription drugs and help children tolerate them better (Frank et al., 2023). Topical creams and varnishes are commonly used for local anesthesia, fluoride delivery, and caries prevention in dental practice. These agents are favored because they are painless and noninvasive, making them especially suitable for pediatric patients (De Freitas et al., 2022).

4.1.5. Key Principles for the Safe and Rational Prescribing of Medications in Pediatric Dental Practice

Proper prescribing practices in pediatric dentistry require careful attention to several essential considerations, including the following:

For children, medication dosage is usually calculated per kilogram of body weight (mg/kg) (Barone et al., 2025). Direct administration of adult doses to children can lead to serious side effects. The child's age, weight, and general health status must be considered when calculating the dose. In infants and young children, immature kidney and liver function can slow the elimination of medications from the body (Goel et al., 2020; Nazar et al., 2023).

Medications used in children must have proven safety and effectiveness. Drugs with a low side effect profile and those approved for pediatric use should be preferred. Furthermore, the medication form (such as syrup, drops, or chewable tablets) should be appropriate for the child's age and swallowing ability. It is also important to follow established pediatric guidelines for antibiotics and analgesics to prevent overuse and misuse (Aly & Elchaghaby, 2021; Goel et al., 2024). Antibiotics should be prescribed only when clearly indicated to prevent resistance (Muhson & Al-Obaidi, 2024; Barone et al., 2025). The shortest effective duration of treatment should be used, and unnecessarily prolonged courses should be avoided (Nazar et al., 2023).

Previous drug reactions, allergies, and current medications should always be reviewed. Beta-lactam allergies, in particular, should be considered when prescribing antibiotics (Goel et al., 2024).

The dosage, method of administration, duration, and potential side effects of the prescribed medication should be clearly and understandably explained to parents. Correct administration by parents is critical to the success of treatment (Kamath & Jawdekar, 2023). It is important to monitor both the effectiveness of the prescribed medication and any potential side effects in the child. If necessary, follow-up appointments should be scheduled to monitor treatment progress.

Finally, when prescribing medications for pediatric patients, it is essential to comply with the legal regulations and ethical standards of the country. Whenever possible, the generic name of the medication should be used rather than the brand name, and both the dosage and duration of treatment should be clearly specified.

4.1.6. Management of Adverse Drug Reactions in Pediatric Dentistry

Adverse drug reactions (ADRs) are a significant clinical concern in pediatric dentistry, as children are more sensitive to medications. Effective management of ADRs requires early recognition, appropriate intervention, and efficient reporting. Dentists should be familiar with clinical signs and symptoms that may indicate an adverse reaction, such as rash, dermatitis, swelling edema, or more sever manifestations like anaphylaxis. If a patient exhibits symptoms of an adverse reaction, the dentist should promptly discontinue the suspected medication. While antihistamines may be sufficient for minor allergic reactions, severe systemic reactions may necessitate the administration of oxygen and a life-saving injection of intramuscular adrenaline. Even in cases of moderate adverse effects or allergic reactions, the patient should be closely monitored and provided with supportive care. All adverse events should be reported to both national authorities and the pharmacovigilance center. It is equally important to fully inform parents about the allergy or adverse reaction and to advise them on what to do if the child experiences another reaction, as such events can recur (Chari et al., 2021).

Additionally, prescribed medications may interact with other drugs or supplements the child is taking for chronic conditions, resulting in drug-drug interactions. This risk is heightened in cases of polypharmacy, which in children is variously defined as the concurrent use of two or more medications for at least one day, the use of multiple medications for 31 days or longer, or the sequential use of multiple medications over the course of a year. As polypharmacy increases the likelihood of drug interactions and adverse medication effects, it is essential to mitigate this risk by obtaining a comprehensive medication and medical history, assessing potential polypharmacy using reputable drug interaction software, and consulting reliable references such as respected web sources or case studies before prescribing medication (Elzagallaai et al., 2017; Ouanounou et al., 2020; Chari et al., 2021; Neininger et al., 2021).

4.1.7. Management of Pediatric Dentistry Patients with Chronic Diseases

Managing dental care for children with chronic conditions requires specialized knowledge and a multidisciplinary approach. This involves assessing the child's oral hygiene, evaluating the potential impact of medical devices or implants, and considering the child's immune status. A comprehensive medical and medication history should be obtained, and consultation with the child's physician is essential when needed. Children with chronic conditions often face a heightened risk of oral diseases; therefore, treatment should integrate medication, behavioral strategies, structured healthcare monitoring, and minimally invasive dentistry (MID). Emphasis should be placed on prevention, risk assessment, and ongoing monitoring, rather than relying solely on surgical interventions (Foster & Fitzgerald, 2005).

Treatment plans must be tailored to the specific needs of each patient, whether they have blood disorders, heart disease, diabetes, or other chronic conditions. After treatment, close monitoring of the child's overall health is crucial, and families should be well-informed about dental care and potential complications (Gupta et al., 2015; Elhusseiny & Saleh, 2024; Edelstein et al., 2025). Chronic systemic diseases often present with distinctive oral manifestations that dental professionals must recognize and manage effectively. For example, children with chronic renal failure may exhibit enamel hypoplasia, delayed tooth eruption, and gingival changes, necessitating careful evaluation and management of bleeding and infection risks. Close collaboration with nephrologists is essential to provide comprehensive care (Beyer et al., 2025).

Dentists also play a vital role in providing palliative care for children with terminal conditions or cancers. These patients frequently experience complex oral health issues that can significantly impact their quality of life. Addressing these challenges requires a coordinated team-based approach to ensure optimal oral and overall health outcomes for this vulnerable population (Svetlakova et al., 2025; Elhusseiny & Saleh, 2024).

4.1.8. Strategies of Education and Communication in Pediatric Dentistry

In addition to providing dental care, pediatric dentistry involves educating children and their families and promoting oral and dental health, as well as ensuring adherence to treatment plans. Thus, the foundations of pediatric dentistry are effective communication and education. Good communication with pediatric patients and their families not only improves treatment outcomes but also helps children develop lifelong dental health habits (Jafarzadeh et al., 2025).

Compared to adults, children are at distinct phases of cognitive, emotional, and social development. As a result, communication between dentists and children should be customized based on the child's age, developmental stage, and unique traits. Children who communicate well are less afraid of the dentist, more confident throughout treatment, and more cooperative. Additionally, effective communication promotes active involvement in care and helps develop positive attitudes toward oral health (Schulz-Weidner et al., 2024).

When it comes to treating pediatric patients, families, especially parents, play a crucial role. Children's oral health habits are strongly influenced by their parents' dental knowledge, attitudes, and behaviors. Treatment success and compliance increase when parents are actively involved, and addressing family concerns helps children feel more secure (Dogan et al., 2025). Therefore, it is important to educate families on fostering good oral hygiene practices, recognizing key aspects of treatment, and protecting their children's dental health.

Age-appropriate, engaging, and easily understood language should be used to teach children about the value of dental care, proper brushing habits, a healthy diet, and the necessity of dental checkups. Simple, concrete terms that children can understand are preferred, and communication should always be tailored to the child's age and developmental level. For young children, role-playing, storytelling, and visual materials can help them grasp the intended message. For older children, establishing cause-and-effect links can help them understand the value of treatment and its stages, improving both their understanding of the procedure and their confidence in the treatment (Schulz-Weidner et al., 2024).

However, using proper language alone is insufficient; additional behavioral management approaches should be applied to promote children's adherence to treatment. These techniques are useful for increasing children's cooperation with treatment. Methods such as tell-show-do, positive reinforcement, modeling, and distraction techniques all help to alleviate children's anxieties and concerns. For example, introducing the device the dentist will use and allowing the child to touch it encourages a more positive attitude toward treatment (Gizani et al., 2022; Alkahtani, 2024).

To ensure these strategies are effective, it is critical to prioritize empathy and active listening in communication. These skills are key to understanding the emotions of both the child and the family. Their concerns and fears should be acknowledged, and they should be allowed to express themselves. Answering their questions patiently helps build trust and improve treatment compliance (Moore, 2022).

Visual and audio materials, such as toothbrushing posters, animations, and hands-on demonstrations, make it easier for children to understand oral health concepts. These materials are especially effective for primary school-aged children, making abstract concepts more concrete and memorable (Media et al., 2025; Pitoy et al., 2021). Additionally, informative brochures and videos for families also support the education process. For these methods to be effective, families must remain actively involved in the treatment journey. Family involvement is crucial for treatment success. Parents should be encouraged to support their child's oral care, help reduce dental anxiety, and promote healthy habits. Positive reinforcement, like praise and small rewards, can motivate children to cooperate during dental visits. While rewards help create positive experiences, consistent monitoring and support for treatment adherence is equally important (Verma et al., 2024). Regular follow-up with families, reminders about medication and oral care, and using digital tools can improve adherence and catch potential issues early (Toma et al., 2020).

Effective communication and education in pediatric dentistry ultimately support both successful treatment and lifelong oral health (Randall & Dhar, 2023; Naeem & Naeem, 2025).

4.2. Geriatric Dentistry: Pharmacotherapy for Elderly Patients

Geriatric dentistry is a specialized discipline focused on the prevention, treatment, and rehabilitation of oral and dental health in geriatric patients. Age-related physiological changes, the rising prevalence of chronic diseases, and polypharmacy (the concurrent use of multiple medications) underscore the critical importance of effective pharmacotherapy management in this population. This section will review the fundamental principles of pharmacotherapy in geriatric patients, highlight common challenges, and provide evidence-based recommendations for clinical practice.

4.2.1. Age-Related Changes in Pharmacokinetics and Pharmacodynamics

Physiological changes associated with aging significantly impact the absorption, distribution, metabolism, and excretion of drugs (pharmacokinetics). While drug absorption is generally unchanged, slowed gastric emptying or alterations in the gastrointestinal tract may affect the absorption of certain medications; however, this effect is of minor clinical significance for most drugs. In terms of distribution, aging is characterized by increased body fat and decreased total body water and lean body mass. These changes increase the volume of distribution for lipophilic (fat-soluble) drugs, thereby prolonging their half-life, while decreasing the volume of distribution for hydrophilic (water-soluble) drugs (Demeester et al., 2023; Gronich, 2024).

Metabolic changes include reduced liver mass and diminished hepatic blood flow, as well as variable enzyme activity, resulting in slower metabolism and excretion of some drugs. Consequently, plasma drug concentrations may increase. Renal function, as measured by glomerular filtration rate (GFR), also declines with age. Notably, even with normal serum creatinine levels, the kidneys' ability to excrete drugs is often impaired, increasing the risk of toxicity for renally excreted medications. Commonly used drugs in dental practice, such as analgesics, antibiotics, and sedatives, may accumulate and increase the risk of adverse effects. Dentists should therefore adjust dosages, either by reducing dose or extending dosing intervals, as appropriate (Ngcobo, 2025; Mangoni et al., 2025).

Additionally, the pharmacodynamic response to drugs may change in older adults. Geriatric patients are particularly sensitive to medications affecting the central nervous system (e.g., sedatives, antipsychotics), anticoagulants, and cardiovascular agents. As a result, the risk of adverse effects such as central nervous system depression, bleeding, or hypotension is higher, even at standard doses and with commonly used dental medications (Pyle & Tolbert, 1994). Furthermore, the efficacy of certain medications (e.g., beta-blockers, diuretics) may be reduced due to age-related changes at the organ or receptor level, potentially diminishing their therapeutic value. Age-related deterioration of homeostatic mechanisms also impairs the body's ability to compensate for drug effects, such as blood pressure drops following administration of local anesthetics or sedatives. This increases the risk of adverse events, including sudden hypotension or electrolyte imbalances (Ngcobo, 2025; Mangoni et al., 2025; Thürmann, 2019).

4.2.2. Polypharmacy and Drug Interaction

Polypharmacy, defined as the simultaneous use of five or more medications, is quite common in geriatrics. It significantly increases the risk of drug-drug interactions and side effects. When planning treatment and prescribing medications for older patients, dentists should carefully review the patient's current medication list, assess potential interactions, and make dosage adjustments if necessary. Furthermore, geriatric patients may use medications with a narrow therapeutic window, meaning that even small dose adjustments can lead to serious side effects. Therefore, it is crucial for dentists to carefully plan pharmacotherapy and closely monitor older adults during treatment (Koren et al., 2019; Ngcobo, 2025; Mangoni et al., 2025).

4.2.3. Cognitive Impairment, Frailty, and Elderly People Living in Nursing Homes

Cognitive and functional abilities decline with age, increasing the risk of medication errors, non-adherence, and complications during dental treatment. Among geriatric patients, those with cognitive impairments such as dementia and Alzheimer's disease, frail individuals, and elderly residents of nursing homes represent high- risk groups for medication mismanagement. Taking medications at the wrong dose or at the wrong time, mixing up medications, and non-adherence to treatment are common in patients with cognitive impairment. Frail individuals have increased susceptibility to medication side effects and toxicity due to diminished physiological reserves. In nursing homes, factors such as multiple illnesses, polypharmacy, and frequent staff turnover further increase the risk of medication errors. Therefore, medication management in these groups should be kept as simple as possible, unnecessary medications should be avoided, and regular medication reviews should be conducted. Furthermore, caregiver education and active involvement in medication management should be prioritized (He et al., 2023; Wang et al., 2024; Ibrahim et al., 2023; Rekatsina et al., 2021).

4.2.4. Sociocultural and Economic Factors Affecting Medication Use in Geriatric Patients

Cultural beliefs, health literacy, and socioeconomic status are key factors influencing medication use in geriatric patients. Low health literacy can result in misunderstandings of instructions, missed doses, and poor adherence to treatment. Financial limitations may also lead to the inaccessibility of prescribed medications, posing another major challenge.

Therefore, patient education and communication should be culturally sensitive, clear, and easy to understand, clearly explaining why and how medications should be used. If necessary, written or visual aids should be provided, and caregivers should be included in the process to reinforce correct medication use (Ibrahim et al., 2020; Punnapurath et al., 2021; Odubanjo et al., 2024).

4.2.5. Non-Pharmacological Alternatives for Geriatric Patients

Non-pharmacological treatment options should also be considered to reduce medication burden and protect geriatric patients from the adverse effects of polypharmacy. Maintaining good oral hygiene, scheduling routine dental checkups, and making appropriate dietary and lifestyle modifications are crucial for preventing dental pain and infections. Methods such as cold application, topical care, and psychological support for acute pain management can help reduce the need for medication. Additionally, physical therapy, relaxation techniques, and cognitive-behavioral approaches can be effective in managing chronic pain or discomfort. These strategies contribute to a holistic approach to treatment, especially for geriatric patients who are taking multiple medications and are at increased risk of side effects (Abdulla et al., 2013; Geziry et al., 2018; Liao et al., 2021).

4.2.6. General Approaches for Managing Medications in Geriatric Patients

When planning medication therapy in dentistry for geriatric patients, it is safest to start treatment with lower doses and gradually increase the dose as the medication's effects are observed. This approach minimizes the risk of side effects and toxicity associated with age-related physiological changes. Furthermore, it is crucial to review all of the patient's current medications and collaborate with the patient's physician and pharmacist to prevent potentially harmful drug interactions. This multidisciplinary collaboration ensures safe treatment, especially in elderly patients with polypharmacy. Patients should be closely monitored for side effects throughout treatment, and any adverse events should be addressed promptly. Finally, both patients and caregivers must be informed about medication schedules, proper dosages, and possible side effects to enhance adherence and reduce risks. This holistic approach establishes the fundamental principles for safe and effective medication management in geriatric patients (Monette & Schwartz, 2023; De Oliveira et al., 2024; Clemens et al., 2024).

4.2.7. Geriatric Dental Medications: Key Considerations

The most frequently utilized medications in dental care for geriatric patients include analgesics, antibiotics, local anesthetics, and antifungal agents. However, due to the physiological changes associated with aging, special care is required when using these medications. Nonsteroidal anti-inflammatory drugs (NSAIDs), in particular, should be used for the shortest possible duration at the lowest dose and sometimes co-administered with proton pump inhibitors to mitigate the risk of of gastrointestinal bleeding, peptic ulcers, and renal dysfunction in geriatric patients. Safer alternatives such as paracetamol should be preferred for pain management (Hyllested et al., 2002;

Abdulla et al.,2013; Freo et al.,2021). Antibiotics should be used with caution in geriatric patients due to age-related declines in renal function. Dosage adjustments should be made, especially for antibiotics such as amoxicillin and cephalosporins, which are primarily renally excreted. Furthermore, the indication for antibiotic use should be carefully evaluated, as unnecessary and prolonged antibiotic use can lead to serious complications such as *Clostridioides difficile* infection (Đukić et al., 2024; Contaldo et al., 2023; Buonavoglia et al., 2021). Although local anesthetics are generally safe, it should be noted that adrenaline-containing preparations may increase the risk of hypertension and arrhythmia in elderly patients with cardiovascular disease. Maximum dosage limits should not be exceeded, and vital signs should be closely monitored during administration (Ahmadi et al., 2015; Kumar et al., 2022; Kadirovna et al., 2024). Antifungal agents are commonly prescribed in geriatric dental care due to the higher prevalence of oral mucosal fungal infections in this population. While topical forms are generally considered safe, liver function and potential drug interactions should be considered when using systemic antifungal drugs (Nikolishyna et al., 2020; Gheorghe et al., 2021). In all these drug groups, treatment should be planned considering the geriatric patient's general health, comorbidities, and concurrent medications. In some cases, even small dose changes can lead to serious side effects due to the narrow therapeutic window of certain drugs, and patients should be closely monitored for side effects and potential drug interactions throughout treatment.

4.2.8. Geriatric Prescribing: Best Practices and Criteria

When planning pharmacotherapy for geriatric patients, it is important to carefully consider the indications, dosages, and duration of medications, avoid unnecessary drug use, and reduce the number of medications whenever possible. Clinicians are guided by various tools and criteria outlined in international guidelines to achieve these goals. Notably, the Beers Criteria (American Geriatrics Society Beers Criteria®) and the START/STOPP Criteria (Screening Tool to Alert to Right Treatment/Screening Tool of Older Persons' Prescriptions) are widely used to identify potentially inappropriate medications and ensure safe prescribing in the elderly (Samuel, 2023; O'Mahony et al., 2023).

The Beers Criteria list drugs and drug groups that should be avoided in older adults, while the START/STOPP Criteria help identify both undertreatment and unnecessary or harmful medications. The Beers Criteria can identify 25–58% of potentially inappropriate medications (PIMs) in various settings. However, they may miss omissions or context-specific issues and are generally recommended as a screening tool for PIMs. The STOPP Criteria detect more PIMs than the Beers Criteria, up to 73%, and are more sensitive for identifying adverse drug events and hospitalizations. The START Criteria, on the other hand, highlight potential prescribing omissions and promote comprehensive, appropriate therapy (Gallagher & O'Mahony, 2008; Thomas & Thomas, 2019; Szoszkiewicz et al., 2024; Samuel, 2023; O'Mahony et al., 2023).

Additionally, the Medication Appropriateness Index (MAI) is a tool used to assess the appropriateness of prescribed medications, considering parameters such as dose, indication, and interactions (Awad & Hanna, 2019; Al-Share et al., 2024; Al-Share et al., 2025). The FORTA (Fit for the Aged) Classification categorizes medications from A to D in terms of efficacy and safety in the elderly, guiding clinicians on which medications should be preferred or avoided. Randomized controlled trials have demonstrated the effectiveness of FORTA-guided prescribing in minimizing medication errors, over- and under-treatment, and adverse drug reactions in hospitalized geriatric patients (Wehling et al., 2016; Pazan et al., 2019).

Furthermore, the PRISCUS List, developed in Germany, identifies potentially inappropriate medications and alternatives for the elderly (Holt et al., 2010). The updated PRISCUS 2.0 includes more substances, new evaluation criteria, and disease-specific considerations, enhancing its relevance and comprehensiveness (Mann et al., 2023; Akyön et al., 2024).

Regular medication reviews conducted by multidisciplinary teams, patient and caregiver education, electronic prescribing systems, and clinical decision support tools are among the methods that support good prescribing practices for geriatric patients. Studies show that such practices reduce drug-related hospitalization rates and the frequency of serious adverse events in the elderly, while significantly improving treatment effectiveness and patient satisfaction (Romskaug et al., 2020; Walsh et al., 2024; Yaacob et al., 2024).

Furthermore, deprescribing, defined as systematically discontinuing unnecessary or harmful medications, reduces side effects and drug interactions related to polypharmacy and improves quality of life and treatment adherence in elderly patients (Page et al., 2016; Reeve et al., 2022). Consequently, it is crucial for patient safety and treatment success that all healthcare professionals, including dentists, utilize criteria such as Beers, START/STOPP, MAI, FORTA, and PRISCUS, as well as deprescribing approaches and current good prescribing practices, when planning pharmacotherapy for elderly patients (Reeve et al., 2017; Scott et al., 2015).

4.2.9. Reporting Adverse Drug Reactions (ADRs)

Adverse drug reactions (ADRs) in elderly patients are both more frequent and often have more serious consequences. The primary reasons for this include age-related physiological changes, polypharmacy, and chronic diseases. Reporting ADRs encountered in clinical practice to national and international pharmacovigilance systems contributes to improving drug safety in the elderly population. Furthermore, ADR reporting expands the database on the safe use of new drugs in older adults and informs updates to clinical guidelines. Physicians and dentists must report these reactions, especially when encountering new or unexpected side effects (Petrovic et al., 2012; Monteiro et al., 2020).

4.2.10. Practical Tools and Electronic Systems

Today, various practical tools and electronic systems are used to improve medication safety and minimize medication errors. Medication reconciliation checklists ensure a regular review of all medications a patient is taking and help identify unnecessary or dangerous medications. Electronic prescribing systems and clinical decision support software support physicians by providing alerts about drug interactions, overdose, and contraindications. The use of these systems reduces medication-related hospitalizations and serious adverse events, especially in elderly patients with polypharmacy (Lagerin et al., 2020; Ailabouni et al., 2021; Rissanen et al., 2023; Gilson et al., 2024).

4.2.11. Patient-Centered Communication and Shared Decision-Making

The success of medication therapy in geriatric patients is closely linked not only to selecting the appropriate medication but also to the active participation of the patient and caregivers in the treatment process. Elderly individuals often face multiple chronic diseases and complex medication regimens. Therefore, the patient's values, life expectancy, treatment expectations, and concerns must be considered when planning medication therapy. A shared decision-making approach fosters open communication between the dentist and the patient (or caregiver), allowing treatment options, potential benefits, and risks to be jointly evaluated. This approach increases patient compliance and reduces misunderstandings and medication errors. Especially for older adults with reduced cognitive capacity or low health literacy, the treatment plan should be simplified and explained in clear, understandable language. Furthermore, involving caregivers in the process facilitates the correct administration of medications at the right time and in the right dose (Shen et al., 2020; Milky & Thomas, 2020; Rostoft et al., 2020; Schuijt et al., 2023).

4.3. Prescribing for Pregnant Patients

The frequency of drug use among women during pregnancy has been examined in numerous studies. Research conducted in the United States found that 62% of pregnant women reported using prescription drugs. One-fourth of these women used narcotic drugs, while 13% used psychotropic drugs (Brocklebank et al., 1978). Another study indicated that women used an average of 3.1 non-vitamin drugs during pregnancy (Piper et al., 1987). A recent survey of French women revealed that 99% of pregnant women received a prescription for at least one medication, with an average of 13.6 prescriptions per woman. Among the participants, 1.6% used a substance designated as Category X by the United States Food and Drug Administration (FDA), indicating that the risks to the fetus outweigh any potential benefits. Additionally, 59% of women received a prescription for a Category D medication, which indicates fetal risk but may be justified in certain circumstances due to potential benefits. The most commonly prescribed drug classes were gastrointestinal drugs (69.4%), dermatological drugs (63.0%), and analgesics (62.3%) (Lacroix et al., 2000). In a Hungarian case-control study, 1–7% of women received drugs classified as possible human teratogens based on the Swedish classification; among 642 drugs used during pregnancy, 18 (2–8%) belonged to this group (Addis et al., 2001). Other research has shown that 97.1% of women took at least one medication during pregnancy, with 95.7% taking a medication in the first trimester (Haas et al., 2018). Data from a recent study in Croatia showed that 56% of pregnant women were taking prescription medication, while 69.5% practiced self-medication, indicating the persistence of this issue (Jovanović & Vulić, 2025).

Despite the increased use of medications, there remains a substantial lack of comprehensive safety information for many drugs taken during pregnancy. For about 25% of commonly prescribed drugs, there is insufficient information to fully assess their safety for the fetus. Pregnant women are often excluded from clinical trials, leading to off-label prescriptions with limited safety data and reliance on outdated or unproven drugs. Although investment in research infrastructure, such as specialized pharmacology centers and improved data collection methods, is increasing, progress remains slow (Pieper, 2015).

The use of various drugs during pregnancy is associated with increased risks of negative outcomes, such as preterm birth, caesarean delivery, fetal demise, and admissions to neonatal intensive care units. A meticulous risk-benefit evaluation is essential, as certain drugs are crucial for maternal health despite limited safety data (Nunge et al., 2025).

4.3.1. Teratogenic Exposure and the Importance of Timing

Exposure to teratogenic chemicals during the initial 2–3 weeks post-conception is typically believed to result in either no consequences or spontaneous pregnancy loss, a phenomenon known as "all or none" (Adam, 2012). Sensitivity to teratogenic agents is generally considered to develop between the 3rd and 8th weeks of gestation, with few defects expected before the 3rd week and a marked decrease in occurrence after the 8th week. The 3–8-week interval corresponds to the phase of organogenesis, during which the rudiments of each organ system are established (Sadler, 2017). Consequently, the first trimester is the most critical period for the onset of teratogenic effects. However, evidence shows that teratogenic effects are not limited to early pregnancy and can also impact later fetal development (Scheuerle & Aylsworth, 2016).

4.3.2. The Food and Drug Administration (FDA)'s Classification System and Teratogenic Risks

A teratogen is an agent capable of causing permanent structural or functional defects in an organism when exposed during embryonic or fetal development.

Identifying human teratogens requires a meticulous analysis of data from various types of studies (Cordero & Oakley Jr, 1983).

In 1979, the FDA implemented a drug classification system to mitigate teratogenicity and prevent unnecessary medication use during pregnancy. According to this system, drugs were classified into categories A, B, C, D, or X:

- A: Controlled studies show no risk
- B: No evidence of risk in humans
- C: Risk cannot be ruled out
- D: Positive evidence of risk, but benefits may outweigh risks
- X: Contraindicated in pregnancy due to clear risks

The FDA discontinued these categories in 2014 and introduced the Pregnancy and Lactation Labeling Rule (PLLR). The previous letter categories were considered confusing and overly simplistic, failing to adequately convey the risks a drug may pose during pregnancy, breastfeeding, and for individuals of reproductive age. The PLLR replaces these letters with detailed narrative summaries describing risks, clinical considerations, and supporting data, providing clearer and more comprehensive information for use during pregnancy and lactation (FDA, 2014).

4.3.3. Teratogenicity in Dental Practice

Given the teratogenic risks associated with pharmacological agents during pregnancy, dentists must be acutely aware of these concerns and carefully plan their treatments. Pharmaceuticals commonly used in dentistry can be categorized into five main groups: analgesics and anti-inflammatory drugs, antibiotics, local anesthetics, sedatives, and emergency drugs. The use of these medications during pregnancy should be evaluated based on the FDA's risk classifications (A, B, C, D, X) and the updated Pregnancy and Lactation Labeling Rule (PLLR) (Osborne et al., 2020).

4.3.4. Analgesics and Anti-inflammatories Use in Pregnancy

Nonsteroidal anti-inflammatory drugs (NSAIDs) such as ibuprofen, aspirin, and naproxen, when used during the third trimester of pregnancy, may result in premature closure of the ductus arteriosus in the fetus, renal impairment, and postnatal complications. These concerns are based on studies involving patients taking high doses of aspirin and have been extrapolated to other NSAIDs (Schoenfeld et al., 1992). Therefore, NSAIDs should be avoided, especially during the third trimester. A case-control study indicated a slightly increased risk of congenital malformations, including heart defects, associated with the use of NSAIDs such as ibuprofen, naproxen, or celecoxib during early pregnancy (Ofori et al., 2006). Further research showed that neonates born to mothers who consumed 5 to 10 grams of aspirin within five days before birth had an increased risk of bleeding tendencies, particularly cerebral hemorrhage. No bleeding tendencies were observed if aspirin was administered at least six days before delivery (Stuart et al., 1982). Paracetamol (acetaminophen) is considered the safest analgesic during pregnancy; however, overdose must be avoided (Guggenheimer & Moore, 2011).

Opioid analgesics should be used judiciously during pregnancy and only when necessary. The Collaborative Perinatal Project, a comprehensive study, assessed the use of opioid analgesics, particularly codeine during pregnancy. The study found that codeine is associated with multiple congenital defects, including heart defects and cleft lip/palate (Heinonen et al., 1977; Klebanoff, 2009). Little is known about the potential fetal risks of oxycodone and hydrocodone. Consequently, opioid analgesics should be used during pregnancy at the minimal effective dose and for the shortest possible duration, always considering the risk-benefit ratio.

4.3.5. Antibiotic Use in Pregnancy

Tetracyclines (including doxycycline) administered during the second and third trimesters of pregnancy can cause permanent discoloration of the fetus's teeth and abnormalities in bone growth. Consequently, they are contraindicated during pregnancy. Penicillins and cephalosporins are considered safe and are the recommended choices for treating dental infections during pregnancy (Muanda et al., 2017).

Regarding metronidazole, although teratogenic effects have been observed in animal studies, the risk to humans is considered negligible with short-term use. Therefore, metronidazole, clindamycin, and erythromycin are generally considered to pose minimal risk. However, the estolate salt of erythromycin is not recommended during pregnancy due to an increased risk of liver toxicity (McCormack et al., 1977). According to FDA classification, azithromycin (Category B) appears to have a lower risk than clarithromycin (Category C); however, its safety during pregnancy requires further evaluation. Azithromycin should be used during pregnancy only when clinically indicated, such as an alternative to beta-lactam antibiotics in cases of severe allergy (Antonucci et al., 2022). Guidelines recommend avoiding aminoglycosides during pregnancy unless no safer alternatives are available due to the potential risk of ototoxicity (Mendia et al., 2012; Rivetti et al., 2023). In summary, the FDA classifies all commonly used dental antibiotics, amoxicillin, azithromycin, cephalexin, clindamycin, erythromycin, metronidazole, and penicillin as pregnancy risk Category B.

4.3.6. Antifungal and Antiviral Drugs Use in Pregnancy

Antifungal agents are not commonly used in dentistry. However, dentists may prescribe antifungal medications such as nystatin and fluconazole to treat oral thrush. Topical azoles (such as clotrimazole and miconazole) and nystatin are considered safe and effective for treating superficial fungal infections during pregnancy. Nystatin is poorly absorbed, which reduces the risk to the fetus. Nystatin is classified as FDA category C (Pilmis et al., 2015).

Systemic azoles (e.g., fluconazole, itraconazole) present dose-dependent teratogenic hazards, particularly at elevated dosages or with extended use during the first trimester. However, single modest doses of fluconazole may be considered safe (King et al., 1998; Moudgal & Sobel, 2003). Fluconazole is listed as FDA Pregnancy Category C for the single-dose vaginal candidiasis regimen, and Category D for all other indications (Donaldson & Goodchild, 2012). A 2008 trial in Denmark showed no overall increased risk of congenital malformations after fetal exposure to short-course treatment with fluconazole in early pregnancy (Nørgaard et al., 2008). Griseofulvin, ketoconazole, voriconazole, flucytosine, and potassium iodide are contraindicated due to their teratogenic or embryotoxic properties (King et al., 1998; Moudgal & Sobel, 2003).

Acyclovir is the most commonly used antiviral in dental practice to treat oral herpes. Numerous studies indicate that acyclovir is generally safe for use during pregnancy, particularly in the second and third trimesters, with no notable side effects reported for mothers or infants. However, one animal study suggests a potential risk of birth abnormalities at elevated doses (Kimberlin et al., 1998; Klein et al., 1991; Ericson et al., 2022).

4.3.7. Local Anesthetics Use During Pregnancy

Generally, local anesthetics must be administered judiciously and in minimal dosages during pregnancy. Most local anesthetics have not demonstrated teratogenic effects in humans and are considered relatively safe for use during pregnancy. Lidocaine preparations are listed by the FDA as Pregnancy Category B, while the others are listed as Category C (Donaldson & Goodchild, 2012). Nevertheless, caution is warranted with certain local anesthetics (e.g., mepivacaine and bupivacaine) due to insufficient data from animal studies (Category C).

The possibility of these substances inducing congenital anomalies in humans cannot be entirely dismissed. In animal research, fetal bradycardia may occur due to elevated levels of lidocaine, bupivacaine, or mepivacaine administered near the umbilical artery (Chestnut, 2004).

All local anesthetics can cross the placenta and cause fetal depression; therefore, it is best to limit the anesthetic dose to the minimum needed for effective pain management. However, the maximum recommended local anesthetic dosages used in dentistry are quite conservative and are unlikely to result in significant fetal blood levels (Fayans et al., 2010). Furthermore, it is advisable to restrict the use of prilocaine and benzocaine due to the potential risk of methemoglobinemia (Mendia et al., 2012). Fetal bradycardia may result from bupivacaine and mepivacaine; additionally, bupivacaine has shown embryocidal effects in rabbits at five times the maximum recommended daily dose and can decrease survival rates in newborn rats at nine times the maximum recommended daily dose. Therefore, the administration of long-acting local anesthetics, such as bupivacaine, in pregnant women is discouraged to reduce the risk of fetal exposure and toxicity (Hilgers et al., 2003; Suresh & Radfar, 2004).

A comprehensive study tracking 55,000 children found no evidence of teratogenicity or other negative effects from the appropriate use of benzocaine, procaine, tetracaine, or lidocaine during pregnancy (Kitson et al., 2000). Specifically, lidocaine is considered safe in controlled doses when combined with epinephrine. It is essential that epinephrine be administered gradually, using repeated aspiration. Vasoconstrictors reduce the toxicity of local anesthetics by decreasing absorption. There are no notable contraindications for the administration of epinephrine at prescribed dosages, provided intravenous injection is avoided. However, levonordefrin is a less potent vasoconstrictor than epinephrine, but its concentration in dental cartridges is five times higher than that of adrenaline, making it more potent and thus posing a greater risk to the fetus (Fayans et al., 2010).

In conclusion, local anesthetics are generally considered safe during pregnancy when administered in appropriate doses and with meticulous application; nonetheless, a risk-benefit analysis should always be conducted. Topical anesthetics (benzocaine, tetracaine) should be used with caution or avoided during pregnancy due to the potential risk of methemoglobinemia (Category C).

4.3.8. Sedative Use During Pregnancy

Sedative drugs exert a depressant influence on the central nervous system and typically cross the placenta, affecting the fetus. Consequently, their use during pregnancy requires particular caution. Benzodiazepines (e.g., diazepam) are among the most extensively researched sedative drugs in the context of pregnancy. Research involving both animals and humans indicates that diazepam administration, particularly during the first trimester, is associated with congenital abnormalities, including oral clefts (Safra et al.,1975; Mazze et al., 1984). Nonetheless, these findings are not consistently reliable, and the teratogenic risk is considered to be quite low with single dose or short term administration. Prolonged or high-dose use may result in developmental issues in the fetus and complications such as respiratory depression in the neonate. Therefore, the use of benzodiazepines during pregnancy is generally discouraged or should only be prescribed during pregnancy when necessary, at the lowest effective dose, as monotherapy, and for the shortest possible duration (Iqbal & Aneja, 2024).

Zolpidem, a non-benzodiazepine, also crosses the placenta and may be associated with increased risks of negative pregnancy outcomes, including low birth weight, preterm delivery, and small for gestational age, particularly at higher doses. However, most studies do not provide robust evidence for significant birth defects at standard doses, and some case reports indicate no adverse effects (Wang et al., 2010; Jurić et al., 2009). The FDA classifies both zaleplon and zolpidem as Category C, making them preferable over benzodiazepines as oral sedatives to help patients relax during dental appointments (Donaldson & Goodchild, 2012).

Animal research has shown that prolonged, high-dose exposure to nitrous oxide in rats can result in skeletal and behavioral teratogenic effects (Koren et al., 1998; Mazze et al., 1984). Additionally, spontaneous abortions and reduced fertility have been linked to occupational exposure to nitrous oxide (Rowland et al., 1992). Nitrous oxide can inactivate vitamin B12, thereby inhibiting the vitamin B12-dependent enzyme methionine synthetase, which is essential for DNA synthesis due to its role in maintaining tetrahydrofolate levels. Short-term, controlled use of nitrous oxide (N2O) is generally considered safe. However, long-term exposure, especially during the first trimester, is not recommended because it can inhibit cell proliferation. Therefore, nitrous oxide use in pregnant women should be kept as brief as possible for the second and third trimester, and long sessions should be avoided. Pregnant dental personnel should avoid nitrous oxide exposure or strictly adhere to safety guidelines, including proper equipment maintenance and air quality monitoring. Respirators are ineffective against nitrous oxide; engineering controls are the primary preventive measures (Van Amsterdam et al., 2022; Wise, 2023).

4.3.9. General Anesthesia Use During Pregnancy

The use of general anesthesia during pregnancy should be carefully evaluated for dental procedures. Non-urgent dental treatments are usually postponed, especially during the first trimester, as fetal organ development is ongoing during this period. The second trimester is considered the safest time for dental procedures. General anesthesia should only be used when necessary and under the supervision of a specialist, as both anesthetic drugs and procedural stress may pose risks to the fetus (ACOG Committee Opinion No. 775, 2019).

According to the American College of Obstetricians and Gynecologists (ACOG Committee Opinion No. 775, 2019) guidelines for nonobstetric surgery during pregnancy, anesthetics used in standard doses have not been shown to cause teratogenic effects, and no adverse fetal brain effects have been observed with exposures shorter than three hours. Necessary surgical procedures for pregnant women should not be postponed, regardless of trimester, while elective surgeries should be scheduled after delivery. Corticosteroids may be considered to reduce the risk of prematurity, and signs of preterm labor should be monitored. The risk of venous thromboembolism should be assessed, and appropriate precautions should be taken. The obstetric care provider should be informed before surgery, and if fetal monitoring is required, appropriate health services and specialists should be available (ACOG Committee Opinion No. 775, 2019). The FDA pregnancy categories and safety considerations for general anesthetic agents used during pregnancy are summarized in Table 19.

4.3.10. Emergency Drugs Used in Pregnancy

Epinephrine is the most important medication used in emergency dental situations. It is the preferred drug for managing cardiovascular and respiratory manifestations of acute allergic reactions. When administered promptly, epinephrine facilitates bronchodilation and increases heart rate and blood pressure. The FDA classifies its use during pregnancy as Category C; however, in emergencies, the benefits to the mother outweigh the potential risks to the fetus. Antidotal medications such as naloxone and flumazenil are used in emergencies to counteract respiratory depression caused by opioids or benzodiazepines. Both are classified as FDA Category C, and in emergencies, the benefits to the mother outweigh the potential risks to the fetus.

Furthermore, nitroglycerin, available in dental offices as a sublingual tablet or spray, is used to treat symptoms of acute myocardial infarction or angina pectoris. During pregnancy, the benefits to the mother outweigh the potential risks to the fetus (Richard et al., 1991; Dixon et al., 1998;; Cholst et al., 1984; Donaldson & Goodchild, 2012).

Antihistamines are used to manage allergic reactions, particularly those that are mild or have a delayed onset. H1 antihistamines used during pregnancy, especially in the first trimester, are generally not associated with an increased risk of congenital anomalies or adverse pregnancy outcomes, and may even be linked to a reduced risk of early-onset pre-eclampsia in women with allergies. Diphenhydramine is often administered intramuscularly at a dose of 50 mg, followed by oral doses of 25–50 mg every 3–4 hours. The FDA classifies diphenhydramine as Category B for use during pregnancy, indicating it is generally considered safe (Donaldson & Goodchild, 2012; Etwel et al., 2017).

4.3.11. Dentists' Role in Managing Drugs During Pregnancy

Dentists must be acutely aware of both the risks and benefits of medications that could adversely affect the fetus when treating pregnant patients. They need to be knowledgeable about the five primary pharmacological categories used during pregnancy: analgesics, antibiotics, local anesthetics, sedatives, and emergency drugs. While most dental procedures can typically be deferred, they should not be postponed in cases of emergencies. When prescribing medications, dentists must carefully weigh the benefits to the mother against the potential risks to the fetus and, if possible, use the lowest effective dose for the shortest duration necessary. Additionally, dentists should ensure a safe treatment protocol by educating patients about medication use during pregnancy (Donaldson & Goodchild, 2012).

4.4. Dental Management of Drug Use During Breastfeeding

More than fifty percent of postpartum women require at least one medication; however, the effects on the initiation and duration of breastfeeding remain inadequately defined due to inconsistent and limited research. Breastfeeding is widely recognized as the optimal method for newborn nutrition, but it may be discontinued due to concerns about the potential adverse effects of maternal medications on the infant. The amount of medication excreted into breast milk varies based on maternal serum levels, the pharmacological properties of the drug, and the mechanism of transfer, such as passive diffusion. Additionally, infant factors including age, health status, feeding frequency, and milk composition can influence the infant's exposure. To assess the risk, both the absolute and relative infant doses should be considered (Ilett & Kristensen, 2005; Auerbach, 1999).

4.4.1. Medication Safety and Risk Assessment in Breastfeeding

Certain drugs should be completely avoided or require careful consideration during breastfeeding because they can potentially harm the infant or reduce milk production. The medications that present the greatest risk include antineoplastic agents, radiopharmaceuticals, and drugs of abuse. Most medications prescribed for conditions such as depression, hypertension, diabetes, and infections are generally safe; however, some require monitoring or substitution with safer alternatives when possible. Therefore, prescribing decisions must balance the benefits for the mother against the potential risks to the infant. Medications with well-established safety profiles and minimal transfer into breast milk should always be prioritized (Chaves & Lamounier, 2004; Spencer et al., 2022; Rowe et al., 2013). Commonly used dental medications during breastfeeding are summarized in Table 20.

Updated prescribing guidelines, including those from the American Academy of Pediatrics (AAP), which encompass the Drugs and Lactation Database and clinical reports, the World Health Organization (WHO) guidelines, and the British National Formulary for Children (BNFC), should always be followed. Resources such as LactMed are valuable aids in clinical decision-making (Sachs, 2013; Spencer et al., 2022).

4.4.2. Dentists' Role in Medication Safety During Breastfeeding

Dentists should prescribe medications to breastfeeding women when the benefits of continuing treatment during lactation outweigh the potential risks. Scheduling feedings or expressing and discarding milk can help minimize the infant's exposure to the medication. Dentists should be aware of medications that require dosage adjustments during lactation and use alternatives when appropriate. Additionally, dentists must identify potential drug effects on the infant and clearly communicate these risks to the patient to ensure proper monitoring and management (Pilgrim et al., 2025).

4.5. Prescribing in Medically Compromised Patients

The increasing prevalence of chronic diseases has heightened the importance of a multidisciplinary approach in healthcare. Chronic diseases such as hypertension, diabetes, stroke, COPD, and cancer are leading determinants of adverse health outcomes and mortality worldwide (Hacker, 2024). The prevalence of chronic diseases ranges from 10–13% in adults, and many individuals have more than one chronic condition (Kovesdy, 2022). These patients are frequently encountered in both dental and medical practices and require special consideration during the prescribing process. Systemic diseases can alter the pharmacokinetic and pharmacodynamic properties of drugs, leading to drug-drug and drug-disease interactions. Many studies have shown high rates of antibiotic prescribing in medically compromised dental patients, generally for prophylaxis or post-procedure, but not always in line with guidelines. This increases the risk of resistance and adverse effects (Cope et al., 2016; Becker et al., 2024; Murphy et al., 2024). In these studies, less than 40% of dentists adhered to international guidelines (Becker et al., 2024; Sbricoli et al., 2024). Patient-related factors such as anxiety and depression can also impact dental treatment outcomes (Abiko et al., 2021). Furthermore, medically compromised patients are at greater risk for complications during dental procedures (Manihani, 2020). Therefore, prescribing in medically compromised patients is critical for patient safety and treatment success.

4.5.1. General Principles and Clinical Approaches

The first step in the prescribing process for patients with systemic diseases is to obtain a thorough medical history. The patient's current medical conditions, all medications used (including over the counter and herbal products), allergies, previous drug reactions, and organ functions should be carefully reviewed. The dentist should be aware of harmful drug interactions with concurrent therapies (Manihani, 2020). Secondly, communication should be established with other healthcare professionals involved in the patient's care, and the treatment plan should be developed in a multidisciplinary manner. Collaboration with specialties such as cardiology, nephrology, endocrinology, and hematology reduces the risk of complications (Mustilwar et al., 2018). Many factors can affect the proper selection of medication and dosage. The patient's age, kidney and liver function, body weight, and comorbidities should all be taken into account when prescribing medications to patients with chronic diseases. For example, dose modification is required for aminoglycoside antibiotics in patients with renal failure to reduce renal toxicity (Nayak-Rao, 2010). Furthermore, current guidelines and drug interaction databases should be used to assess potential drug side effects and interactions (Sbricoli et al., 2024). Managing anxiety and stress is also crucial to minimize the risk of medical emergencies during dental care (Abiko et al., 2021).

4.5.2. Prescribing in Patients with Cardiovascular Disease

Cardiovascular diseases particularly hypertension, heart failure, arrhythmia, and ischemic heart disease, are among the most common systemic conditions encountered during the prescribing process. The use of NSAIDs in these patients should be carefully considered. Multiple large studies and meta-analyses have shown that NSAID use increases the risk of hospitalization for heart failure by 20–40%. The risk is dose-dependent and varies according to the type of NSAID, with drugs like ketorolac, etoricoxib, and indomethacin associated with the highest risks (Arfè et al., 2016). Additionally, patients with other comorbidities such as diabetes, kidney failure, and elderly individuals are more vulnerable (Holt et al., 2023). If NSAIDs are required for their antiinflammatory effect, dentists should prescribe the lowest effective dose for the shortest possible duration and monitor closely for signs of fluid retention or decompensation (Schjerning et al., 2020). To mitigate the unintentional use of NSAIDs in this population, patient education and routine medication assessment are essential (Levine et al., 2020).

Furthermore, the use of vasoconstrictors such as adrenaline in local anesthetics should be limited in patients with serious arrhythmias or uncontrolled hypertension. Research comparing 1:80,000 and 1:200,000 concentrations revealed that 1:200,000 adrenaline induces fewer hemodynamic alterations (reduced increases in heart rate and blood pressure) while maintaining comparable anesthetic efficacy (Managutti et al., 2015; Soman et al., 2021). In dental practice, blood pressure and heart rate must be monitored during procedures in individuals with cardiac disease. Local anesthetics should be used at the lowest possible effective adrenaline concentration, ideally not exceeding 1:100,000, and lower concentrations such as 1:200,000, should be considered for high-risk patients. It is crucial to avoid unnecessary adrenaline use, especially in patients with unstable or severe cardiac disease. This approach helps prevent potential cardiovascular complications and improves patient safety (Soman et al., 2021; Da Silveira et al., 2021).

According to the American Heart Association (AHA) and European Society of Cardiology (ESC) recommendations, antibiotic prophylaxis with amoxicillin is generally recommended for high-risk patients before invasive procedures. However, studies have shown that these recommendations are not fully adhered to in practice. Only half to three-quarters of high-risk patients receive appropriate prophylaxis, which may result in some patients not being adequately protected against serious, preventable infections such as infective endocarditis (Brandão et al., 2023; Gong et al., 2024; Sperotto et al., 2024).

4.5.3. Prescribing in Diabetic Patients

Diabetes mellitus causes persistently high blood sugar levels, which reduce the effectiveness of the immune system and negatively impact new blood vessel formation and tissue healing. This increases the risk of infection and prolongs wound healing in individuals with diabetes. There is a two-way relationship between diabetes and periodontitis: diabetes increases the risk for periodontitis, and periodontal inflammation negatively affects glycaemic control (Preshaw et al., 2012). Medications that can impair glycemic control, especially systemic corticosteroids, should be avoided if possible. Blood glucose should be monitored closely, and insulin or antidiabetic doses should be adjusted as needed. Procedures should be scheduled in the morning and after the patient has eaten (Dasari et al., 2021). Furthermore, because renal function is frequently affected in diabetic patients, medication doses should be adjusted accordingly (Deng et al., 2021).

Medications commonly used in diabetes treatment, such as metformin, sulfonylureas, and insulin, can cause side effects including dry mouth (xerostomia), taste changes, and delayed wound healing. These medications can negatively impact oral health by causing blood sugar fluctuations, decreased salivary flow, and impaired immune function. Although sodium-glucose co-transporter 2 (SGLT2) inhibitors increase the risk of genital infections due to their mechanism of increasing glucose excretion in the urine, the current literature does not clearly link SGLT2 inhibitors to an increased risk of oral fungal infections such as oral candidiasis (Palmer et al., 2021; Li et al., 2022). Glucagon-Like Peptide-1 (GLP-1) receptor agonists can also cause side effects such as taste changes and dry mouth; the gastrointestinal side effects of these medications can further affect taste perception (Li et al., 2022). No specific oral mucosal lesions or significant increases in oral infections have been identified as common adverse effects of GLP-1 receptor agonists in large meta-analyses and studies (Xie et al., 2025). All oral antidiabetic medications increase the risk of periodontal disease, tooth decay, and oral mucosal lesions. Poor glycemic control, in particular, further increases these risks, and some medications can exacerbate dry mouth.

Dentists should consider these potential side effects in patients with diabetes, regularly assess for signs of dry mouth and infection, provide detailed oral hygiene education, and offer suggestions for increasing saliva flow when necessary. Furthermore, it is important to remember that wound healing may be delayed, and treatment plans should be tailored accordingly. Regular dental checkups and preventative measures are crucial in this patient group, which is at high risk for periodontal disease and tooth decay (Verhulst et al., 2019; Ahmad & Haque, 2021; Duarte et al., 2025).

4.5.4. Prescribing in Epileptic Patients

Certain fundamental approaches stand out for successful and safe treatment in dental practice for patients with epilepsy. First, a detailed medical history should be obtained, including the patient's epilepsy type, seizure frequency, triggers, and medications used. It is crucial to verify that seizures are under control. Contacting the patient's neurologist before treatment can be particularly helpful in complex cases. Appointments should be short and scheduled in the morning to minimize patient stress, provide a calm environment, and encourage relaxation through behavioral approaches. Known triggers, such as flashing lights, should be avoided in patients with photosensitive epilepsy (Goswami et al., 2023).

Being prepared for emergencies is essential. During a potential seizure, oral instruments should be removed quickly, the patient should be placed in a supine position, protected from injury, and an open airway should be ensured. If the seizure is prolonged or the airway is compromised, medical intervention may be necessary. It should be noted that medications used in dentistry, such as antibiotics and analgesics, can interact with antiepileptics, and the patient's doctor should be consulted if necessary. Antiepileptic drugs, particularly phenytoin and valproate, can lead to gingival enlargement, delayed healing, and an increased risk of cavities and periodontal disease. Therefore, patients should be provided with detailed oral hygiene instructions, and regular dental checkups and professional cleanings should be recommended (Nashkova et al., 2017).

In restorative treatments, solid, fixed restorations should be preferred to reduce the risk of fracture or dislocation during seizures, and removable dentures should be avoided if possible. When sedation is necessary, conscious sedation (e.g., nitrous oxide) is generally considered safe; however, IV local anesthetics, which can lower the seizure threshold, should be avoided. General anesthesia may also be an option for uncooperative or high-risk patients. All of these approaches contribute to both maintaining oral health in patients with epilepsy and ensuring safety during treatment (Svsg & Degala, 2020; Goswami et al., 2023; Santos et al., 2024; Tindall et al., 2025).

4.5.5. Prescribing in Patients with Renal Failure

Kidney failure slows the elimination of many drugs from the body by reducing the glomerular filtration rate (GFR). This can lead to drug accumulation and increase the risk of toxicity, especially for drugs that are primarily excreted by the kidneys, such as aminoglycoside antibiotics and certain painkillers (Naud et al., 2011). Similarly, many nephrotoxic drugs, such as NSAIDs and aminoglycoside antibiotics, can cause kidney damage or worsen existing kidney dysfunction. Therefore, these medications should be avoided whenever possible or used with extreme caution. Because NSAIDs pose a particular risk to the kidneys, dentists should prescribe safer options like acetaminophen for pain management. Adjustment of dosage based on the patient's GFR is essential to prevent medication toxicity. This adjustment is especially crucial for drugs with a narrow therapeutic index, as even small fluctuations in drug concentration can result in significant toxicity (Proctor et al., 2005; Naud et al., 2011). In complex cases, or when medications that are heavily excreted by the kidneys are necessary, consultation with the patient's physician is essential. Findings such as oral mucosal lesions and slow-healing wounds, which may occur due to renal failure, should be carefully evaluated and considered in treatment planning. Furthermore, this patient group requires closer monitoring and increased attention to medication-related side effects (Proctor et al., 2005; Perazella, 2009).

4.5.6. Prescribing in Patients with Hepatic Failure

Drugs that are heavily metabolized in the liver, such as erythromycin and paracetamol, greatly increase the risk of hepatotoxicity and other adverse effects in people with liver disease. This risk is particularly high when high doses or multiple drugs metabolized in the liver are used. For pain management in dentistry, NSAIDs are generally not recommended because they increase the risk of bleeding and renal complications. Paracetamol can be used in low doses not exceeding 2 grams per day in patients with non-alcoholic liver disease. For dental and interventional procedures, doses of drugs metabolized in the liver should be reduced or dosing intervals extended to prevent drug accumulation and toxicity. Drugs with high hepatotoxic potential, such as high doses of paracetamol, erythromycin, and some opioids (such as pethidine), should be avoided. Because the risk of coagulopathy is increased in patients with liver failure, coagulation tests should be performed before invasive procedures, and, if necessary, correction should be made with fresh frozen plasma or vitamin K. Furthermore, because liver disease can alter drug distribution and excretion, all treatments should be carefully reviewed for potential drug-drug interactions (Lammert et al., 2010; Bosilkovska et al., 2012; Tang & Varma, 2025; Armani et al., 2023).

4.5.7. Prescribing in Immunosuppressed Patients

Patients receiving immunosuppressive therapy for cancer, organ transplantation, or autoimmune diseases have a significantly increased risk of oral infections and complications following dental treatment. These patients frequently experience problems such as fungal, bacterial, and viral infections (e.g., oral hairy leukoplakia, stomatitis, periodontitis), delayed wound healing, and dry mouth. A meta-analysis has shown that infection rates after dental treatment can be as high as 15% in immunosuppressed patients. These findings emphasize the importance of preventive approaches and careful monitoring (Glück et al., 2005; Manak & Metelitsa, 2021).

Studies of dental implants performed under antibiotic prophylaxis in organ transplant patients have shown high success and low complication rates. These findings support the importance of prophylactic antibiotic use before invasive dental treatments in immunosuppressed patients. Furthermore, close monitoring for infection and healing disorders, regular dental checkups, and early intervention for developing oral lesions are recommended. Live vaccines and additional immunosuppressive medications should be avoided during dental treatment, and all prescriptions should be carefully reviewed for drug interactions and side effects. Finally, monitoring immune status indicators, particularly CD4+ T lymphocyte counts, can help guide infection risk prediction and treatment planning (Glück et al., 2005; Burtscher & Torre, 2021; Manak & Metelitsa, 2021).

4.5.8. Patient Education and Communication

Patient education is essential for treatment success and safety. Patients should be clearly informed about medication selection, potential side effects, and necessary precautions. It is frequently observed that patients are not adequately informed about the side effects and precautions associated with medication use. Research shows that while the majority of patients receive verbal explanations about their medications, the proportion who are informed about side effects is quite low, and even fewer receive written information. Therefore, providing easy-to-understand and readable written materials (e.g., information leaflets or drug information sheets) alongside verbal explanations significantly improves patients' correct medication use, retention, and adherence to treatment (Talbot, 2018). Color-coded or simplified documents enhance information retention, especially in elderly patients or those taking multiple medications. Furthermore, encouraging patients to repeat the information in their own words (teach-back) and tailoring instructions to their literacy level and learning style ensures accurate understanding (Alkatheri & Albekairy, 2013). Finally, providing patients with emergency contact information and encouraging them to share an up-to-date list of their medications with all healthcare professionals is crucial for a safe and coordinated treatment process (Alghamdi, 2021).

Table 19. FDA pregnancy category and safety notes for general anesthesia

Agent	FDA Pregnancy Category	Safety Notes
Sevoflurane	C	Safe for short use; monitor maternal-fetal status
Isoflurane	C	Similar to sevoflurane
Desflurane	C	Limited data; short use considered safe
Nitrous Oxide	C	Use cautiously; avoid prolonged exposure
Propofol	B	Safe for induction
Thiopental	C	Limited use; generally safe
Fentanyl	C	Use cautiously; risk near delivery
Rocuronium	C	Safe; minimal placental transfer
Succinylcholine	C	Safe for rapid sequence induction
Midazolam	D (1st trimester)	Avoid in 1st trimester; use cautiously later

Table 20. Common drugs used in dentistry during breastfeeding

Drug	Use in Dentistry	Safety During Breastfeeding	Dentist Considerations for Patient Counseling
Acetaminophen (Paracetamol)	Analgesic	Safe	Generally safe; Low concentrations of paracetamol are absorbed into breast milk and can be identified in the urine of nursing infants; nevertheless, adverse responses have generally not been recorded. However rashes have been recognaized in other study which recommended monitor for rare rash in infant (Matheson et al.,1985)
Ibuprofen and other NSAIDs	Analgesic/ Anti-inflammatory	Use with caution; avoid high doses	Avoid cyclooxygenase selective inhibitors; avoid aspirin >100 mg due to risk of Reye syndrome. (AAP, 2001)
Codeine	Narcotic analgesic	Generally Avoided. FDA Black Box Warning due to risk of rapid metabolism and infant death. (FDA,2013,2017)	If used, monitor infant closely for sedation or respiratory depression.
Hydrocodone and Oxycodone	Narcotic analgesics	A higher risk of causing sedation and respiratory depression in the infant than codeine (Hendrickson et al., 2012)	Use caution; risk of infant sedation and withdrawal symptoms. (Madadi 2009; berlin 2009)
Penicillins (e.g., Amoxicillin)	Antibiotic	Compatible	Full adult dose; monitor infant for diarrhea or fever
Cephalosporins (e.g., Cephalexin)	Antibiotic	Compatible	Use higher dose regimens due to increased clearance in mother
Metronidazole	Antibiotic	Use with caution; recommend 12-24 hr breastfeeding interruption after single dose	Advise patient to pump and discard milk for 12-24 hours after treatment. May give milk an unpleasant taste
Erythromycin Azithromycin Clarithromycin	Macrolides Antibiotic	Compatible but use caution (Arbor Pharmaceuticals, 2011) Compatible (Pfizer, 2011) Use caution; limited data (Abbott, 2011)	Monitor for pyloric stenosis in infant; use caution due to concentration in milk Considered safe during breastfeeding; monitor infant as with other macrolides Avoid unless no alternatives; manufacturer advises caution

Drug	Use in Dentistry	Safety During Breastfeeding	Dentist Considerations for Patient Counseling
Tetracyclines (including Doxycycline)	Antibiotic	Manufacturer advises against breastfeeding Pfizer; 2007; AAP considers compatible (AAP, 2001)	Avoid due to risk of tooth staining; Doxycycline binds less to calcium in tooth enamel resulting in lower risk of tooth staining compared to other tetracyclines.
Nystatin	Antifungal	Safe	Poor absorption; safe for oral thrush treatment (Czeizel et al., 2003)
Fluconazole	Antifungal	Safe (AAP, 2001)	Considered safe; used for vaginal candidiasis; short-course treatment preferred
Acyclovir	Antiviral	Compatible	Considered safe during breastfeeding; minimal excretion in milk
Local Anesthetics, (Bupivacaine, Lidocaine with/without epinephrine, Mepivacaine with/without levonordefrin, Prilocaine), Articaine. Dyclonine topical Lidocaine topical, Benzocaine topical, Tetracaine topical	Local anesthesia	Generally safe (AAP, 2001)	Use minimal effective dose; monitor patient. because of its short half-life, it is unlikely that epinephrine distributes into breast milk and, therefore, it is not contraindicated for use during lactation (Rieken & Terezhalmy, 2006; Porter, 2002; Hale, 2010). Articaine local and Benzocaine Tetracaine (topical) used with caution.
Benzodiazepines Nonbenzodiazepines Zaleplon Zolpidem	Sedatives	Avoid Use with caution (not reviewed) (AAP, 2001) Considered safe (AAP, 2001)	Most benzodiazepines should be avoided. Pump and discard for short half lives drugs such midazolam and triazolam were successful for some patients (Howie et al., 2006) monitor infant for sedation
Emergency Drugs (Albuterol, Epinephrine, Flumazenil, Naloxone, Nitroglycerin) Diphenhydramine	Emergency medications	Albuterol and Epinephrine Generally safe. Use the others with caution	Use as needed; monitor mother and infant; minimal excretion in milk (Lindberg et al., 1984; Ito et al., 1993). Although the AAP has no official stance, small occasional doses of diphenhydramine are unlikely to harm breastfed infants. according to Ito et al., A mother's need for naloxone does not necessitate the cessation of breastfeeding. (Cholst et al., 1984). Flumazenil possesses a short elimination half-life (mean, 54 minutes) and exhibits poor oral bioavailability, which further reduces its transfer into breast milk. (Donaldson& Goodchild, 2012).

Conclusion

In summary, safe and effective medication management in dental practice requires a patient-centered, individualized approach that takes into account the unique physiological, psychological, and social characteristics of each patient group whether pediatric, geriatric, pregnant, breastfeeding, or those with systemic diseases. Adherence to current evidence-based guidelines, careful selection and dosing of medications, and vigilant monitoring for side effects and interactions are essential for optimizing treatment outcomes and minimizing risks. Equally important are clear communication, patient and caregiver education, and multidisciplinary collaboration among healthcare professionals. By integrating these principles, dental practitioners can ensure the highest standards of care, promote patient safety, and support long-term oral and overall health across diverse patient populations.

Chapter 5

Prescribing for Specific Dental Conditions

Abstract

Different clinical conditions encountered in dentistry necessitate tailored pharmacological strategies to optimize patient management and outcomes. For specific dental conditions such as periodontal disease, endodontic infections, surgical procedures, and temporomandibular joint disorders, medication selection and treatment planning should be carefully adapted to the nature and severity of the disease, as well as the individual characteristics and needs of the patient. The use of antimicrobials and supportive medications in periodontal treatment, the choice of appropriate antibiotics and analgesics for endodontic infections, medications prescribed for pain and infection control during and after surgical procedures, and pharmacotherapy for temporomandibular joint disorders are all critical to achieving treatment success and ensuring patient comfort and safety. This chapter will discuss current evidence-based approaches to medication use in these specific conditions frequently encountered in dental practice, as well as key considerations, clinical guidelines, and practical recommendations for their safe and effective management in diverse patient populations.

Keywords: periodontal disease, endodontic infections, surgical procedures, temporomandibular joint disorders, pharmacological strategies

5.1. Periodontal Diseases: Pharmacotherapy for Periodental Treatment

Pharmacotherapy for periodontal diseases has evolved to encompass both traditional and novel approaches targeting microbial biofilms and the host's inflammatory response. Standard treatment typically begins with mechanical plaque removal; however, when this is insufficient, adjunctive pharmacological agents such as systemic or locally delivered antibiotics (e.g., clindamycin, metronidazole, tetracyclines) are employed to reduce pathogenic bacteria and inflammation. Nevertheless, no single antimicrobial has emerged as the gold standard due to concerns regarding resistance and side effects

(Luchian et al., 2021; Leszczyńska et al., 2011). Local drug delivery systems (LDDS), including hydrogels, fibers, and nanoparticles, have gained prominence for their ability to provide site-specific, sustained drug release, thereby improving efficacy and minimizing systemic exposure (Wei et al., 2021; Joshi et al., 2016; Xu et al., 2019). Host modulation therapies, such as disease-modifying antirheumatic drugs, monoclonal antibodies (e.g., rituximab, tocilizumab), statins, and nutritional supplements like n-3 fatty acids, show promise in reducing inflammation and promoting tissue regeneration, although some agents, such as TNF-α inhibitors, have demonstrated inconsistent results (Balta et al., 2021). Natural bioactive compounds, including curcumin, resveratrol, and polyphenols, are being investigated for their anti-inflammatory, antimicrobial, and tissue-regenerative properties, with advanced delivery systems under development to address challenges such as poor bioavailability (Hashim et al., 2025; Hashim et al., 2024; Kim et al., 2024). Probiotics and certain nutritional supplements have also demonstrated anti-inflammatory benefits when combined with conventional therapy (Balta et al., 2021). While these pharmacotherapies offer new avenues for managing periodontitis, further research and large-scale clinical trials are needed to establish their long-term effectiveness and optimal integration with standard care (Balta et al., 2021; Wei et al., 2021; Hashim et al., 2025; Hashim et al., 2024).

Plaque removal is essential for maintaining oral health and preventing gum disease. Mechanical plaque removal, primarily through toothbrushing and interdental cleaning, is the cornerstone of oral hygiene and the prevention of periodontal diseases. Evidence consistently shows that both manual and powered toothbrushes are effective at reducing plaque and gingival inflammation, with powered brushes offering a slight additional benefit in some cases, particularly for individuals with limited dexterity or a higher risk of disease (Chapple et al., 2015; Slot et al., 2020; Van der Weijden et al., 2023). Interdental brushes are generally more effective than floss for cleaning between teeth, except in areas where brushes cannot fit, in which case floss is recommended (Chapple et al., 2015; Slot et al., 2020; Stana et al., 2023). Professional mechanical plaque removal (PMPR), when combined with thorough oral hygiene instruction (OHI), can further improve gingival health; however, repeated and well-reinforced self-care may achieve results similar to professional cleaning alone (Needleman et al., 2015; Needleman et al., 2005; Sanz et al., 2015). Long-term supportive therapy that includes PMPR is associated with low rates of tooth loss and minimal clinical attachment loss in patients treated for periodontitis, although the direct impact on long-term periodontal outcomes requires further study (Trombelli et al., 2015; Sanz et al., 2015). The effectiveness of self-performed plaque removal is often limited by technique, underscoring the importance of patient education and motivation (Van Der Weijden & Hioe, 2005; Westfelt et al., 1996; Van der Weijden et al., 2023). Overall, the best outcomes are achieved by combining regular toothbrushing, interdental cleaning, and professional care tailored to individual needs (Stana et al., 2023; Chapple et al., 2015; Slot et al., 2020; Van der Weijden et al., 2023).

Effective plaque control requires overcoming the complex protective defenses of the microbial biofilm, specifically the extracellular polymeric substance (EPS) matrix which shields bacteria from antimicrobial agents. Consequently, pharmacological strategies in this phase are designed not only to exert bactericidal effects but also to disrupt biofilm structural integrity and inhibit bacterial adhesion to tooth surfaces. Agents capable of penetrating the EPS matrix or interfering with bacterial attachment mechanisms are critical for accessing pathogens in retention sites that mechanical devices may miss. Recent research highlights the utility of specific chemical additives that function synergistically with mechanical debridement to destabilize this matrix (Jakubovics et al., 2021; Liu et al., 2018; Wang et al., 2020). For instance, additives like taurolidine enhance mechanical plaque removal efficiency and implant maintenance (John et al., 2025). Emerging strategies also target biofilm maturation pathways (quorum sensing) and surface modification to prevent colonization. By addressing biofilm stability, these interventions bridge the gap between mechanical hygiene and chemical antisepsis, optimizing long-term oral health (Jiao et al., 2019; Juszczuk-Kubiak, 2024; Sionov & Steinberg, 2022)

Furthermore, the pharmacological management of periodontitis increasingly considers the systemic link to cardiovascular health. Agents like statins, while primarily prescribed for atherosclerosis, exhibit pleiotropic anti-inflammatory effects that may concurrently reduce periodontal inflammation. This highlights a dual therapeutic potential where managing systemic inflammation complements local mechanical and chemical strategies for optimal plaque control and tissue stability (Kligman et al.,2021; Polizzi et al., 2022).

Adjunctive pharmacological agents, such as antiseptics and antibiotics, are commonly used alongside mechanical plaque removal to enhance plaque control and reduce gingivitis. Systematic reviews and meta-analyses consistently show that chemical agents particularly chlorhexidine (in both mouthrinses and dentifrices), triclosan-copolymer dentifrices, and essential oil mouthrinse provide significant additional reductions in plaque and gingival inflammation compared to mechanical methods alone, with mouthrinses generally outperforming dentifrices in plaque reduction (Boyle & Duke, 2021; Escribano et al., 2016; Figuero et al., 2019; Serrano et al., 2015). Locally applied antibiotics, such as piperacillin plus tazobactam gel, may offer further improvements in specific cases like peri-implant mucositis, though their benefits appear limited to certain clinical parameters and are not universally superior to standard care (Abdulkareem et al., 2021; Ilyes et al., 2024; Leszczyńska et al., 2011; Seymour et al., 2005). While adjunctive chemical agents are especially beneficial for high-risk or less compliant patients, no single pharmacological agent is considered a gold standard, and their use should be tailored to individual needs and risk profiles (Chapple et al., 2015; Leszczyńska et al., 2011; Newman, 1998). Overall, adjunctive pharmacological agents are effective in improving plaque control and gingival health, but optimal results are achieved when combined with consistent mechanical cleaning and personalized oral hygiene strategies (Chapple et al., 2015; Escribano et al., 2016; Figuero et al., 2019; Serrano et al., 2015).

5.2. Endodontic Infections: Antibiotics and Analgesics in Endodontic Therapy

Endodontic infections are primarily managed by mechanical cleaning and disinfection of the root canal, with antibiotics reserved for specific situations such as systemic involvement, spreading infections, or in medically compromised patients. Routine use of antibiotics for localized infections or pain is not recommended due to the risk of antibiotic resistance and limited efficacy in these cases (Segura-Egea et al., 2017; Segura-Egea et al., 2017b; Segura-Egea et al., 2018). Amoxicillin, often combined with clavulanic acid, is the most commonly prescribed antibiotic, while clindamycin is preferred for patients with penicillin allergies (Deniz-Sungur et al., 2020; Parirokh et al., 2023; Segura-Egea et al., 2017; Segura-Egea et al., 2017b).

Despite clear guidelines, studies show that antibiotics are frequently overprescribed for conditions such as irreversible pulpitis or localized abscesses, where they offer little benefit. This highlights the need for better education among dentists and dental students (Deniz-Sungur et al., 2020; Maslamani et al., 2017; Salvadori et al., 2019; Segura-Egea et al., 2017b). Analgesics such as ibuprofen and diclofenac are widely used and are appropriate for pain control in endodontic therapy (Maslamani & Sedeqi, 2017; Shenoy et al., 2016).

Local application of antibiotics and steroid-containing medicaments, such as triple antibiotic paste or Ledermix, can be effective in reducing pain and inflammation, especially in cases of symptomatic irreversible pulpitis. However, further research is needed to establish their optimal use. Drainage, when possible, significantly improves outcomes and may reduce the need for antibiotics (Alkhamsan et al., 2023; Mohammadi & Abbott, 2009).

The European Society of Endodontology and other expert bodies emphasize evidence-based, judicious use of antibiotics to prevent resistance and ensure patient safety (Segura-Egea et al., 2017; Segura-Egea et al., 2018). Overall, best practice is to reserve antibiotics for cases with systemic symptoms or risk factors, use analgesics for pain, and focus on local infection control through endodontic procedures (Parirokh et al., 2023; Segura-Egea et al., 2017; Segura-Egea et al., 2017b).

5.3. Oral Surgery: Medication Management in Surgical Procedures

Medication management in oral surgery is crucial to minimize complications and optimize patient outcomes, especially given the increasing complexity of patients' medical histories and drug regimens. Preoperative optimization involves careful consideration of anticoagulants, antiplatelet agents, antihypertensives, and diabetes medications. Current guidelines generally recommend the continuation of anticoagulant and antithrombotic therapy during minor oral surgery, alongside local hemostatic measures, to avoid the thromboembolic risks associated with drug interruption (Allyn et al., 2023; Cancino et al., 2023; Johnston, 2016).

For patients at high risk of complications due to polypharmacy, protocols emphasize pre- and postoperative antibiotic coverage, local interventions, and monitoring of coagulation status, particularly in those on anticoagulants or antiresorptive drugs (Morgado-Sevillano et al., 2024; Saleem et al., 2021). Pain management should be tailored to the procedure and the individual patient, with evidence supporting the use of nonsteroidal anti-inflammatory drugs (NSAIDs) and acetaminophen as first-line agents. Opioids should be reserved for select cases, as overprescribing can be avoided without compromising pain control (Al-Bayati et al., 2020; Cheung et al., 2017; Tatch,

2019). Oral oxycodone, when used, is effective for acute postoperative pain but should be part of a multimodal regimen to minimize side effects and opioid consumption (Cheung et al., 2017; Tatch, 2019). Additionally, preoperative corticosteroids may be considered for more painful procedures to reduce inflammation (Ghasemi & Vahidi, 2021).

Overall, individualized medication management that balances the risks of bleeding, infection, and pain improves safety and outcomes in oral surgery (Allyn et al., 2023; Morgado-Sevillano et al., 2024; Saleem et al., 2021).

5.4. Antiplatelet Management Before Dental Surgical Procedures

Current evidence strongly supports continuing antiplatelet therapy, including both single and dual regimens, before dental surgical procedures, as the risk of significant bleeding is low and can almost always be managed with local hemostatic measures (Calcia et al., 2021; Doganay et al., 2018; Li et al., 2018; Lillis et al., 2011; Medeiros et al., 2017; Wahl, 2014). Discontinuing antiplatelet medications increases the risk of potentially life-threatening thromboembolic events, while the bleeding risk from dental surgery is generally minor and rarely requires more than local intervention (Dézsi et al., 2017; Lillis et al., 2011; Wahl, 2018).

Meta-analyses and large clinical studies show that although patients on dual antiplatelet therapy may experience a higher incidence of intraoperative or immediate postoperative bleeding, these events are typically mild and controllable (Calcia et al., 2021; Doganay et al., 2018; Li et al., 2018; Lillis et al., 2011; Medeiros et al., 2017). There is no significant difference in bleeding rates between different types of dental surgeries, and no evidence suggests that stopping antiplatelet therapy reduces bleeding complications (Calcia et al., 2021; Doganay et al., 2018; Li et al., 2018).

For more complex or prolonged procedures, individualized risk assessment and consultation with the patient's physician are recommended, but routine discontinuation of antiplatelet agents is not advised (Aminoshariae et al., 2021; Dézsi et al., 2017). The consensus is that dental extractions and minor oral surgeries can be safely performed without altering antiplatelet regimens, provided that appropriate local hemostatic techniques are used (Calcia et al., 2021; Doganay et al., 2018; Lillis et al., 2011; Medeiros et al.,

2017). This approach minimizes the risk of thrombotic complications and ensures patient safety (Dézsi et al., 2017; Lillis et al., 2011; Wahl, 2014).

5.5. Anticoagulant Management Before Dental Procedures

Current evidence suggests that most dental procedures, including extractions and minor oral surgeries, can be safely performed in patients taking oral anticoagulants such as warfarin or direct oral anticoagulants (DOACs) without altering or discontinuing their medication. The risk of thromboembolic events from stopping anticoagulation outweighs the risk of bleeding, which is generally low and manageable with local hemostatic measures such as sutures, gauze, or tranexamic acid mouthwash (Bacci et al., 2010; Chahine et al., 2019; Costa-Tort et al., 2021; Manfredi et al., 2019; Manfredini et al., 2021).

Systematic reviews and large studies have found no significant increase in bleeding complications when anticoagulation is continued, and any bleeding that does occur is typically controlled with local interventions (Bacci et al., 2010; Chahine et al., 2019; Costa-Tort et al., 2021; De Andrade et al., 2019; Manfredi et al., 2019; Manfredini et al., 2021). For patients on warfarin, ensuring the INR is within the therapeutic range (usually 1.8–4) is recommended, and for those on DOACs, evidence does not support routine discontinuation before dental procedures (Bacci et al., 2010; Costa-Tort et al., 2021; De Andrade et al., 2019; Manfredi et al., 2019; Manfredini et al., 2021).

Antifibrinolytic agents like tranexamic acid may further reduce bleeding risk, especially in warfarin users, though high-quality evidence for their use with DOACs is still lacking (Engelen et al., 2018). Importantly, heparin bridging is not recommended due to the increased risk of bleeding. Therefore, consultation with the patient's physician and individualized risk assessment are advised, particularly for complex or prolonged procedures (Aminoshariae et al., 2021; Lin et al., 2021).

Overall, the consensus is to maintain anticoagulation for most dental procedures, use local measures to manage bleeding, and avoid unnecessary interruption of therapy (Bacci et al., 2010; Chahine et al., 2019; Costa-Tort et al., 2021; Manfredi et al., 2019; Manfredini et al., 2021).

5.6. Antihypertensive and Antidiabetic Medication Management Before Dental Surgical Procedures

Before dental surgical procedures, careful management of antihypertensive and antidiabetic medications is essential to minimize perioperative risks and optimize patient outcomes. For antihypertensive drugs, current guidelines recommend continuing most medications up to and including the day of surgery, as abrupt withdrawal can lead to rebound hypertension and increased cardiovascular risk. Maintaining blood pressure control is crucial for safe anesthesia and surgical outcomes (Allyn et al., 2023).

For patients with diabetes, preoperative assessment should include recent Hemoglobin A1c (HbA1c) and blood glucose levels to evaluate glycemic control and adjust therapy as needed (Allyn et al., 2023; Cheisson et al., 2018). Insulin is typically continued at the usual dose the evening before surgery, but oral antidiabetic drugs (except possibly metformin) are usually withheld on the morning of the procedure, with metformin often stopped from the evening before to reduce the risk of lactic acidosis. Newer agents such as Sodium-Glucose Co-Transporter 2 (SGLT2) inhibitors should be discontinued at least 3 days prior to surgery to prevent perioperative ketoacidosis. Glucagon-Like Peptide-1 (GLP-1) receptor agonists should also be withheld daily doses on the day of the procedure and weekly doses for one week prior to prevent pulmonary aspiration (Allyn et al., 2023; Dhatariya et al., 2024; Ghorbani et al., 2024; Romain et al., 2025; Ramanathan et al.,2025).

The scientific literature shows a wide range of recommendations and inconsistency regarding the need to administer antibiotics prior to dental surgery in patients with diabetes, and there is no scientific evidence demonstrating its effectiveness as a precautionary measure (Sykara et al., 2022). Good glycemic control reduces the risk of postoperative infections and impaired wound healing, and both hypoglycemia and hyperglycemia should be avoided perioperatively (Allyn et al., 2023; Cheisson et al., 2018; Tan et al., 2022).

For minor dental procedures, most antihypertensive and antidiabetic medications can be safely continued, but individualized assessment is important, especially for patients with comorbidities or complex regimens (Allyn et al., 2023). Close perioperative monitoring of blood pressure and glucose is recommended, and collaboration between dental, anesthesia, and medical teams is key for safe management (Allyn et al., 2023; Cheisson et al., 2018; Kuzulugil et al., 2019; Wu et al., 2016).

5.7. Antiresorptive Such as Bisphosphanate Drug Management before Dental Surgical Procedure

Management of patients on antiresorptive drugs such as bisphosphonates before dental surgical procedures, especially tooth extractions, centers on minimizing the risk of medication-related osteonecrosis of the jaw (MRONJ). Current evidence suggests that a routine "drug holiday" (temporary discontinuation of antiresorptives) before dental surgery does not significantly reduce the risk of MRONJ and may not be necessary, particularly for bisphosphonates and denosumab, though recommendations may vary depending on the drug type, dose, and patient risk factors (Liu et al., 2022; Ottesen et al., 2020; Takeda et al., 2023).

Multiple systematic reviews and meta-analyses, as well as randomized and observational studies, have found no clear evidence that a drug holiday lowers MRONJ incidence after tooth extraction or other dentoalveolar procedures. Some studies even suggest it may negatively impact patient health or delay necessary dental care without providing benefit (Aboalela et al., 2022; Morishita et al., 2022; Omori et al., 2022; Ottesen et al., 2020; Ottesen et al., 2021; Zhu et al., 2023). Animal studies also show that while a drug holiday may partially restore bone cell activity, it does not prevent MRONJ-like lesions (Hadaya et al., 2021). Histological investigations reveal that even extended drug holidays (up to several months) do not reliably restore normal bone cell function or improve surgical outcomes.

Instead, preventive strategies focus on thorough preoperative dental assessment, treating existing oral infections, maintaining excellent oral hygiene, and using minimally invasive surgical techniques with primary closure when possible (Aminoshariae et al., 2022; Liu et al., 2022; Morgado-Sevillano et al., 2024; Tilotta et al., 2023). Antibiotic prophylaxis and careful postoperative monitoring are also recommended to further reduce complications (Liu et al., 2022; Morgado-Sevillano et al., 2024).

Patients receiving antiresorptives for cancer (especially intravenously) are at higher risk for MRONJ than those treated for osteoporosis, and additional risk factors such as diabetes, immunosuppression, or concurrent antiangiogenic therapy should be considered (Aminoshariae et al., 2022). Multidisciplinary collaboration between prescribers and dental professionals is essential for optimal care (Takeda et al., 2023; Tilotta et al., 2023).

Overall, while evidence quality is low and more high-quality studies are needed, current guidelines generally advise against routine drug holidays and emphasize preventive dental care and risk assessment before invasive procedures (Liu et al., 2022; Ottesen et al., 2020; Takeda et al., 2023).

5.8. Temporomandibular Joint Disorders: Pharmacotherapy for TMJ Pain and Dysfunction

Pharmacotherapy for temporomandibular joint (TMJ) disorders targets pain relief and improved joint function, using a range of medications such as non-steroidal anti-inflammatory drugs (NSAIDs), corticosteroids, muscle relaxants, antidepressants, and anticonvulsants, often as part of a broader, multidisciplinary approach (Garstka et al., 2023; Ouanounou et al., 2017; Wu et al., 2021). NSAIDs are commonly prescribed for acute pain, while muscle relaxants and low-dose antidepressants may help with chronic or myofascial pain (Khattab & Malik, 2020; Ouanounou et al., 2017).

Intra-articular injections, particularly of hyaluronic acid and corticosteroids, can provide additional pain relief, with some evidence suggesting that hyaluronic acid injections may offer longer-lasting benefits compared to oral pharmacotherapy or physical therapy, though all approaches can improve pain and function (Derwich et al., 2021; Okumuş et al., 2013). Platelet-rich plasma injections and oral glucosamine have also been explored, but evidence for their effectiveness remains inconsistent or limited, and further research is needed (Derwich et al., 2021; Derwich et al., 2023).

Novel drug delivery systems and tissue engineering strategies are emerging, aiming for sustained intra-articular release to enhance pain management and joint regeneration (Mountziaris et al., 2009; Wu et al., 2021). Importantly, no single pharmacological treatment is universally superior, and therapy should be tailored to the individual, often in combination with non-pharmacological interventions such as physical therapy, occlusal splints, and behavioral modifications (Ferrillo et al., 2022; Garstka et al., 2023).

Accurate diagnosis is essential to guide appropriate pharmacotherapy, and long-term management may require psychological assessment and imaging to address the multifactorial nature of TMJ disorders (Garstka et al., 2023; Khattab & Malik, 2020). Overall, while pharmacotherapy plays a key role in symptom management, it is most effective when integrated into a comprehensive, patient-specific treatment plan (Garstka et al., 2023; Ouanounou et al., 2017; Wu et al., 2021).

Conclusion

Effective pharmacological management in dentistry requires a condition-specific, evidence-based approach that considers both the nature of the disease and individual patient factors. Advances in drug delivery, host modulation, and targeted therapies are expanding treatment options for periodontal disease, endodontic infections, oral surgery, and temporomandibular joint disorders. However, optimal outcomes are achieved when pharmacotherapy is integrated with mechanical interventions, preventive strategies, and multidisciplinary collaboration. Ongoing research and individualized care remain essential to ensure patient safety, minimize complications, and improve overall treatment success in dental practice.

Chapter 6

Alternative and Adjunctive Therapies in Dentistry

Abstract

Today's dental practice incorporates alternative and adjunctive therapies, not only to complement traditional treatment methods but also to address patients' evolving needs and expectations. These therapies encompass a wide variety of approaches, including herbal treatments, acupuncture, aromatherapy, laser applications, ozone therapy, homeopathy, and probiotics. Such methods are gaining increasing traction, particularly in areas like chronic pain management, oral healing, accelerating the recovery process, and enhancing patients' quality of life. In modern dentistry, evidence-based practices remain the foundation of care, and ongoing research continues to evaluate the effectiveness, safety, and long-term outcomes of alternative and adjunctive therapies. As the prevalence of patient disabilities and complex health conditions rises, dentists' awareness of these modalities, as well as appropriate patient selection, individualized application, and monitoring, will become increasingly important. This chapter provides a comprehensive review of the current literature on alternative and adjunctive treatment methods used in dentistry, including their indications, therapeutic applications, and safety profiles.

Keywords: alternative therapies, adjunctive therapies, evidence-based dentistry, chronic pain management, patient selection

6.1. Herbal Dentistry

Herbal dentistry is a key component of natural or holistic dentistry, involves the use of medicinal herbs, plant extracts, and natural remedies to prevent and treat oral health issues. This approach has gained renewed interest due to its potential to provide effective, sustainable, and safer alternatives to conventional dental treatments, aligning with the principles of holistic wellness (Duggal et al., 2024).

6.1.1. The Historical Perspective

The use of herbs for oral health dates back to ancient civilizations such as the Egyptians, Greeks, and Chinese, who utilized herbal remedies to maintain oral hygiene and treat dental problems. Furthermore, traditional systems like Ayurveda and Traditional Chinese Medicine have recognized the oral health benefits of various herbs for centuries (Duggal et al., 2024).

6.1.2. Uses of Herbal Remedies in Dentistry

Herbal and alternative remedies are increasingly explored in dentistry as potential treatments for a range of oral health issues, including dental caries, periodontal disease, oral infections, and inflammation. Many medicinal plants and their extracts have demonstrated antimicrobial, anti-inflammatory, antioxidant, analgesic, and even anticancer properties, making them attractive alternatives or adjuncts to conventional dental therapies, especially due to their lower cost and reduced side effects compared to synthetic drugs. Applications in oral health conditions are broad: herbal remedies are used to manage common dental issues such as gingivitis, periodontitis, dental caries, oral ulcers, mucositis, and postoperative wound healing, and they also help alleviate symptoms related to systemic diseases affecting oral health (Anwar et al., 2025).

Commonly used herbs and natural products in dental care include bloodroot, chamomile, myrrh, peppermint, sage, aloe vera, and propolis, which have been shown to help manage conditions like gingivitis, periodontitis, and oral ulcers. While traditional and cultural use of herbal remedies is widespread, particularly in developing countries, scientific validation through rigorous clinical studies remains limited, and more research is needed to confirm their efficacy, safety, and mechanisms of action.

The incorporation of herbal medicine into dental practice provides a holistic approach to oral health care. It offers numerous benefits, such as fewer side effects compared to synthetic drugs, cost-effectiveness, and greater patient acceptance. Additionally, many medicinal plants possess multiple therapeutic properties including antimicrobial, anti-inflammatory, analgesic, and antioxidant effects that support overall oral health. However, it is crucial for practitioners to be well informed about proper dosages and potential side effects, as the potency of herbal products can vary and they are not without risks. Overall, herbal remedies hold promise for enriching dental care, but evidence-based guidelines and further clinical trials are essential for their broader acceptance and safe use in dentistry (Moghadam et al., 2020; Martínez et al., 2017; Anwar et al., 2025; Abdolahinia et al., 2022; Taheri et al., 2011; Duggal et al., 2024; Mehrotra et al., 2023; Sahney, 2022; Yadav et al., 2021; Refaey et al., 2024). Table 21 highlights the most commonly used herbal medicines in dentistry, along with their respective benefits and limitations.

6.1.3. Herbal Remedies' Mechanisms of Action

Herbal compounds exert their effects through various biochemical pathways. For example, eugenol from clove inhibits prostaglandin synthesis, thereby reducing inflammation and pain (Prashar et al., 2006). Neem's antimicrobial activity is attributed to its ability to disrupt bacterial cell walls and inhibit biofilm formation (Subapriya & Nagini, 2005). Curcumin, found in turmeric, modulates inflammatory cytokines and oxidative stress pathways, contributing to its anti-inflammatory and antioxidant effects (Aggarwal & Harikumar, 2009). Understanding these mechanisms helps optimize the use of herbal remedies in dental care.

6.1.4. Dosage and Formulations

Herbal remedies in dentistry are available in various forms, such as mouthwashes, gels, pastes, drops and essential oils. For example, clove oil is typically used topically in a diluted form to avoid mucosal irritation (Duggal et al., 2024). Neem extracts are commonly incorporated into toothpastes and mouth rinses at concentrations ranging from 0.2% to 5% for plaque control (Sugiarta et al., 2019; Dhingra & Vandana, 2017). Aloe vera is usually applied two to four times daily, with most patients experiencing significant improvement within five to seven days (Mansour et al., 2014; Tariq et al., 2023). For instance, a typical formulation for gingival infections includes Myrrh, Niaouli (Nioli), and Clove, each known for their potent antimicrobial and anti-inflammatory properties. Similarly, herbal blends for halitosis (bad breath) often contain Patchouli, Peppermint, Clove, Lemon, and Cinnamon, which work synergistically to reduce oral malodor through antibacterial and aromatic effects. In cases of bruxism (teeth grinding), essential oils such as Marjoram, Lavender, and Vetiver are used for their calming and muscle-relaxing properties. For tooth and gum sensitivity, Clove oil is a well-established remedy due to its analgesic and anti-inflammatory actions (Refaey et al., 2024). In Türkiye, these herbal formulations are commonly prepared as liquid dosage forms like drops, which allow for accurate dosing and convenient use. For instance, the suggested formulation for treating gingival infections is 1 ml (about 20 drops) of each herbal extract, whereas for halitosis, smaller amounts of 0.15 ml (approximately 3 drops) per herb are typically administered. This adaptability helps dental professionals tailor treatments to the specific needs of each patient.

6.1.5. Herbs Most Widely Used in Modern Dental Care

Clove (*Syzygium aromaticum*) has a long history of use in dentistry, primarily due to its main active compound, eugenol, which possesses analgesic, antibacterial, antifungal, and anti-inflammatory properties. Traditionally, clove oil has been applied directly to the gums to relieve toothache and dental pain, and it is a common ingredient in toothpastes and mouthwashes. Research highlights clove's effectiveness against oral pathogens such as *Streptococcus mutans*, which are responsible for dental caries and gum disease (Gupta et al., 2011). Its antimicrobial and antiplaque effects make it a promising alternative or adjunct to conventional dental treatments, especially in regions where access to modern medicine is limited or where antibiotic resistance is a concern. Clove is also valued for its ability to reduce gum inflammation, treat oral ulcers, and combat halitosis. While clove and its extracts are generally considered safe and cost-effective, some studies note the need for further research to fully establish their clinical efficacy and safety profiles in dental care. Overall, clove remains a vital herbal remedy in dentistry, offering natural pain relief and infection control, and continues to be explored for broader applications in oral health (Khbrani et al., 2022; Mittal et al., 2014; Shankar et al., 2022; Ahuja & Singh, 2022; Gambhir, 2016).

Neem (*Azadirachta indica*) extracts, when incorporated into toothpastes and mouth rinses at concentrations typically ranging from 0.2% to 5%, have demonstrated significant efficacy in controlling dental plaque and improving gingival health. Multiple randomized controlled trials and systematic reviews have shown that neem-based products can reduce plaque and gingivitis scores comparably to standard agents like chlorhexidine, without the common side effects such as staining or taste alteration associated with chemical mouthwashes. Neem-containing toothpastes and gels have been found to significantly lower plaque indices and bacterial counts, including

Streptococcus mutans, a key contributor to dental caries, over periods ranging from one week to six months. Studies in both adults and children indicate that neem mouth rinses and toothpastes are as effective as conventional products in reducing oral bacteria and improving oral hygiene, making them a promising, cost-effective, and well-tolerated alternative for long-term use. However, while the results are promising, some reviews note that the quality of evidence is limited by small sample sizes and methodological flaws, and call for more rigorous, high-quality trials to confirm these findings. Overall, neem extracts in oral care products appear to be effective for plaque control and gingivitis prevention, supporting their traditional use in dental hygiene (Dhivya, 2018; Dhingra & Vandana, 2017; Sugiarta et al., 2019). Additionally, a randomized controlled trial showed that a neem-based mouthrinse is equally effective in reducing periodontal indices as chlorhexidine (Chatterjee et al., 2011).

Aloe vera gel, when applied directly to the oral mucosa, has been shown to be effective and safe for the treatment of oral ulcers, including recurrent aphthous stomatitis. Systematic reviews and randomized controlled trials indicate that aloe vera can accelerate healing, reduce ulcer size, and decrease pain and inflammation, with some studies finding it as effective or even superior to standard treatments like amlexanox and topical steroids, but with fewer side effects and a higher safety profile. Aloe vera is typically applied two to four times daily, and most patients experience significant improvement within five to seven days. While aloe vera's pain relief and reduction in ulcer size are comparable to other interventions, its main advantages are faster healing and minimal adverse effects. Studies also highlight aloe vera's anti-inflammatory and wound healing properties, making it a promising alternative or adjunct to conventional therapies. No significant side effects have been reported, and aloe vera gels are generally well tolerated. Overall, aloe vera gel is a safe, effective, and accessible option for managing oral ulcers, especially for those seeking natural or non-steroidal treatments (Zou et al., 2022; Mansour et al., 2014; Tariq et al., 2023; Yousef et al., 2022).

Turmeric (*Curcuma longa*) has gained significant attention in dentistry due to its anti-inflammatory, antimicrobial, and antioxidant properties, primarily attributed to its active component, curcumin. Research shows that turmeric can be beneficial in managing various oral health conditions. For example, a study found that turmeric gel applied to gingival tissues reduced inflammation and bleeding in patients with gingivitis (Pradeep et al., 2012; Umapathy et al., 2022).

Table 21. Herbal medicines in dentistry: Properties, clinical use, advantages, and disadvantages (Duggal et al., 2024; Anwar et al., 2025)

Herb	Properties	Clinical Use	Advantages	Disadvantages	Reference
Clove (*Syzygium aromaticum* (L.) Merr. & L. M. Perry)	Analgesic, Antibacterial, Antimicrobial	Alleviates toothaches and gum pain; used as a topical application	Natural anesthetic (eugenol), effective pain relief	May cause irritation if used undiluted	Duggal et al., 2024; Anwar et al., 2025
Chamomile (*Matricaria chamomilla* L.)	Anti-inflammatory, Calming	Soothes gum irritation and promotes relaxation	Natural anti-inflammatory, gentle	Limited clinical trials	Duggal et al., 2024
Neem (*Azadirachta indica* A. Juss.)	Antimicrobial, Anti-inflammatory	Prevents gum disease, reduces plaque formation	Effective in oral hygiene, traditional use	Potential allergic reactions	Duggal et al., 2024
Aloe vera (*Aloe vera* (L.) Burm. f.)	Soothing, Healing, Anti-inflammatory	Treats oral sores, reduces gum inflammation	Promotes healing, natural soothing agent	Quality varies by product	Duggal et al., 2024
Tea tree oil (*Melaleuca alternifolia* Maiden & Betche) Cheel	Antimicrobial, Antibacterial, Antifungal	Used in mouthwash and topical application for gum disease and bad breath	Powerful antimicrobial	Toxic if ingested, must be diluted	Duggal et al., 2024
Peppermint oil (*Mentha × piperita* L.)	Antimicrobial, Cooling, Numbing	Used in mouthwash to freshen breath and alleviate pain	Refreshing, natural analgesic	May cause irritation in some individuals	Duggal et al., 2024
Marigold (*Calendula officinalis* L.)	Anti-inflammatory, Antimicrobial	Used as mouth rinse or gel to soothe gums and promote healing	Promotes healing, gentle on tissues	Limited clinical evidence	Duggal et al., 2024
Sage (*Salvia officinalis* L.)	Antimicrobial, Astringent	Reduces oral bacteria and promotes gum health	Natural antiseptic	Limited data on long-term use	Duggal et al., 2024
Myrrh (*Commiphora myrrha*)	Antimicrobial, Anti-inflammatory, Astringent	Used for gum health and to reduce inflammation	Promotes healing and reduces plaque	Limited clinical trials	Anwar et al., 2025
Turmeric (*Curcuma longa* L.)	Anti-inflammatory, Antioxidant, Antimicrobial	Used to reduce gum inflammation and plaque	Natural anti-inflammatory and antioxidant	May stain teeth if used excessively	Anwar et al., 2025
Tulsi (Holy Basil) (*Ocimum tenuiflorum* L.)	Antimicrobial, Anti-inflammatory, Antioxidant	Used to reduce plaque and promote oral hygiene	Natural antiseptic and antioxidant	Limited clinical evidence	Anwar et al., 2025

Herb	Properties	Clinical Use	Advantages	Disadvantages	Reference
Sesame seeds (*Sesamum indicum* L.)	Antioxidant, Anti-inflammatory	Used as natural chewables to improve oral health	Accessible and affordable	Limited direct clinical evidence	Anwar et al., 2025
Fennel seeds (*Foeniculum vulgare* Mill.)	Antimicrobial, Antioxidant	Used as natural chewables to freshen breath and reduce plaque	Natural breath freshener	Limited clinical trials	Anwar et al., 2025

6.1.6. Integration with Conventional Dentistry

Herbal dentistry is often used as a complement to conventional dental care. Dentists may incorporate herbal remedies alongside standard treatments to provide a holistic and personalized approach to oral health. This integration requires dental professionals to be knowledgeable about herbal products, their appropriate use, potential interactions, and the monitoring of outcomes (Duggal et al., 2024).

6.1.7. Patient Education and Acceptance

Patient acceptance of herbal dentistry varies, with many individuals attracted to natural therapies because of their perceived safety and fewer side effects (Almas & Al-Zeid, 2004). However, education is crucial to inform patients about proper use, potential allergies, and the importance of integrating herbal remedies with conventional care. Herbal therapies should always be used under professional supervision to ensure safety, minimize side effects, and avoid interactions with other medications. Moreover, standardization and quality control of herbal products are critical to guarantee their efficacy and consistency (Refaey et al., 2024). Dental professionals play a key role in guiding patients and dispelling myths to ensure the safe and effective use of these therapies (Elmaghraby et al., 2023).

6.1.8. Challenges and Limitations

Despite its promising benefits, herbal dentistry faces challenges such as limited rigorous scientific evidence, variability in the composition and potency of herbal products, lack of standardization, and regulatory issues. More clinical trials and research are needed to establish evidence-based guidelines for safe and effective use (Duggal et al., 2024; Anwar et al., 2025).

6.1.9. Environmental and Safety Considerations

Herbal dentistry aligns with environmental sustainability by using renewable plant sources and biodegradable products. However, caution is necessary as some herbal products can cause adverse reactions or toxicity if misused (Duggal et al., 2024; Anwar et al., 2025).

6.1.10. Future Directions

Recent research in herbal dentistry is increasingly focused on isolating and characterizing the specific active phytochemicals responsible for the therapeutic effects of medicinal plants. Scientists are working to identify these bioactive compounds such as flavonoids, alkaloids, and polyphenols to better understand their mechanisms of action and potential benefits in oral health care. In addition, there is a strong emphasis on developing standardized herbal formulations to ensure consistency, safety, and efficacy across different products. Standardization helps address the variability often seen in herbal preparations due to differences in plant sources, extraction methods, and concentrations of active ingredients.

Furthermore, the integration of nanotechnology is opening new avenues for improving the delivery and bioavailability of herbal agents. Nanoparticle-based delivery systems can enhance the penetration of phytochemicals into oral tissues, provide controlled release, and increase therapeutic effectiveness while minimizing side effects. These technological advancements are complemented by progress in molecular biology, which allows for a deeper investigation into how herbal compounds interact with cellular and molecular targets in the oral cavity.

Ongoing and future clinical trials are essential for evaluating the safety and efficacy of these novel herbal formulations in real-world dental practice. The accumulation of robust clinical evidence will support the development of evidence-based protocols and guidelines for the use of herbal products in dentistry. As a result, these scientific advances are expected to foster greater acceptance and integration of herbal therapies into mainstream dental care, offering patients more natural and potentially safer alternatives for oral health management (Patel et al., 2019).

6.2. Integrative Approaches to Pain Management

Pain is one of the most common reasons for patient consultation in dentistry and can present in both acute and chronic forms. Tooth decay, pulpitis, periodontal disease, post-surgical pain, temporomandibular joint (TMJ) disorders, and orofacial pain syndromes are core areas of pain management in dental practice. Traditionally, dental pain management has relied largely on pharmacological agents such as analgesics, nonsteroidal anti-inflammatory drugs, and local anesthetics as well as surgical interventions. However, in recent years, integrative approaches have become increasingly important. Recent reviews indicate a shift toward combining classic pharmacological treatments (analgesics, antibiotics, corticosteroids) with non-pharmacological and emerging therapies, particularly in endodontics and chronic oral pain (Falatah et al., 2023).

Integrative approaches recognize that dental pain is not only a biological issue but is also influenced by psychological, social, and environmental factors. Therefore, complementary and alternative methods, lifestyle changes, and psychosocial support are now being integrated into treatment plans alongside pharmacological therapies. A multidisciplinary and patient-centered approach is especially necessary for patients with chronic orofacial pain, TMJ disorders, and dental phobia (Aggarwal et al., 2021; Labanca et al., 2023).

Holistic pain management in dentistry includes pharmacological treatments, physical therapy and rehabilitation, psychological approaches, acupuncture, laser therapy, relaxation techniques, nutritional adjustments, and exercise programs. For example, TMJ disorders may be managed with muscle relaxation exercises (such as supervised jaw exercises, post-isometric relaxation, and self-therapy), individually fabricated occlusal splints, hot and cold applications, manual therapy, massage, and stress management techniques. For post-dental pain, in addition to medication, cold compresses, proper nutrition, and oral hygiene recommendations can support the healing process (Wänman & Marklund, 2019).

Psychological approaches are also an important part of pain management in dentistry. For patients with dental anxiety or phobia, methods such as cognitive-behavioral therapy (CBT), relaxation exercises, and hypnosis can positively impact pain perception and treatment compliance. CBT helps patients change negative thoughts about dental treatment and develop healthier coping strategies. Additionally, relaxation techniques applied before and during dental procedures can reduce anxiety and raise the pain threshold (Penlington et al., 2022; Santini, 2025; Vambheim et al., 2021; Weisfeld et al., 2021).

Complementary and alternative medicine practices are increasingly used in holistic dental pain management. Acupuncture is a proven complementary treatment for reducing both dental pain and patient anxiety, with strong scientific support in this field. Low-level laser therapy (LLLT) has been found particularly effective in reducing pain and inflammation during endodontic and periodontal procedures. Cryotherapy and platelet-rich fibrin (PRF) applications can accelerate healing and improve pain control when used alongside conventional treatments. Mind-body therapies such as relaxation, mindfulness, and hypnosis also contribute significantly to managing dental anxiety and pain perception (Falatah et al., 2023; Lin et al., 2017; Kilgore, 2019).

Nutrition should not be overlooked in dental pain management. After surgery, choosing soft and nutritious foods can accelerate healing and reduce pain intensity. Anti-inflammatory diets are also thought to reduce chronic pain and support oral health, though further research specific to dentistry is needed (Taekman & Bonakdar, 2018). Physical and manual therapies, especially for TMJ disorders, can provide additional relief through massage and manipulation. These holistic and adjunctive approaches are important tools in managing pain and supporting healing in dentistry.

One of the key advantages of holistic pain management is that it encourages patients to take an active role in their treatment. Patients become more responsible for their own pain management, contributing through lifestyle changes and complementary practices. This increases treatment adherence and allows for more sustainable, long-term outcomes. Clinical studies show that holistic approaches in dentistry can reduce pain intensity and pain-related functional loss, particularly in chronic orofacial pain and TMJ disorders. Furthermore, these methods can decrease medication-related side effects and improve patients' overall quality of life. Reducing the use of opioids and other potent analgesics is another significant benefit of holistic approaches (Algarni, 2024; Taylor et al., 2024; Moreno-Ligero et al., 2023).

6.3. Role of Adjunctive Therapies in Enhancing Treatment Outcomes

In dentistry, adjuvant treatments are used alongside primary treatment methods to enhance treatment success. These supportive practices increase the effectiveness of the main therapy and accelerate the healing process. Adjuvant methods play a significant role, particularly in surgical procedures, periodontal treatments, implant placements, and conditions with a high risk of infection.

In periodontal therapy, combining systemic antibiotics with scaling and root planing (SRP) has been shown to result in statistically significant improvements in probing pocket depth (PPD), clinical attachment level (CAL), and bleeding on probing (BOP) compared to SRP alone. Locally administered antibiotics offer similar benefits with fewer side effects (Teughels et al., 2020; Kondreddy et al., 2025; Ramanauskaite et al., 2020; Herrera et al., 2020). Photodynamic therapy (PDT) and certain laser therapies have also been investigated as adjuncts in periodontal disease, with results indicating improved clinical outcomes in periodontitis, particularly in reducing PPD and improving CAL. However, the findings are heterogeneous and require further research for confirmation. There is limited data available for other agents such as ozone therapy, additional antibiotics, and vitamin D (Salvi et al., 2019; Ramanauskaite et al., 2020; Wang et al., 2024).

Furthermore, biomaterials such as bone grafts, membranes, and growth factors enhance treatment success, especially in bone and soft tissue regeneration. Probiotics help maintain the balance of the oral flora by suppressing pathogenic microorganisms. Pharmacological agents used for pain and edema control also increase patient comfort and support the healing process. For example, adjunctive corticosteroids after third molar surgery reduce pain, swelling, and trismus, improving patient-reported outcomes regardless of the drug or administration route (Parhizkar et al., 2022). Adjunctive surgical procedures can also enhance both functional and aesthetic outcomes in orthodontic and orthognathic cases (Fatima et al., 2019).

All these adjuvant approaches work through mechanisms such as preventing infection, accelerating tissue healing, reducing pain and inflammation, and maintaining microbial balance.

Conclusion

In summary, herbal medicine in dentistry offers a natural and holistic approach to oral health care, utilizing the therapeutic properties of herbs to promote oral hygiene and treat various dental conditions. The integration of herbal and other complementary therapies into clinical practice is promising, but it requires careful attention to scientific validation, quality control, and patient-specific needs to ensure optimal outcomes. Holistic (integrative) approaches to pain management further exemplify a multidisciplinary and patient-centered model, addressing not only the physical aspects of pain but also the psychological, social, and environmental dimensions. This comprehensive approach leads to more effective and lasting results. Additionally, the appropriate selection and implementation of adjuvant treatments whether herbal, pharmacological, or procedural significantly enhance treatment outcomes and patient satisfaction in both the short and long term. Together, these evolving strategies represent a new paradigm in modern dentistry, where traditional methods are thoughtfully combined with complementary practices to provide safer, more effective, and patient-centered oral health care.

Chapter 7

Future Trends and Developments in Dental Management

Abstract

This chapter explores the transformative impact of emerging pharmacotherapies, digital technologies, and precision medicine on dental prescribing and clinical practice. It highlights advances such as nanomaterial-based drug delivery systems, artificial intelligence (AI) for diagnostics and treatment planning, and the integration of telehealth, virtual reality, and mobile health applications. The discussion covers the promise of antimicrobial peptides and phytochemicals as novel therapeutics, as well as the growing role of personalized and precision dental care informed by genomics and data science. The chapter also addresses the challenges of clinical translation, including safety, regulatory, and ethical considerations, and the need for robust evidence and equitable access. Perspectives from both patients and practitioners are considered, emphasizing the benefits and barriers associated with digital innovation. Ultimately, the chapter underscores the importance of balancing technological advancement with patient-centered care, professional education, and ethical oversight to ensure safe, effective, and inclusive dental drug management in the future.

Keywords: pharmacotherapy, digital dentistry, precision medicine, artificial intelligence drug delivery systems

7.1. Transformative Trends Shaping the Future of Dentistry

Dentistry is experiencing a period of rapid transformation, propelled by technological innovation, shifting demographics, and evolving models of care. Notable trends include the integration of artificial intelligence (AI) and machine learning for diagnostics, treatment planning, and office management, as well as the adoption of digital tools such as three-dimensional (3D) printing, augmented and virtual reality, and telehealth (Spielman, 2024; Joda et al., 2020; Alam et al., 2023; Chen et al., 2020; Sharma & Kadu, 2024; Kinariwala et al., 2020). These advancements are enhancing both clinical outcomes and patient experiences.

Personalized and precision dental care, informed by advances in genomics, molecular biology, and data science, is expected to become increasingly prevalent, enabling tailored prevention and treatment strategies (DaSilva et al., 2022; Rasool, 2019). The COVID-19 pandemic accelerated the adoption of teledentistry and remote care, underscoring the importance of digital communication and hybrid models of care delivery (Gordon et al., 2022; Spielman, 2024; DaSilva et al., 2022; Leresche, 2022).

Value-based care and interprofessional collaboration are also gaining momentum, aiming to improve access, reduce disparities, and enhance population oral health (Gordon et al., 2022; Leresche, 2022). Dental education is evolving in parallel, with competency-based, hybrid, and virtual learning environments preparing future practitioners for a technology-rich landscape (Spielman, 2024). While these innovations promise greater efficiency and improved outcomes, experts emphasize the need for evidence-based implementation, attention to equity, and the preservation of the human connection in patient care (Joda et al., 2020; DaSilva et al., 2022; Leresche, 2022). Ultimately, the future of dentistry will be defined by a balance between cutting-edge technology and compassionate, patient-centered practice.

7.2. Emerging Pharmacotherapies in Dentistry

Emerging pharmacotherapies in dentistry increasingly use biomaterial-based local drug delivery systems (DDS), many leveraging nanotechnologies to release active compounds directly at sites of dental disease. Natural polymers (chitosan, alginate, gelatin) and synthetic carriers (hydrogels, nanofibers, nanoparticles, bioactive coatings) are formed into gels, fibers, microspheres, films, and scaffolds tailored for periodontal therapy, periimplantitis, caries prevention, endodontics, anesthesia, restorative treatments, and pediatric dentistry. These approaches improve local bioavailability, enable controlled release, and reduce systemic side effects, and they are being applied to enhance osseointegration and infection control around implants (Hakim et al., 2021; Lou et al., 2023; Costa et al., 2021; Alavi et al., 2024; Katsarov et al., 2021). Tatullo et al., (2024) reported that a spray formulation based on PLGA poly(lactic-co-glycolic acid) microparticles loaded with sodium amoxicillin (AMX-Na), amoxicillin trihydrate (AMX-Tri), and metronidazole (Met) may provide a promising approach for precision dentistry and personalized therapeutic strategies (Tatullo et al., 2024).

Systematic reviews and preclinical studies indicate substantial promise for nanomaterial-based delivery systems to improve outcomes in periodontitis, caries prevention, and implantology (Hakim et al., 2024; Chandran et al., 2024). However, most evidence remains preclinical: high-quality clinical trials are limited. Key challenges include long-term safety and biocompatibility, variability in release profiles, potential toxicity and microbial resistance from subtherapeutic dosing, and practical barriers to clinical translation such as manufacturing, sterilization, regulatory approval, and cost (Kaur et al., 2019; Kunrath et al., 2022; Costa et al., 2021). Robust human studies and standardized safety evaluations are therefore needed before widespread clinical adoption.

Furthermore, the increasing problem of antibiotic resistance has prompted a search for novel alternatives to overcome this challenge, leading to the exploration of antimicrobial peptides (AMPs) and phytochemicals such as curcumin to combat drug resistance (Griffith et al., 2022; Bapat et al., 2023).

Antimicrobial peptides (AMPs), also known as host defense peptides (HDPs), are short, typically cationic peptides produced by a variety of cell types including neutrophils, epithelial cells, and other immune cells that play key roles in innate immunity. AMPs exert broad spectrum antimicrobial effects against bacteria, fungi, and viruses, primarily by disrupting microbial membranes. They also have immunomodulatory functions (modulating inflammation, chemoattraction, and wound healing) and, in some cases, reported antitumor activity. These combined properties make AMPs attractive candidates for local therapeutic use in the oral cavity, where mucosal innate defenses are especially important (Griffith et al., 2022; Niu et al., 2021).

In dentistry, both natural and synthetic AMPs have shown promising activity against oral pathogens such as *Streptococcus* mutans, a major cause of dental caries. Some AMPs inhibit bacterial adhesion and biofilm formation, and a subset has been reported to promote remineralization in vitro (Niu et al., 2020; Niu et al., 2021). AMPs can also reduce or eliminate pathogens in root canals and periodontal pockets, and their immunomodulatory effects may aid tissue repair. Importantly, several studies indicate that AMPs can modulate oral biofilms in ways that may help reverse dysbiosis while preserving beneficial commensals (Mai et al., 2017; Griffith et al., 2022). However, most evidence to date is preclinical; challenges that must be addressed before clinical translation include peptide stability, potential cytotoxicity at high doses, delivery and sustained release in the oral environment, manufacturing costs, and thorough safety testing (Kimura, 2021; Pei et al., 2022; Musaimi et al., 2022; Szefczyk et al., 2025; Chen et al., 2025).

Notably, curcumin is a natural polyphenol extracted from the rhizome of the medicinal plant Curcuma longa. It exhibits antibacterial, antiinflammatory, anticancer, antimutagenic, antioxidant, and antifungal activities, making it an attractive target for clinical research in both oral and systemic diseases. However, curcumin's poor aqueous solubility, low bioavailability, and rapid metabolic degradation limit its clinical usefulness and have driven the development of nanoformulations (nanocurcumin, nCur) to improve stability, solubility, and delivery (Roy et al., 2020; Bapat et al., 2023) .

Multiple in-vitro investigations have demonstrated antibacterial effects of nanocurcumin formulations against *Streptococcus mutans*, *Porphyromonas gingivalis*, and *Enterococcus faecalis*, pathogens linked to dental caries, periodontitis, and endodontic infections. Although some clinical studies report improved outcomes for conditions such as periodontitis and oral lichen planus, larger controlled trials are required to confirm efficacy and safety (Bapat et al., 2023).

7.3. The Potential Impact of Precision Medicine on Dental Prescribing Practices

Precision medicine, which tailors care to an individual's genetic, biological, and behavioral characteristics is poised to transform dental prescribing by enabling more precise, effective, and safer treatments. Advances in genomics, pharmacogenomics, and artificial intelligence now make it possible to predict patient responses to medications, reduce adverse drug reactions, and optimize drug selection and dosing, particularly for analgesics and antibiotics (Garcia et al., 2013; Pudakalkatti et al., 2017; Kumar et al., 2015; Hung et al., 2022).

For example, pharmacogenomic testing can help dentists identify patients at increased risk for opioid dependence or adverse drug reactions, supporting more responsible opioid prescribing and potentially reducing misuse (Kumar et al., 2015; Rindal et al., 2023). Similarly, knowledge of genetic and microbiome variation can guide targeted antibiotic use, helping to combat antimicrobial resistance and avoid unnecessary treatments (Săndulescu et al., 2024; Patini, 2020; Jamaldini, 2020). At the same time, the integration of digital workflows, virtual articulators, and artificial intelligence (AI) powered diagnostic tools is improving precision, predictability, and efficiency in prosthodontics, orthodontics, and surgical planning (Lobo et al., 2025). Complementary approaches including salivary and microbiome biomarkers for early diagnosis and monitoring, and emerging immunotherapies and microbiome-directed treatments for oral cancers and chronic conditions are further enabling personalized, targeted interventions (Steigmann et al., 2024; Marinelli et al., 2021).

Despite this promise, significant barriers remain. Large-scale data integration and international databases are essential to advance precision dentistry but raise ethical and privacy concerns that require robust governance, secure data handling, and clear consent frameworks. Most precision approaches also need prospective clinical validation and rigorous predictive modeling to demonstrate reliability, clinical utility, and cost effectiveness before routine implementation. Finally, ensuring equitable access to precision dental care represents a major ethical and practical challenge; without policies addressing affordability, infrastructure, and digital literacy, these innovations risk widening existing oral health disparities (Erdmann et al., 2021; Malcangi et al., 2023; Schwendicke & Krois, 2022).

7.4. Current Perspectives in Dentistry Practice and Education

Teledentistry, the remote delivery of dental care using digital technologies, became an essential tool during the COVID-19 pandemic, enabling remote consultations, diagnosis, monitoring, and patient education when in-person visits were limited. This approach allowed dentists to maintain continuity of care and manage urgent dental needs despite lockdowns and social-distancing measures. However, greater reliance on remote management also increased dependence on pharmacological interventions, particularly analgesics and antibiotics. Although teledentistry improved access and patient safety, it may have inadvertently contributed to higher rates of opioid and antibiotic prescribing, raising concerns about medication misuse and antimicrobial resistance (Ather et al., 2020; Gurzawska-Comis et al., 2020; Janakiram et al., 2020; Dar-Odeh et al., 2020).

Virtual (VR) and augmented reality (AR) are also reshaping dentistry, bringing innovation to both education and patient care. In dental schools, VR and AR are now essential tools for training, allowing students to practice procedures in a safe, controlled, and repeatable environment. These immersive technologies, especially when paired with haptic feedback, enhance students' knowledge and confidence, often outperforming traditional teaching methods.

Clinically, dentists use VR and AR to plan and execute complex surgeries with greater precision, overlaying real-time data and visualizations to improve communication and outcomes. VR is also making dental visits less stressful for patients, particularly children, by providing calming distractions that significantly reduce pain and anxiety. While challenges such as cost, standardization, and the need for further research persist, the positive impact of VR and AR in dentistry is increasingly evident. As adoption grows and technology advances, these tools are poised to become integral components of both dental education and clinical practice, ultimately enhancing outcomes for practitioners and patients alike (Moussa et al., 2021; Ahmad et al., 2025; De Barros Padilha et al., 2023; Koolivand et al., 2024).

Similarly, the integration of wearable devices, digital therapeutics, and mobile health (mHealth) applications (apps) is rapidly transforming dental care by enabling continuous, patient-centered management beyond traditional clinical settings. Wearable innovations such as smart toothbrushes, retainers, intraoral sensors, and oral health trackers now allow for real-time monitoring of oral hygiene, device usage, and even implant health. Mobile health apps, like iGAM, empower patients to photograph and track their gum health remotely, facilitating professional oversight and continuity of care when in-person visits are not feasible. These digital tools support early disease detection, improve patient engagement, and enhance communication between patients and dental professionals, while also reducing the need for frequent clinic visits, an especially significant benefit for individuals with mobility or access challenges (Tobias & Spanier, 2020; Tobias et al., 2020).

However, the adoption of these technologies introduces important ethical, technical, and implementation challenges. The generation and storage of large volumes of sensitive health data raise significant concerns about privacy, security, and informed consent. Additionally, disparities in digital literacy and access risk exacerbating existing health inequalities, creating a digital divide in oral healthcare. There are also concerns about algorithmic bias, over-reliance on technology, and the usability of these tools for diverse patient populations. To address these issues, robust ethical frameworks and regulatory guidelines are essential to ensure the reliability, transparency, and accountability of digital dental health solutions. As these technologies evolve, their successful integration into dental care will depend on careful, equitable implementation (McGrath et al., 2015; Tobias & Spanier, 2020).

Furthermore, AI tools integrate patient data and assist in clinical decision-making, although their real-world impact on prescribing and outcomes is still under evaluation (Hung et al., 2022). Studies have shown that AI can enable early and precise detection of dental caries, periodontal diseases, and oral cancers, with diagnostic accuracy comparable to or surpassing that of experienced clinicians (Schwendicke et al., 2020; Ding et al., 2023; Rokaya et al., 2024). AI has also proven effective in treatment planning, outcome prediction, and patient education, contributing to more personalized, predictive, and preventive dentistry (Shan et al., 2020; Bonny et al., 2023; Khurshid, 2023; Folly, 2024).

Despite these advances, challenges such as lack of standardization, limited interpretability, and ethical considerations remain barriers to widespread adoption (Schwendicke et al., 2020; Mörch et al., 2021; Ahmed et al., 2021b). Realizing the full potential of AI-driven and Precision dental care will require further research, clinician training, and seamless integration of these technologies into daily practice (Garcia et al., 2013; Reddy et al., 2019; Kornman & Duff, 2012).

7.5. Patient and Practitioner Perspectives Toward Digital Innovations

Patients are experiencing significant improvements in their dental care as a result of technological advancements. Enhanced diagnostic accuracy, more comfortable digital impressions, and personalized treatment planning contribute to better clinical outcomes and higher satisfaction. Digital tools such as smile design software, aligner treatment simulations and mobile health apps empower patients to visualize potential results and actively participate in their care, increasing motivation and acceptance of recommended treatments. However, these benefits are accompanied by concerns regarding data privacy, informed consent, and the security of personal health information. Additionally, disparities in access to technology and varying levels of digital literacy the so-called digital divide may prevent some vulnerable populations from fully benefiting from these innovations (Srivastava et al., 2023; Schierz et al., 2023; Elmarakeby et al., 2025).

On the other hand, practitioners appreciate these digital tools not only for their impact on patient care but also for their value in professional development, education, and training, particularly through innovations like the metaverse and AR/VR simulation. Despite these advantages, significant barriers remain, including high implementation costs, steep learning curves, and the necessity for ongoing training. Additionally, practitioners express concerns about over-reliance on technology, ethical considerations, and the pressing need for clear regulatory guidelines to ensure safe and effective integration into clinical practice (Wang et al., 2024; Barakat, 2023; Ahmad et al., 2025).

Conclusion

The future of dental drug management is being shaped by rapid advancements in pharmacotherapy, digital technologies, and precision medicine. Innovations such as nanomaterial-based drug delivery systems, AI-driven diagnostics, and personalized prescribing practices promise to enhance treatment efficacy, safety, and patient experience. However, these opportunities are accompanied by challenges, including the need for robust clinical evidence, ethical oversight, and strategies to ensure equitable access. As dentistry continues to evolve, a balanced approach that integrates technological progress with patient-centered care and ongoing professional development will be essential for maximizing benefits and addressing emerging risks.

Chapter 8

Conclusion

This book comprehensively covers the fundamental principles of drug prescribing in dentistry, their clinical approaches, and key points to consider in light of current guidelines. Medication use in dentistry is crucial not only for addressing a patient's current symptoms but also for maintaining overall health, preventing complications, and enhancing treatment success. Therefore, selecting the right medication, adjusting dosage appropriately, determining the duration of treatment, and managing potential side effects are among the fundamental responsibilities of dentists.

8.1. Summary of Key Points

The main chapters of the book provide a detailed examination of the most commonly encountered pharmacological agents in dentistry: antibiotics, analgesics, antifungals, antivirals, and local anesthetics. Extensive coverage is provided on topics such as the rational use of antibiotics, combating antimicrobial resistance, the safe and effective use of analgesics, prescribing medications for special patient groups (children, the elderly, pregnant women, and those with systemic diseases), drug interactions, and the prevention of adverse reactions. It also addresses the ethical and legal responsibilities dentists must consider in their clinical decision-making processes, in line with current national and international guidelines.

Drug prescribing in dentistry requires a careful assessment of the patient's medical history, considering existing systemic diseases and other medications used. Medication selection and dosage adjustments should be made with great care, especially in elderly patients, pregnant women, and children exposed to polypharmacy. Furthermore, pharmacokinetic and pharmacodynamic parameters, patients' potential allergic reactions to medications and kidney and liver function should also be considered.

The book also provides information on medication management in common dental emergencies, legal and ethical principles to consider when prescribing, prescription examples, and practical tips. This information aims to help dentists more easily overcome the challenges they may encounter in their daily practice.

8.2. The Importance of Continuing Education and Adhering to Guidelines

Drug prescribing in dentistry is a dynamic and constantly evolving field. The rapid advancement of scientific research and technological advancements facilitates the emergence of new drugs and treatment approaches. Therefore, it is crucial for dentists to participate in continuing education activities throughout their professional lives, keep up-to-date with current literature, and closely monitor changes in guidelines. Prioritizing patient safety and public health, not only by acquiring fundamental knowledge but also by adhering to ethical principles, is an integral part of their professional responsibility.

Continuous professional development enables dentists to keep their knowledge and skills current, learn new treatment approaches, and achieve optimal outcomes in their clinical practice. The unnecessary and misuse of antibiotics, in particular, is one of the primary causes of the increasing problem of antimicrobial resistance worldwide. Therefore, dentists must meticulously adhere to antibiotic prescribing guidelines, using antibiotics only when indicated and at the appropriate dosage. Similarly, unnecessary and excessive use of analgesics and other medications should be avoided, and patients should be informed about potential side effects and drug interactions.

Ethical and legal responsibilities are also integral to prescribing practices in dentistry. Respecting patient rights when writing prescriptions, maintaining confidentiality, and ensuring the patient's active participation in the treatment process contribute to the strengthening of the patient-doctor relationship. Furthermore, it should be remembered that errors made while writing prescriptions can negatively impact both patient health and the professional reputation of dentists. Therefore, dentists must be careful and meticulous in writing prescriptions and act in accordance with legal regulations and professional ethics.

8.3. Future Directions

Drug prescribing practices in dentistry are expected to develop further in the future. In particular, the integration of digital health technologies, the widespread use of electronic prescribing systems, and the use of artificial intelligence-supported clinical decision support systems will reduce the margin of error in prescribing processes and increase patient safety. Electronic prescribing systems will enable instant visibility of drug interactions and allergy warnings, and patients' medication history can be easily tracked. Furthermore, artificial intelligence and machine learning-based applications will support dentists' clinical decision-making processes, contributing to the creation of more personalized and effective treatment plans. With the integration of personalized medicine approaches into dentistry, treatment outcomes will be optimized using patients' genetic information.

References

Abdolahinia, E., Hajisadeghi, S., Banan, Z., Dadgar, E., Delaramifar, A., Izadian, S., Sharifi, S., & Dizaj, S. (2022). Potential applications of medicinal herbs and phytochemicals in oral and dental health: Status quo and future perspectives. *Oral Diseases*. https://doi.org/10.1111/odi.14276.

Abdulkareem, A., Abdulbaqi, H., Gul, S., Milward, M., Chasib, N., & Alhashimi, R. (2021). Classic vs. novel antibacterial approaches for eradicating dental biofilm as adjunct to periodontal debridement: An evidence-based overview. *Antibiotics, 11*(1), Article 9. https://doi.org/10.3390/antibiotics11010009.

Abdulla, A., Adams, N., Bone, M., Elliott, A., Gaffin, J., Jones, D., Knaggs, R., Martin, D., Sampson, L., & Schofield, P. (2013). Guidance on the management of pain in older people. Age and Ageing, 42(Suppl 1), i1–i57. https://doi.org/10.1093/ageing/afs200.

Abdulla, A., Bone, M., Adams, N., Elliott, A., Jones, D., Knaggs, R., Martin, D., Sampson, E., & Schofield, P. (2013). Evidence-based clinical practice guidelines on management of pain in older people. *Age and Ageing*, 42(2), 151–153. https://doi.org/10.1093/ageing/afs199.

Abebe, M., Arefayne, N., Temesgen, M., & Admass, B. (2022). Incidence and predictive factors associated with hemodynamic instability among adult surgical patients in the post-anesthesia care unit, 2021: A prospective follow up study. *Annals of Medicine and Surgery*, 74. https://doi.org/10.1016/j.amsu.2022.103321.

Abiko, Y., Paudel, D., Matsuoka, H., Moriya, M., & Toyofuku, A. (2021). Psychological backgrounds of medically compromised patients and its implication in dentistry: A narrative review. *International Journal of Environmental Research and Public Health,* 18(16), 8792. https://doi.org/10.3390/ijerph18168792.

Aboalela, A., Farook, F., Alqahtani, A., Almousa, M., Alanazi, R., & Almohammadi, D. (2022). The effect of antiresorptive drug holidays on medication-related osteonecrosis of the jaw: A systematic review and meta-analysis. *Cureus, 14*, e30485. https://doi.org/10.7759/cureus.30485.

Abusalah, M., Gan, S., Al-Hatamleh, M., Irekeola, A., Shueb, R., & Yean, C. (2020). Recent advances in diagnostic approaches for Epstein–Barr virus. *Pathogens*, 9(3), 226. https://doi.org/10.3390/pathogens9030226.

Abusalim, G. (2022). Prevalence and investigations of bacterial contamination in dental healthcare associated environments. *Journal of King Saud University - Science*, 102153. https://doi.org/10.1016/j.jksus.2022.102153.

Adam, M. P. (2012). The all-or-none phenomenon revisited. *Birth Defects Research Part A: Clinical and Molecular Teratology*, 94(8), 664–669. https://doi.org/10.1002/bdra.23051.

Addis, A., Magrini, N., & Mastroiacovo, P. (2001). Drug use during pregnancy. The Lancet, 357(9258), 800. https://doi.org/10.1016/S0140-6736(05)71800-2.

Addy, L., & Martin, M. (2005). Clindamycin and dentistry. *British Dental Journal, 199*, 23–26. https://doi.org/10.1038/sj.bdj.4812535.

Aderonke, I. (2025). Infection control measures in dental practice. *Journal of Medical and Dental Science Research*. https://doi.org/10.35629/076x-12016574.

Aggarwal, B. B., & Harikumar, K. B. (2009). Potential therapeutic effects of curcumin, the anti-inflammatory agent, against neurodegenerative, cardiovascular, pulmonary, metabolic, autoimmune and neoplastic diseases. *The International Journal of Biochemistry & Cell Biology, 41*(1), 40–59. https://doi.org/10.1016/j.biocel.2008.06.010.

Aggarwal, V., Wu, J., Fox, F., Howden, D., Guthrie, E., & Mighell, A. (2021). Implementation of biopsychosocial supported self-management for chronic primary orofacial pain including temporomandibular disorders: A theory, person and evidence-based approach. *Journal of Oral Rehabilitation*. https://doi.org/10.1111/joor.13229.

Agnihotri, R., & Gaur, S. (2012). Chemically modified tetracyclines: Novel therapeutic agents in the management of chronic periodontitis. *Indian Journal of Pharmacology, 44*(2), 161–167. https://doi.org/10.4103/0253-7613.93841.

Aguilera, G., Tabilo, C., Jara, Á., & Aliste, J. (2024). 0.25% bupivacaine–1% lidocaine vs 0.5% bupivacaine for ultrasound-guided infraclavicular brachial plexus block: a randomized controlled trial. *Regional Anesthesia & Pain Medicine*. https://doi.org/10.1136/rapm-2024-105511.

Ahmad, F., Ahmad, W., Xiong, J., & Xia, Z. (2025). AR and MR in dentistry: Developments, applications, and prospects. *IEEE Transactions on Medical Robotics and Bionics, 7*, 171–188. https://doi.org/10.1109/TMRB.2024.3503999.

Ahmad, R., & Haque, M. (2021). Oral health messiers: Diabetes mellitus relevance. *Diabetes, Metabolic Syndrome and Obesity: Targets and Therapy*, 14, 3001–3015. https://doi.org/10.2147/DMSO.S318972.

Ahmadi, H., Ebrahimi, A., & Ahmadi, F. (2021). Antibiotic therapy in dentistry. *International Journal of Dentistry, 2021*(1), 6667624.

Ahmadi, S., Streja, E., Zahmatkesh, G., Streja, D., Kashyap, M., Moradi, H., Molnar, M., Reddy, U., Amin, A., Kovesdy, C., & Kalantar-Zadeh, K. (2015). Reverse epidemiology of traditional cardiovascular risk factors in the geriatric population. *Journal of the American Medical Directors Association*, 16(11), 933–939. https://doi.org/10.1016/j.jamda.2015.07.014.

Ahmed, M., Rao, T., Saeed, A., Mutahir, Z., Hameed, S., Inayat, S., Shahzad, H., Ullah, N., Abaid-Ullah, M., Ibrahim, M., Munir, S., Javed, A., Khan, J., Khalid, M., & Ahmed, S. (2021a). Antifungal drugs: Mechanism of action and resistance. In *Biochemistry of Drug Resistance* (pp. 109–134). Springer. https://doi.org/10.1007/978-3-030-76320-6_5.

Ahmed, N., Abbasi, M., Zuberi, F., Qamar, W., Halim, M., Maqsood, A., & Alam, M. (2021b). Artificial intelligence techniques: Analysis, application, and outcome in dentistry—A systematic review. *BioMed Research International, 2021*. https://doi.org/10.1155/2021/9751564.

Ahuja, A., & Singh, S. (2022). Impact of the current scenario and future perspectives for management of oral diseases: Remarkable contribution of herbs in dentistry. *Anti-Infective Agents*. https://doi.org/10.2174/2211352520666220405124929.

Ahuja, M., Bishnoi, M., & Chopra, K. (2008). Protective effect of minocycline, a semi-synthetic second-generation tetracycline against 3-nitropropionic acid (3-NP)-induced neurotoxicity. *Toxicology, 244*(2–3), 111–122. https://doi.org/10.1016/j.tox.2007.11.003.

Ailabouni, N., Marcum, Z., Schmader, K., & Gray, S. (2021). Medication use quality and safety in older adults: 2019 update. *Journal of the American Geriatrics Society*, 69(S3), S7–S14. https://doi.org/10.1111/jgs.17018.

Aires, A., Barreto, A., & Semedo-Lemsaddek, T. (2020). Antimicrobial effects of essential oils on oral microbiota biofilms: The toothbrush *in vitro* model. *Antibiotics, 10*(1), Article 21. https://doi.org/10.3390/antibiotics10010021

Akpan, A., & Morgan, R. (2002). Oral candidiasis. *Postgraduate Medical Journal, 78*(922), 455–459. https://doi.org/10.1136/pmj.78.922.455.

Aksoy, N. (2022a). Penisilinler. In Z. Gören, B. Yeğen, B. Okuyan, & G. Şener (Eds.), *Güncel farmakoloji: Fizyoloji temelinde hasta odaklı yaklaşım* (pp. 721–724). Güneş Tıp Kitabevi.

Aksoy, N. (2022b). Sefalosporinler. In Z. Gören, B. Yeğen, B. Okuyan, & G. Şener (Eds.), *Güncel farmakoloji: Fizyoloji temelinde hasta odaklı yaklaşım* (pp. 724–727). Güneş Tıp Kitabevi.

Aksoy, N. (2022c). Tetrasiklinler. In Z. Gören, B. Yeğen, B. Okuyan, & G. Şener (Eds.), *Güncel farmakoloji: Fizyoloji temelinde hasta odaklı yaklaşım* (pp. 730–733). Güneş Tıp Kitabevi.

Aksoy, N., & Dumlu M. R. (2022). Antiseptikler ve Dezenfektanlar. In Z. Gören, B. Yeğen, B. Okuyan, & G. Şener (Eds.), *Güncel farmakoloji: Fizyoloji temelinde hasta odaklı yaklaşım* (pp. 730–733). Güneş Tıp Kitabevi.

Akyön, Ş., Sılay, K., & Thürmann, P. (2024). Tools to reduce inappropriate drug use in geriatric patients: PRISCUS 2.0 list updates. *Archives of Gerontology and Geriatrics Plus*, 4, 100052. https://doi.org/10.1016/j.aggp.2024.100052.

Al-Bayati, O., Font, K., Soldatos, N., Carlson, E., Parsons, J., & Powell, C. (2020). Evaluation of the need to prescribe opioid medication to control post-surgical pain of different periodontal/oral surgeries. *Journal of Periodontology*. https://doi.org/10.1002/JPER.20-0315.

Al-Ogaili, N., Rasheed, A., & Al-Beldawi, A. (2024). Effectiveness of disinfection with 70% isopropyl alcohol to reduce bacterial contamination of mobile phones carried by medical personnel in Baghdad Teaching Hospital. *Journal of Al-Farabi for Medical Sciences, 1*(1), Article 87. https://doi.org/10.59746/jfms.v1i1.87.

Al-Share, Q., Khasawneh, R., Rababa'h, A., Asfar, F., & Mohammad, Y. (2024). Evaluation of medication appropriateness index in cardiovascular outpatient clinic: A cross-sectional study. *Currents in Pharmacy Teaching & Learning*, 17(2), 102262. https://doi.org/10.1016/j.cptl.2024.102262.

Al-Share, Q., Tahrawi, A., Khasawneh, D., Alshare, A., & Alkhasawneh, S. (2025). Retrospective evaluation of medication appropriateness in older adults with hepatic cirrhosis. *Science Progress*, 108, 00368504251330037. https://doi.org/10.1177/00368504251330037.

Al-Harbawee, A., Kassam, K., Patel, A. N., Cottom, H., & Cheng, L. (2021). Oral pemphigus vulgaris: Dentists take-home message. *Clinical Case Reports, 9*(7).

Alajlan, N., Carrasco-Labra, A., Karabucak, B., & Lee, S. (2024). Systemic corticosteroid uses in endodontics- Part 1: Managing postoperative pain. *Journal of Endodontics*. https://doi.org/10.1016/j.joen.2024.03.004.

Alam, F., Tufail, A., Ullah, S., Junaid, S., Ahmad, Z., Ullah, N., & Ahmed, F. (2024). Prescribing patterns of analgesics for dental pain in tertiary care hospitals of Khyber Pakhtunkhwa (KP). *International Journal of Pharmacy & Integrated Health Sciences*. https://doi.org/10.56536/ijpihs.v6i1.173.

Alam, M., Abutayyem, H., Kanwal, B., & Shayeb, M. (2023). Future of orthodontics—A systematic review and meta-analysis on the emerging trends in this field. *Journal of Clinical Medicine, 12*(2), 532. https://doi.org/10.3390/jcm12020532.

Alavi, S., Malik, L., Matti, R., Al-Najafi, F., Shahmabadi, H., & Sharma, L. (2024). Bioresponsive nanotechnology in pediatric dental drug delivery. *Journal of Drug Delivery Science and Technology*. https://doi.org/10.1016/j.jddst.2024.105436.

Algarni, H. (2024). A holistic approach to postendodontic pain management: A narrative review. *Journal of Pharmacy & Bioallied Sciences, 16*, S4262–S4270. https://doi.org/10.4103/jpbs.jpbs_1301_24.

Alghamdi, A. (2021). Delivery of information and explanation of side effects of drug to the patients; real situation, obstacles and solutions: A review. *International Journal of Medicine in Developing Countries*, 5(1), 1–6 https://doi.org/10.24911/ijmdc.51-1629194661.

Ali, A., & Hammuda, A. (2019). Local Anesthesia Effects on Postoperative Pain After Pediatric Oral Rehabilitation Under General Anesthesia. *Pediatric dentistry*, 41 3, 181-185.

Ali, R., M., Adom, S., Khatun, R., Khan, K., & Paul, D. (2018). Bronchospasm during general anaesthesia-an alarming threat. *KYAMC Journal*, 8, 27-30. https://doi.org/10.3329/KYAMCJ.V8I2.35701.

Ali, R., Bartholomew, J., Coffey, R., Carrico, C., Kitten, T., & Madurantakam, P. (2021). Peracetic acid: A practical alternative to formalin for disinfection of extracted human teeth. *Bioengineering, 8*(12), Article 217. https://doi.org/10.3390/bioengineering8120217.

Alitalo, O., Kohtala, S., Rosenholm, M., Saarreharju, R., González-Hernández, G., Sarparanta, M., Rozov, S., & Rantamäki, T. (2024). Nitrous oxide induces hypothermia and TrkB activation: Maintenance of body temperature abolishes antidepressant-like effects in mice. *Neuropharmacology*, 261. https://doi.org/10.1016/j.neuropharm.2024.110172.

Aljohani, H., Albalawi, R., Orri, F., Alshammari, K., Shikdar, N., Sayhab, B., Alkahtani, H., Alwably, A., Algazlan, A., Alghamdi, A., & Alqahtani, A. (2021). Types of sedation used in pediatric dentistry. *International Journal Of Community Medicine And Public Health*. https://doi.org/10.18203/2394-6040.ijcmph20214797.

Alkahtani, Z. (2024). Comparative study of different behavioral management techniques in treating anxious pediatric dental patients. *Journal of Pharmacy & Bioallied Sciences, 16*(Suppl 2), S2679–S2681. https://doi.org/10.4103/jpbs.jpbs_362_24.

Alkatheri, A., & Albekairy, A. (2013). Does the patients' educational level and previous counseling affect their medication knowledge? *Annals of Thoracic Medicine*, 8(2), 105–108. https://doi.org/10.4103/1817-1737.109823.

Alkhamsan, R., Aldaiji, R., Aldhahri, A., Alsaljah, W., Alotaibi, A., Alqahtani, K., & Khawaji, M. (2023). Efficacy of antibiotics and steroids as intra-canal medicament in endodontics: A systematic review. *Annals of Dental Specialty*. https://doi.org/10.51847/usx8ugepcr.

Allyn, S., Bentov, N., & Dillon, J. (2023). Perioperative optimization and management of the oral and maxillofacial surgical patient: A narrative review on updates in anticoagulation, hypertension and diabetes medications. *Journal of Oral and Maxillofacial Surgery*. https://doi.org/10.1016/j.joms.2023.11.015.

Almas, K. (1993). Miswak (chewing stick) and its role in oral health. *Postgraduate Dent, 3*, 214–218.

Almas, K., & Al-Zeid, Z. (2004). The immediate antimicrobial effect of a toothbrush and miswak on cariogenic bacteria: A clinical study. *The Journal of Contemporary Dental Practice, 5*(1), 105–114.

Almenrader, N., Passariello, M., Coccetti, B., Haiberger, R., & Pietropaoli, P. (2007). Premedication in children: A comparison of oral midazolam and oral clonidine. *Paediatric Anaesthesia, 17*(11), 1143–1149.

Alonazi, N., Alshaer, S., Alanazi, F., Aljuraid, S., Alanzi, A., Alsuwaylimi, B., Albalawi, H., & Alotaibi, T. (2023). Non-pharmacological approaches to manage pain and anxiety in pediatric dentistry. Journal of Population Therapeutics and Clinical Pharmacology, 30(2), e4724. https://doi.org/10.53555/jptcp.v30i2.4724.

Alqhtani, A., Mohammed, A., Al-Ghazaly, F., Alareqi, A., & Irmawati, A. (2024). Prevention of oral cross-infection by using povidone-iodine compared with other antiseptic agents for orally transmitted diseases: A review. *Health Dynamics, 10*(5), Article 6. https://doi.org/10.33846/hd10506.

Alshamoosi, M. (2021). *Efficacy and Safety of Propofol as Compare to Other Anesthetics: A Systematic Review and Meta-Analysis*, 5. https://doi.org/10.32553/IJMBS.V5I3.1810.

Altınışık, H., & Nezir, M. (2025). Clinical evaluation of in-office bleaching with low, medium, and high concentrate hydrogen peroxide: A 6-month double-blinded randomized controlled trial. *Clinical Oral Investigations, 29*. https://doi.org/10.1007/s00784-025-06348-8.

Altman, J., Everitt, B. J., Robbins, T. W., Glautier, S., Markou, A., Nutt, D., ... & Phillips, G. D. (1996). The biological, social and clinical bases of drug addiction: Commentary and debate. *Psychopharmacology, 125*, 285–345.

Aly, M., & Elchaghaby, M. (2021). The prescription pattern and awareness about antibiotic prophylaxis and resistance among a group of Egyptian pediatric and general dentists: A cross-sectional study. *BMC Oral Health*, 21, 16. https://doi.org/10.1186/s12903-021-01685-y.

American Academy of Pediatrics Committee on Drugs. (2001). Transfer of drugs and other chemicals into human milk. *Pediatrics*, 108(3), 776–789. https://doi.org/10.1542/peds.108.3.776.

American College of Obstetricians and Gynecologists. (2003). ACOG practice bulletin number 47, October 2003: Prophylactic antibiotics in labor and delivery. *Obstetrics and Gynecology, 102*(4), 875–882.

American Dental Association. (2016). Guidelines for the use of sedation and general anesthesia by dentists. *Adopted by the ADA House of Delegates*, 1–15.

Aminimanizani, A., Beringer, P., & Jelliffe, R. (2001). Comparative pharmacokinetics and pharmacodynamics of the newer fluoroquinolone antibacterials. *Clinical Pharmacokinetics, 40*, 169–187. https://doi.org/10.2165/00003088-200140030-00003.

Aminoshariae, A., Donaldson, M., Horan, M., Kulild, J., & Baur, D. (2021). Perioperative antiplatelet and anticoagulant management with endodontic microsurgical techniques. *Journal of Endodontics*. https://doi.org/10.1016/j.joen.2021.07.006.

Aminoshariae, A., Donaldson, M., Horan, M., Mackey, S., Kulild, J., & Baur, D. (2022). Emerging antiresorptive medications and their potential implications for dental surgeries. *Journal of the American Dental Association*. https://doi.org/10.1016/j.adaj.2021.12.008.

Amrita, A., Agarwal, P., Agarwal, M., Agarwal, A., Garg, J., & Mehra, P. (2024). Comparative evaluation of octenidine with chlorhexidine mouthwash in gingivitis and periodontitis patients: A randomized clinical trial. *Journal of Pharmacy & Bioallied Sciences, 16*(S789–S791). https://doi.org/10.4103/jpbs.jpbs_1011_23.

Amsden, G. (1996). Erythromycin, clarithromycin, and azithromycin: Are the differences real? *Clinical Therapeutics, 18*(1), 56–72. https://doi.org/10.1016/S0149-2918(96)80179-2.

Anderson, N., Schultz, A., Ditcham, W., & Von Ungern-Sternberg, B. (2020). Assessment of different techniques for the administration of inhaled salbutamol in children breathing spontaneously via tracheal tubes, supraglottic airway devices, and tracheostomies. *Pediatric Anesthesia*, 30, 1363 - 1377. https://doi.org/10.1111/pan.14028.

Andrade, C. (2022). The practical importance of half-life in psychopharmacology. *The Journal of Clinical Psychiatry, 83*(4). https://doi.org/10.4088/jcp.22f14584.

Angelette, A., Rando, L., Wadhwa, R., Barras, A., Delacroix, B., Talbot, N., Ahmadzadeh, S., Shekoohi, S., Cornett, E., Kaye, A., & Kaye, A. (2023). Tetracycline-, doxycycline-, minocycline-induced pseudotumor cerebri and esophageal perforation. *Advances in Therapy, 40*, 1366–1378. https://doi.org/10.1007/s12325-023-02435-y.

Antel, R., & Ingelmo, P. (2022). Local anesthetic systemic toxicity. *CMAJ: Canadian Medical Association Journal*, 194, E1288 - E1288. https://doi.org/10.1503/cmaj.220835.

Antonucci, R., Cuzzolin, L., Locci, C., Dessole, F., & Capobianco, G. (2022). Use of azithromycin in pregnancy: More doubts than certainties. *Clinical Drug Investigation,* 42(11), 921–935. https://doi.org/10.1007/s40261-022-01182-2.

Anwar, M., Sayed, G., Hal, D., Hafeez, M., Shatat, A., Salman, A., Eisa, N., Ramadan, A., El-Shiekh, R., Hatem, S., & Aly, S. (2025). Herbal remedies for oral and dental health:

A comprehensive review of their multifaceted mechanisms including antimicrobial, anti-inflammatory, and antioxidant pathways. *Inflammopharmacology*. https://doi.org/10.1007/s10787-024-01631-8.

Aquilanti, L., Mascitti, M., Togni, L., Contaldo, M., Rappelli, G., & Santarelli, A. (2022). A Systematic Review on Nerve-Related Adverse Effects following Mandibular Nerve Block Anesthesia. *International Journal of Environmental Research and Public Health*, 19. https://doi.org/10.3390/ijerph19031627.

Arbitman, L., Chen, S., Kim, B., Lee, M., Zou, P., Doughty, B., Li, Y., & Zhang, T. (2024). Assessment of Infant Exposure to Antidepressants through Breastfeeding: A Literature Review of Currently Available Approaches. *Pharmaceutics*, 16. https://doi.org/10.3390/pharmaceutics16070847.

Arduino, P., & Porter, S. (2006). Oral and perioral herpes simplex virus type 1 (HSV-1) infection: Review of its management. *Oral Diseases*, 12(3), 254–270. https://doi.org/10.1111/j.1601-0825.2006.01202.x.

Arezzo, F., Cormio, G., La Forgia, D., Santarsiero, C. M., Mongelli, M., Lombardi, C., Cazzato, G., Cicinelli, E., Loizzi, V. (2022). A machine learning approach applied to gynecological ultrasound to predict progression-free survival in ovarian cancer patients. *Archives of Gynecology and Obstetrics, 306*, 2143–2154. https://doi.org/10.1007/s00404-022-06578-1.

Arfè, A., Scotti, L., Varas-Lorenzo, C., Nicotra, F., Zambon, A., Kollhorst, B., Schink, T., Garbe, E., Herings, R., Straatman, H., Schade, R., Villa, M., Lucchi, S., Valkhoff, V., Romio, S., Thiessard, F., Schuemie, M., Pariente, A., Sturkenboom, M., & Corrao, G. (2016). Non-steroidal anti-inflammatory drugs and risk of heart failure in four European countries: Nested case-control study. *BMJ*, 354, i4857. https://doi.org/10.1136/bmj.i4857.

Arfeen, M., Srivastava, A., Srivastava, N., Khan, R., Almahmoud, S., & Mohammed, H. (2024). Design, classification, and adverse effects of NSAIDs: A review on recent advancements. *Bioorganic & Medicinal Chemistry, 112*, 117899. https://doi.org/10.1016/j.bmc.2024.117899.

Armani, S., Geier, A., Forst, T., Merle, U., Alpers, D., & Lunnon, M. (2023). Effect of changes in metabolic enzymes and transporters on drug metabolism in the context of liver disease: Impact on pharmacokinetics and drug–drug interactions. *British Journal of Clinical Pharmacology*, 90, 942–958. https://doi.org/10.1111/bcp.15990.

Arnal, M., Hijos-Mallada, G., & Lanas, Á. (2021). Gastrointestinal and cardiovascular adverse events associated with NSAIDs. *Expert Opinion on Drug Safety, 21*, 373-384. https://doi.org/10.1080/14740338.2021.1965988.

Aronson, J. (2004). Rational prescribing, appropriate prescribing. *British Journal of Clinical Pharmacology, 57*(3), 229–230. https://doi.org/10.1111/j.1365-2125.2004.02090.x.

Aronson, J. (2007). Concentration-effect and dose-response relations in clinical pharmacology. *British Journal of Clinical Pharmacology, 63*(3), 255–257. https://doi.org/10.1111/j.1365-2125.2007.02871.x.

Arthur, G., & Covino, B. (1991). Pharmacokinetics of local anaesthetics. *Baillière's Clinical Anaesthesiology*, 5, 635-658. https://doi.org/10.1016/S0950-3501(05)80047-9.

Ashley, P., Anand, P., & Anderson, K. (2021). Best clinical practice guidance for conscious sedation of children undergoing dental treatment: An EAPD policy document. *European Archives of Paediatric Dentistry, 22*, 989–1002. https://doi.org/10.1007/s40368-021-00660-z.

Ashley, P., Chaudhary, M., & Lourenço-Matharu, L. (2018). Sedation of children undergoing dental treatment. *The Cochrane Database of Systematic Reviews, 12*, CD003877. https://doi.org/10.1002/14651858.CD003877.pub5.

Ashnagar, A., Naseri, N., & Alboghobesh, S. (2016). Synthesis and study of antibacterial effects of pentanedial (glutaraldehyde). *Biosciences, Biotechnology Research Asia, 4*, 65–70. https://doi.org/10.13005/bbra.

Ather, A., Patel, B., Ruparel, N., Diogenes, A., & Hargreaves, K. (2020). Coronavirus disease 19 (COVID-19): Implications for clinical dental care. *Journal of Endodontics, 46*, 584–595. https://doi.org/10.1016/j.joen.2020.03.008.

Auerbach, K. (1999). Breastfeeding and maternal medication use. Journal of Obstetric, Gynecologic, and Neonatal Nursing, 28(5), 554–563. https://doi.org/10.1111/j.1552-6909.1999.tb02029.x.

Auerbacher, M., Gebetsberger, L., Hickel, R., & Kaisarly, D. (2023). Chairside oral prophylaxis for people with profound intellectual or multiple disabilities—a retrospective feasibility study. *Clinical Oral Investigations*, 27, 6747 - 6756. https://doi.org/10.1007/s00784-023-05287-6.

Aulestia-Viera, P., Braga, M., & Borsatti, M. (2018). The effect of adjusting the pH of local anaesthetics in dentistry: a systematic review and meta-analysis. International Endodontic Journal, 51, 862–876. https://doi.org/10.1111/iej.12899.

Awad, A., & Hanna, O. (2019). Potentially inappropriate medication use among geriatric patients in primary care setting: A cross-sectional study using the Beers, STOPP, FORTA and MAI criteria. *PLoS ONE*, 14, e0218174. https://doi.org/10.1371/journal.pone.0218174.

Bacci, C., Maglione, M., Favero, L., Perini, A., Lenarda, R., Berengo, M., & Zanon, E. (2010). Management of dental extraction in patients undergoing anticoagulant treatment. *Thrombosis and Haemostasis, 104*, 972–975. https://doi.org/10.1160/TH10-02-0139.

Bahar, E., & Yoon, H. (2021). Lidocaine: A Local Anesthetic, Its Adverse Effects and Management. *Medicina*, 57. https://doi.org/10.3390/medicina57080782.

Bailey, T. C., Little, J. R., Littenberg, B., Reichley, R. M., & Dunagan, W. C. (1997). A meta-analysis of extended-interval dosing versus multiple daily dosing of aminoglycosides. *Clinical Infectious Diseases, 24*(5), 786–795.

Bajwa, S. F., & Mohammed, R. H. (2023). *Type II Hypersensitivity Reaction*. In StatPearls. StatPearls Publishing.

Bakshi, S., & Bakshi, S. (2021). Povidone–iodine: An essential antiseptic in the COVID-19 pandemic. *Saudi Journal of Otorhinolaryngology Head and Neck Surgery, 23*, 126. https://doi.org/10.4103/sjoh.sjoh_34_21.

Balsalobre, L., Blanco, A., & Alarcón, T. (2019). Beta-lactams. In *Antibiotic Drug Resistance* (pp. 57–72).

Balta, M., Papathanasiou, E., Blix, I., & Van Dyke, T. (2021). Host modulation and treatment of periodontal disease. *Journal of Dental Research, 100*, 798–809. https://doi.org/10.1177/0022034521995157.

Bambini, F., De Stefano, C. A., Giannetti, L., Memè, L., & Pellecchia, M. (2003). Influence of biphosphonates on the integration process of endosseous implants evaluated using single photon emission computerized tomography (SPECT). *Minerva Stomatologica, 52*, 331–338.

Bambini, F., Giannetti, L., Memè, L., Pellecchia, M., & Selvaggio, R. (2005). Comparative analysis of direct and indirect implant impression techniques: An *in vitro* study. *Minerva Stomatologica, 54*, 395–402.

Bansal, R., & Jain, A. (2014). Overview on the current antibiotic containing agents used in endodontics. *North American Journal of Medical Sciences, 6*(8), 351–358. https://doi.org/10.4103/1947-2714.139277.

Bapat, R., Bedia, S., Bedia, A., Yang, H., Dharmadhikari, S., Abdulla, A., Chaubal, T., Bapat, P., Abullais, S., Wahab, S., & Kesharwani, P. (2023). Current appraises of therapeutic applications of nanocurcumin: A novel drug delivery approach for biomaterials in dentistry. *Environmental Research, 116971*. https://doi.org/10.1016/j.envres.2023.116971.

Barakat, H. (2023). Artificial intelligence and digital dentistry: 7 takeaways. *International Dental Journal*. https://doi.org/10.1016/j.identj.2023.07.181.

Barbosa, E., Clift, H., Olson, L., Zhu, L., & Liu, W. (2024). Structural insights into dopamine receptor-ligand interactions: From agonists to antagonists. *ACS Chemical Neuroscience*. https://doi.org/10.1021/acschemneuro.4c00295.

Bardol, M., Pan, S., Walker, S., Standing, J., & Dawes, J. (2023). Pharmacokinetic pharmacodynamic modeling of analgesics and sedatives in children. Paediatric Anaesthesia, 33(2), 147–162. https://doi.org/10.1111/pan.14712.

Barkin, R., Beckerman, M., Blum, S., Clark, F., Koh, E., & Wu, D. (2010). Should Nonsteroidal Anti-Inflammatory Drugs (NSAIDs) be Prescribed to the Older Adult?. *Drugs & Aging*, 27, 775-789. https://doi.org/10.2165/11539430-000000000-00000.

Barone, M., Basilicata, M., Bruno, G., Bacci, C., Bollero, P., Docimo, R., ... & Cavallari, F. (2025). Antibiotics use for dental or oral cavity infections in pediatric dentistry: Knowledge and prescribing practices between Italian dentists. *Antibiotics, 14*(4), 357.

Barone, M., Basilicata, M., Bruno, G., Bacci, C., Bollero, P., Docimo, R., Gracco, A., & De Stefani, A. (2025). Antibiotics use for dental or oral cavity infections in pediatric dentistry: Knowledge and prescribing practices between Italian dentists. *Antibiotics*, 14(4), 357. https://doi.org/10.3390/antibiotics14040357.

Bascones Martínez, A., Aguirre Urízar, J. M., Bermejo Fenoll, A., Blanco Carrión, A., Gay-Escoda, C., González-Moles, M. A., ... & de Vicente Rodríguez, J. C. (2004). Consensus statement on antimicrobial treatment of odontogenic bacterial infections. *Medicina Oral, Patologia Oral y Cirugia Bucal, 9*(5), 369–376.

Bates, D. W. (1997). The costs of adverse drug events in hospitalized patients. *JAMA: The Journal of the American Medical Association, 277*(4), 307. https://doi.org/10.1001/jama.1997.03540280045032.

Batista, N., De Paula, C., Poiate, I., Poiate, E., Zuza, E., & Camargo, G. (2021). Evaluation of periodontal indices in young adults submitted to chlorhexidine 0.12% mouthwash:

a randomized clinical trial. *Revista de Odontologia da UNESP*. https://doi.org/10.1590/1807-2577.04521.

Becker D. E. (2010). Pain management: Part 1: Managing acute and postoperative dental pain. *Anesthesia progress, 57*(2), 67–80. https://doi.org/10.2344/0003-3006-57.2.67.

Becker, K., Gurzawska-Comis, K., Klinge, B., Lund, B., & Brunello, G. (2024). Patterns of antibiotic prescription in implant dentistry and antibiotic resistance awareness among European dentists: A questionnaire-based study. *Clinical Oral Implants Research*. https://doi.org/10.1111/clr.14285.

Bem, J. L., & Mann, R. D. (1988). Drug point: Danger of interaction between ciprofloxacin and theophylline. *British Medical Journal (Clinical Research Ed.), 296*(6629), 1131.

Bender, R. P., Lindsey, R. H., Burden, D. A., & Osheroff, N. (2004). N-acetyl-p-benzoquinone imine, the toxic metabolite of acetaminophen, is a topoisomerase II poison. *Biochemistry, 43*(12), 3731–3739.

Bent, S. (2008). Herbal medicine in the United States: Review of efficacy, safety, and regulation: Grand rounds at University of California, San Francisco Medical Center. *Journal of General Internal Medicine, 23*, 854–859.

Bentley, J., Heard, K., Collins, G., & Chung, C. (2015). Mixing medicines: how to ensure patient safety. *The Pharmaceutical Journal*. https://pharmaceutical-journal.com/article/ld/mixing-medicines-how-to-ensure-patient-safety.

Benyamin, R., Trescot, A. M., Datta, S., Buenaventura, R., Adlaka, R., Sehgal, N., Glaser, S. E., & Vallejo, R. (2008). Opioid complications and side effects. *Pain Physician, 11*(2 Suppl), S105–S120.

Berlin, C. M., Paul, I. M., & Vesell, E. S. (2009). Safety issues of maternal drug therapy during breastfeeding. *Clinical Pharmacology & Therapeutics,* 85(1), 20–22. https://doi.org/10.1038/clpt.2008.183.

Bernard, P., & Charneux, J. (2011). Bullous pemphigoid: A review. *Annales de Dermatologie et de Vénéréologie, 138*, 173181.

Bertossi, D., Barone, A., Iurlaro, A., Marconcini, S., De Santis, D., Finotti, M., & Procacci, P. (2017). Odontogenic orofacial infections. *Journal of Craniofacial Surgery, 28*, 197–202. https://doi.org/10.1097/SCS.0000000000003250.

Betz, S. (2019). HPV-related papillary lesions of the oral mucosa: A review. *Head and Neck Pathology*, 13, 80–90. https://doi.org/10.1007/s12105-019-01003-7.

Beyer, A., Ebach, F., Reutter, H., Sauerstein, K., Hilger, A., Krickau, T., Tzschoppe, A., Woelfe, J., Galiano, M., & Schaefer, J. (2025). Oral health status in children with chronic kidney disease, kidney transplantation, and nephrotic syndrome: A cross-sectional study. *Pediatric Nephrology*, 40, 2287–2293. https://doi.org/10.1007/s00467-025-06698-1.

Bhanot, R., & Mago, J. (2016). Corticosteroids in dentistry. *Indian Journal of Dental Sciences, 8*, 252-254.

Bhattacharya, S. (2010). The facts about penicillin allergy: A review. *Journal of Advanced Pharmaceutical Technology & Research, 1*(1), 11–17.

Bhuvaraghan, A., King, R., Larvin, H., & Aggarwal, V. (2021). Antibiotic use and misuse in dentistry in India—A systematic review. *Antibiotics, 10*, Article 1459. https://doi.org/10.3390/antibiotics10121459.

Bindu, S., Mazumder, S., & Bandyopadhyay, U. (2020). Non-steroidal anti-inflammatory drugs (NSAIDs) and organ damage: A current perspective. *Biochemical Pharmacology, 180*, 114147. https://doi.org/10.1016/j.bcp.2020.114147.

Black, D. J., Kunze, K. L., Wienkers, L. C., Gidal, B. E., Seaton, T. L., McDonnell, N. D., ... & Trager, W. F. (1996). Warfarin-fluconazole. II. A metabolically based drug interaction: In vivo studies. *Drug Metabolism and Disposition, 24*(4), 422–428.

Bogari, A., Aldakhil, I., Alsuwaidan, M., Alhassani, N., Alroudan, D., Aljuaid, O., Alqarni, M., Alzahrani, O., Alolayan, A., Jawhar, Z., Saba, A., & Badri, S. (2022). Inhalation anaesthetics: types, mechanism of action and adverse effects. *International Journal Of Community Medicine And Public Health*. https://doi.org/10.18203/2394-6040.ijcmph 20223230.

Böhle, S., Röhner, E., Zippelius, T., Jacob, B., Matziolis, G., & Rohe, S. (2021). Cytotoxic effect of sodium hypochlorite (Lavanox 0.08%) and chlorhexidine gluconate (Irrisept 0.05%) on human osteoblasts. *European Journal of Orthopaedic Surgery & Traumatology, 32*, 81–89. https://doi.org/10.1007/s00590-021-02907-3.

Bonny, T., Nassan, W., Obaideen, K., Mallahi, M., Mohammad, Y., & El-Damanhoury, H. (2023). Contemporary role and applications of artificial intelligence in dentistry. *F1000Research, 12*. https://doi.org/10.12688/f1000research.140204.1.

Bookstaver, P., Bland, C., Griffin, B., Stover, K., Eiland, L., & McLaughlin, M. (2015). A review of antibiotic use in pregnancy. *Pharmacotherapy: The Journal of Human Pharmacology and Drug Therapy, 35*, 1052–1062. https://doi.org/10.1002/phar.1649.

Bosilkovska, M., Walder, B., Besson, M., Daali, Y., & Desmeules, J. (2012). Analgesics in patients with hepatic impairment. *Drugs*, 72, 1645–1669. https://doi.org/10.2165/11635500-000000000-00000.

Boubacar, B., Cheikh, F., Makhtar, N., Abibou, N., Ulimata, D., Victoire, S., Birane, S., Malick, D., Thiéyacine, B., Saad, B., & Oumar, K. (2025). Evaluation of the Anesthetic Management of Patients Operated for Maxillofacial Reconstruction Surgery in a Sub-Saherian Country: About Six Observed Cases. *Scholars Journal of Medical Case Reports*. https://doi.org/10.36347/sjmcr.2025.v13i01.038.

Bourgeois, B. F. (1988). Pharmacologic interactions between valproate and other drugs. *The American Journal of Medicine, 84*(1), 29–33.

Boyle, S., & Duke, A. (2021). Are adjunctive therapies effective in reducing gingivitis and plaque? *Evidence-Based Dentistry, 22*, 98–99. https://doi.org/10.1038/s41432-021-0204-0

Brailo, V., Janković, B., Lozić, M., Gabrić, D., Kuna, T., Stambolija, V., & Verzak, Ž. (2019). Dental Treatment Under General Anesthesia in a Day Care Surgery Setting. *Acta Stomatologica Croatica*, 53, 64 - 71. https://doi.org/10.15644/asc53/1/7.

Brandão, M., Latado, L., Oliveira, L., Sarmento, V., & Latado, A. (2023). Evaluation of antibiotic prophylaxis prescriptions for infectious endocarditis before oral procedures between cardiologists and dentists. *International Journal of Cardiovascular Sciences*. https://doi.org/10.36660/ijcs.20230034.

Brocklebank, J. C., Ray, W. A., Federspiel, C. F., & Schaffner, W. (1978). Drug prescribing during pregnancy: A controlled study of Tennessee Medicaid recipients. *American Journal of Obstetrics and Gynecology*, 132(3), 235–244. https://doi.org/10.1016/0002-9378(78)90213-2.

Brookes, Z., Bescos, R., Belfield, L., Ali, K., & Roberts, A. (2020). Current uses of chlorhexidine for management of oral disease: A narrative review. *Journal of Dentistry, 103*, 103497. https://doi.org/10.1016/j.jdent.2020.103497.

Brown, E. G. (2002). Effects of coding dictionaries on signal generation: A consideration of use of MedDRA compared with WHO-ART. *Drug Safety, 25*, 445–452.

Brown, E., Pavone, K., & Naranjo, M. (2018). Multimodal General Anesthesia: Theory and Practice. *Anesthesia and Analgesia*, 127, 1246 - 1258. https://doi.org/10.1213/ANE.0000000000003668.

Brunton, L. L., Chabner, B. A., & Knollmann, B. C. (Eds.). (2011). *Goodman & Gilman's: The pharmacological basis of therapeutics* (12th ed., p. 17). McGraw Hill.

Brzezinski-Sinai, Y., Zwang, E., Plotnikova, E., Halizov, E., Shapira, I., Zeltser, D., Rogowski, O., Berliner, S., Matot, I., & Shenhar-Tsarfaty, S. (2021). Cholinesterase activity in serum during general anesthesia in patients with or without vascular disease. *Scientific Reports*, 11. https://doi.org/10.1038/s41598-021-96251-5.

Bsg, E. (1998). Cleaning and disinfection of equipment for gastrointestinal endoscopy. Report of a Working Party of the British Society of Gastroenterology Endoscopy Committee. *Gut, 42*, 585–593. https://doi.org/10.1136/gut.42.4.585.

Budtz-Jørgensen, E. (1981). Oral mucosal lesions associated with the wearing of removable dentures. *Journal of Oral Pathology, 10*(2), 65–80. https://doi.org/10.1111/j.1600-0714.1981.tb01251.x.

Bukhnikashvili, E., Abashidze, N., Iverieli, A., & Gogishvili, K. (2021). HIV/AIDS related oral manifestations and their statistics in Georgia 2016. *TSMU Collection of Scientific Works*. https://doi.org/10.52340/csw.2021.13.

Buonavoglia, A., Leone, P., Solimando, A., Fasano, R., Malerba, E., Prete, M., Corrente, M., Prati, C., Vacca, A., & Racanelli, V. (2021). Antibiotics or no antibiotics, that is the question: An update on efficient and effective use of antibiotics in dental practice. *Antibiotics*, 10, 5050. https://doi.org/10.3390/antibiotics10050550.

Burns, M. (1999). Management of narrow therapeutic index drugs. *Journal of Thrombosis and Thrombolysis, 7*, 137–143.

Burtscher, D., & Torre, D. (2021). Dental implant procedures in immunosuppressed organ transplant patients: A. systematic review. *International Journal of Oral and Maxillofacial Surgery*. https://doi.org/10.1016/j.ijom.2021.06.008.

Bushra, R., Aslam, N., & Khan, A. Y. (2011). Food-drug interactions. *Oman Medical Journal, 26*(2), 77.

Buxton, I. O. (2023). Pharmacokinetics: The dynamics of drug absorption, distribution, metabolism, and elimination. In L. L. Brunton & B. C. Knollmann (Eds.), *Goodman & Gilman's: The pharmacological basis of therapeutics* (14th ed.). McGraw-Hill Education. https://accesspharmacy.mhmedical.com/content.aspx?bookid=3191&sectionid=267905627.

Cairns, R., Schaffer, A. L., Brown, J. A., Pearson, S. A., & Buckley, N. A. (2020). Codeine use and harms in Australia: Evaluating the effects of re-scheduling. *Addiction, 115*(3), 451-459.

Calcia, T., Oballe, H., De Oliveira Silva, A., Friedrich, S., & Muniz, F. (2021). Is alteration in single drug anticoagulant/antiplatelet regimen necessary in patients who need minor oral surgery? A systematic review with meta-analysis. *Clinical Oral Investigations, 25*, 3369–3381. https://doi.org/10.1007/s00784-021-03882-z.

Caldwell, J., Gardner, I., & Swales, N. (1995). An introduction to drug disposition: The basic principles of absorption, distribution, metabolism, and excretion. *Toxicologic Pathology, 23*(2), 102–114.

Campagna, J., Bond, M., Schabelman, E., & Hayes, B. (2012). The use of cephalosporins in penicillin-allergic patients: A literature review. *The Journal of Emergency Medicine, 42*(5), 612–620. https://doi.org/10.1016/j.jemermed.2011.05.035.

Cancino, J., Fonseca, D., & Parada, F. (2023). Stomatological management of anticoagulated patients undergoing oral surgery: A narrative review. *Odontología Vital*. https://doi.org/10.59334/rov.v2i39.590.

Carrasco-Labra, A., Polk, D. E., Urquhart, O., Aghaloo, T., Claytor Jr, J. W., Dhar, V., ... & Moore, P. A. (2024). Evidence-based clinical practice guideline for the pharmacologic management of acute dental pain in adolescents, adults, and older adults: A report from the American Dental Association Science and Research Institute, the University of Pittsburgh, and the University of Pennsylvania. *The Journal of the American Dental Association, 155*(2), 102-117.

Carta, M. G., Cossu, G., Pintus, E., Zoccheddu, R., Callia, O., Conti, G., Pintus, M., Gonzalez, C. I. A., Massidda, M. V., Mura, G., et al., (2021). Active elderly and health—Can moderate exercise improve health and wellbeing in older adults? Protocol for a randomized controlled trial. *Trials, 22*, 331. https://doi.org/10.1186/s13063-021-05278-6.

Casale, M., Moffa, A., Vella, P., Sabatino, L., Capuano, F., Salvinelli, B., Lopez, M., Carinci, F., & Salvinelli, F. (2016). Hyaluronic acid: Perspectives in dentistry. A systematic review. *International Journal of Immunopathology and Pharmacology*, 29, 572 - 582. https://doi.org/10.1177/0394632016652906.

Cascorbi, I. (2012). Drug interactions—Principles, examples and clinical consequences. *Deutsches Ärzteblatt International, 109*(33–34), 546.

Castelló, C., Zamora-Martínez, N., Tarazona-Álvarez, B., & Paredes-Gallardo, V. (2024). Comparative evaluation of two cetylpyridinium chloride-based mouthwashes on the mechanical properties and strength loss of elastomeric chains used in dentistry: An in vitro study. *Heliyon, 10*, e27721. https://doi.org/10.1016/j.heliyon.2024.e27721.

Chahine, J., Khoudary, M., & Nasr, S. (2019). Anticoagulation use prior to common dental procedures: A systematic review. *Cardiology Research and Practice, 2019*, 9308631. https://doi.org/10.1155/2019/9308631.

Chandran, M., & Usha, R. (2024). Novel biomaterial assisted drug delivery systems for the management of oral diseases–Future therapeutic approaches. *International Journal of Applied Pharmaceutics*. https://doi.org/10.22159/ijap.2024v16i1.49448.

Chang, Y., Tai, K., Huang, F., & Huang, M. (2000). Cytotoxic and nongenotoxic effects of phenolic compounds in human pulp cell cultures. *Journal of Endodontics, 26*(8), 440–443. https://doi.org/10.1097/00004770-200008000-00002.

Chapman, P. B., Hauschild, A., Robert, C., Haanen, J. B., Ascierto, P., Larkin, J., ... & McArthur, G. A. (2011). Improved survival with vemurafenib in melanoma with BRAF V600E mutation. *New England Journal of Medicine, 364*(26), 2507–2516.

Chapple, I., Van Der Weijden, F., Doerfer, C., Herrera, D., Shapira, L., Polak, D., Madianos, P., Louropoulou, A., Machtei, E., Donos, N., Greenwell, H., Van Winkelhoff, A., Kuru, E., Arweiler, N., Teughels, W., Aimetti, M., Molina, A., Montero, E., & Graziani, F. (2015). Primary prevention of periodontitis: Managing gingivitis. *Journal of Clinical Periodontology, 42*(Suppl 16), S71–S76. https://doi.org/10.1111/jcpe.12366.

Chari, D., Dave, B., Bargale, S., Deshpande, A., Shah, S., & Shah, P. (2021). Adverse drug reaction: Knowledge, attitude and practice amongst paediatric dentists in India: An electronic survey. *Advances in Human Biology*, 11(1), 44–48. https://doi.org/10.4103/AIHB.AIHB_107_20.

Chase, H., Fuller, C., & Reynolds, P. (1981). The role of penicillin-binding proteins in the action of cephalosporins against *Escherichia coli* and *Salmonella typhimurium*. *FEBS Journal, 117*, 301–310. https://doi.org/10.1111/J.1432-1033.1981.TB06337.X.

Chate, R. A. C., White, S., Hale, L. R. O., Howat, A. P., Bottomley, J., Barnet-Lamb, J., Lindsay, J., Davies, T. I., & Heath, J. M. (2006). The impact of clinical audit on antibiotic prescribing in general dental practice. *British Dental Journal, 201*(10), 635–641. https://doi.org/10.1038/sj.bdj.4814261.

Chatterjee, A., Saluja, M., Singh, N., & Kandwal, A. (2011). To evaluate the antigingivitis and antiplaque effect of an *Azadirachta indica* (neem) mouthrinse on plaque-induced gingivitis: A double-blind, randomized, controlled trial. *Journal of Indian Society of Periodontology, 15*(4), 398–401. https://doi.org/10.4103/0972-124X.92578.

Chatzistefanou, I., Zikos, P., Venetis, G., Vahtsevanos, K., & Antoniades, K. (2015). Melkersson-Rosenthal syndrome. *World Journal of Stomatology, 4*(1), 8-11.

Chaudhary, K., Bagharwal, P., & Wadhawan, S. (2017). Anesthesia for intellectually disabled. *Journal of Anaesthesiology, Clinical Pharmacology*, 33, 432 - 440. https://doi.org/10.4103/joacp.JOACP_357_15.

Chaudhry, S. B., Veve, M. P., & Wagner, J. L. (2019). Cephalosporins: A focus on side chains and β-lactam cross-reactivity. *Pharmacy (Basel), 7*, 103.

Chauhan, A., & Jindal, T. (2020). Methods of sterilization and disinfection. In *Microbiological Methods for Environment, Food and Pharmaceutical Analysis* (pp. 67–92). Springer. https://doi.org/10.1007/978-3-030-52024-3_4.

Chaurand-Lara, J., & Facio-Uma, J. A. (2013). *Methylprednisolone injection following the surgical extraction of impacted lower third molars: A split-mouth study.*

Chaves, R. G., & Lamounier, J. A. (2004). Breastfeeding and maternal medications. *Jornal de Pediatria*, 80(5 Suppl), s189–s198. https://doi.org/10.1590/S0021-75572004000700009.

Cheisson, G., Jacqueminet, S., Cosson, E., Ichai, C., Leguerrier, A., Nicolescu-Catargi, B., Ouattara, A., Tauveron, I., Valensi, P., & Benhamou, D. (2018). Perioperative management of adult diabetic patients. Preoperative period. *Anaesthesia, Critical Care & Pain Medicine, 37*(Suppl 1), S9–S19. https://doi.org/10.1016/j.accpm.2018.02.020.

Chen, R., Wang, T., Song, J., Pu, D., He, D., Li, J., Yang, J., Li, K., Zhong, C., & Zhang, J. (2021). Antiviral drug delivery system for enhanced bioactivity, better metabolism and pharmacokinetic characteristics. *International Journal of Nanomedicine*, 16, 4959–4984. https://doi.org/10.2147/IJN.S315705.

Chen, X., Cui, S., Chen, Y., Wang, C., Liu, Q., Qi, Y., & Du, S. (2025). Efficient delivery of oncolytic peptide LTX315 by ZIF8: pHresponsive release, improved stability, and reduced hemolysis. *Molecular Pharmaceutics*. https://doi.org/10.1021/acs.molpharmaceut.4c01144.

Chen, Y., Foster, J., Wang, M., Rohmah, I., Tseng, Y., & Chiu, H. (2024). Global prevalence and risk factors of emergence delirium in pediatric patients undergoing general anesthesia: A systemic review and meta-analysis.. *Journal of pediatric nursing*, 77, 74-80 . https://doi.org/10.1016/j.pedn.2024.03.010.

Chen, Y., Stanley, K., & Att, W. (2020). Artificial intelligence in dentistry: Current applications and future perspectives. *Quintessence International, 51*(3), 248–257. https://doi.org/10.3290/j.qi.a43952.

Chen, Z., Lin, M., Huang, Z., Zeng, L., Huang, L., Yu, D., & Zhang, L. (2019). Efficacy of chloral hydrate oral solution for sedation in pediatrics: a systematic review and meta-analysis. *Drug Design, Development and Therapy*, 13, 2643 - 2653. https://doi.org/10.2147/DDDT.S201820.

Chestnut, D. (2004). *Obstetric anesthesia: Principles and practice* (3rd ed.). Elsevier Mosby.

Cheung, C., Wong, S., Qiu, Q., & Wang, X. (2017). Oral oxycodone for acute postoperative pain: A review of clinical trials. *Pain Physician, 20*(2S), SE33–SE52. https://doi.org/10.36076/ppj.2017.se52.

Chidambaran, V., Costandi, A., & D'Mello, A. (2015). Propofol: A Review of its Role in Pediatric Anesthesia and Sedation. *CNS Drugs*, 29, 543-563. https://doi.org/10.1007/s40263-015-0259-6.

Chiu, P., Bottino, P., & Patterson, G. (2006). Sterol composition of nystatin and amphotericin B resistant tobacco calluses. *Lipids, 15*(1), 50–54. https://doi.org/10.1007/BF02534118.

Choi, K. H., Kim, A. J., Son, I. J., Kim, K. H., Kim, K. B., Ahn, H., & Lee, E. B. (2010). Risk factors of drug interaction between warfarin and nonsteroidal anti-inflammatory drugs in practical setting. *Journal of Korean Medical Science, 25*(3), 337–341.

Cholst, I. N., Wardlaw, S. L., Newman, C. B., & Frantz, A. G. (1984). Prolactin response to breast stimulation in lactating women is not mediated by endogenous opioids. *American Journal of Obstetrics and Gynecology*, 150(5 Pt 1), 558–561. https://doi.org/10.1016/S0002-9378(84)80177-2.

Chopra, R., Merali, R., Paolinelis, G., & Kwok, J. (2014). An audit of antimicrobial prescribing in an acute dental care department. *Primary Dental Journal, 3*(4), 24–29. https://doi.org/10.1308/205016814813877270.

Chow, A. W. Complications, diagnosis, and treatment of odontogenic infections. In T. W. Post (Ed.), *UpToDate*. Waltham, MA: UpToDate Inc. http://www.uptodate.com. Accessed August 9, 2025.

Christrup, L. L. (1997). Morphine metabolites. *Acta Anaesthesiologica Scandinavica*, 41(1), 116-122. https://doi.org/10.1111/j.1399-6576.1997.tb04625.x.

Chua, K.-P., Hu, H.-M., Waljee, J. F., Brummett, C. M., & Nalliah, R. P. (2021). Opioid prescribing patterns by dental procedure among US publicly and privately insured patients, 2013 through 2018. *The Journal of the American Dental Association, 152*(4), 309–317. https://doi.org/10.1016/j.adaj.2021.01.001.

Clemens, S., Iglseder, B., Alzner, R., Kogler, M., Rose, O., Kutschar, P., Krutter, S., Kanduth, K., Dückelmann, C., Flamm, M., & Pachmayr, J. (2024). Effects of medication management in geriatric patients who have fallen: Results of the EMMA mixed-methods study. *Age and Ageing*, 53, afae070. https://doi.org/10.1093/ageing/afae070.

Cohen, S. P., Vase, L., & Hooten, W. M. (2021). Chronic pain: An update on burden, best practices, and new advances. *The Lancet, 397*(10289), 2082-2097.

Cohen, S., & Hargreaves, K. M. (2014). *Pathways of the pulp* (11th ed.). Mosby.

Colburn, W. A., & Lee, J. W. (2003). Biomarkers, validation and pharmacokinetic-pharmacodynamic modelling. *Clinical Pharmacokinetics, 42*, 997–1022.

Colloca, L., & Miller, F. G. (2011). The nocebo effect and its relevance for clinical practice. *Psychosomatic Medicine, 73*(7), 598–603.

Conaghan, P. G. (2012). A turbulent decade for NSAIDs: Update on current concepts of classification, epidemiology, comparative efficacy, and toxicity. *Rheumatology International, 32*, 1491-1502.

Connor, A., Hutton, P., Severn, P., & Masri, I. (2011). Electronic Prescribing and Prescription Design in Ophthalmic Practice. *European Journal of Ophthalmology*, 21, 644 - 648. https://doi.org/10.5301/EJO.2011.6225.

Contaldo, M., D'Ambrosio, F., Ferraro, G., Di Stasio, D., Di Palo, M., Serpico, R., & Simeone, M. (2023). Antibiotics in dentistry: A narrative review of the evidence beyond the myth. *International Journal of Environmental Research and Public Health, 20*, Article 6025. https://doi.org/10.3390/ijerph20116025.

Conti, P. C. R., Bonjardim, L. R., Stuginski-Barbosa, J., Costa, Y. M., & Svensson, P. (2021). Pain complications of oral implants: Is that an issue? *Journal of Oral Rehabilitation, 48*(2), 195-206.

Cooper, L., Stankiewicz, N., Sneddon, J., Seaton, R. A., & Smith, A. (2022). Indications for the use of metronidazole in the treatment of non-periodontal dental infections: A systematic review. *JAC-Antimicrobial Resistance, 4*(4), dlac072.

Cope, A. L., & Chestnutt, I. G. (2014). Inappropriate prescribing of antibiotics in primary dental care: Reasons and resolutions. *Primary Dental Journal, 3*(4), 33–37. https://doi.org/10.1308/205016814813877333.

Cope, A., Francis, N., Wood, F., & Chestnutt, I. (2016). Antibiotic prescribing in UK general dental practice: A cross-sectional study. *Community Dentistry and Oral Epidemiology*, 44(2), 145–153. https://doi.org/10.1111/cdoe.12199.

Cope, A., Francis, N., Wood, F., Mann, M. K., & Chestnutt, I. G. (2014). Systemic antibiotics for symptomatic apical periodontitis and acute apical abscess in adults. *Cochrane Database of Systematic Reviews*, (6).

Corcuera-Flores, J., Silvestre-Rangil, J., Cutando-Soriano, A., & López-Jiménez, J. (2016). Current methods of sedation in dental patients: A systematic review of the literature. *Medicina Oral, Patología Oral y Cirugía Bucal, 21*, e579–e586. https://doi.org/10.4317/medoral.20981.

Corder, G., Castro, D., Bruchas, M., & Scherrer, G. (2018). Endogenous and exogenous opioids in pain. *Annual Review of Neuroscience, 41*, 453-473. https://doi.org/10.1146/annurev-neuro-080317-061522.

Cordero, J. F., & Oakley, G. P., Jr. (1983). Drug exposure during pregnancy: Some epidemiologic considerations. *Clinical Obstetrics and Gynecology*, 26(2), 418–428. https://doi.org/10.1097/00003081-198306000-00019.

Corrie, K., & Hardman, J. G. (2011). Mechanisms of drug interactions: Pharmacodynamics and pharmacokinetics. *Anaesthesia & Intensive Care Medicine, 12*(4), 156–159.

Costa-Tort, J., Flaviano, V., González-Navarro, B., Jané-Salas, E., Estrugo-Devesa, A., & López-López, J. (2021). Update on the management of anticoagulated and antiaggregated patients in dental practice: Literature review. *Journal of Clinical and Experimental Dentistry, 13*, e948–e956. https://doi.org/10.4317/jced.58586.

Costa, B., Reichenbach, S., Keller, N., Nartey, L., Wandel, S., Jüni, P., & Trelle, S. (2017). Effectiveness of non-steroidal anti-inflammatory drugs for the treatment of pain in knee and hip osteoarthritis: A network meta-analysis. *The Lancet, 390*, e21-e33. https://doi.org/10.1016/S0140-6736(17)31744-0.

Costa, J., Portugal, J., Neves, C., & Bettencourt, A. (2021). Should local drug delivery systems be used in dentistry? *Drug Delivery and Translational Research, 12*, 1395–1407. https://doi.org/10.1007/s13346-021-01053-x.

Cote, C. J., Wilson, S., & American Academy of Pediatrics Committee on Drugs. (2016). Guidelines for monitoring and management of pediatric patients during and after sedation for diagnostic and therapeutic procedures: An update. *Pediatrics, 138*(1), e20161212. https://doi.org/10.1542/peds.2016-1212.

Craft, J. C., Feldman, W. E., & Nelson, J. D. (1979). Clinicopharmacological evaluation of amoxicillin and probenecid against bacterial meningitis. *Antimicrobial Agents and Chemotherapy, 16*(3), 346–352.

Croons, V., Martinet, W., & De Meyer, G. (2010). Selective removal of macrophages in atherosclerotic plaques as a pharmacological approach for plaque stabilization: Benefits versus potential complications. *Current Vascular Pharmacology, 8*(4), 495–508. https://doi.org/10.2174/157016110791330816.

Cunha, B. A. (2006). The atypical pneumonias: Clinical diagnosis and importance. *Clinical Microbiology and Infection, 12* Suppl 3, 12–24. https://doi.org/10.1111/j.1469-0691.2006.01393.x.

Currie, G. M. (2018). Pharmacology, part 2: Introduction to pharmacokinetics. *Journal of Nuclear Medicine Technology, 46*(3), 221–230. https://doi.org/10.2967/jnmt.117.199638.

Curtis, N., Orr, D., Ross, G., & Boulton, M. (1979). Affinities of penicillins and cephalosporins for the penicillin-binding proteins of *Escherichia coli* K-12 and their antibacterial activity. *Antimicrobial Agents and Chemotherapy, 16*, 533–539. https://doi.org/10.1128/AAC.16.5.533.

Cusenza, I., Pensa, V., Rastelli, S., Galati, C., Cogotzi, S., D'Orto, B., & Nagni, M. (2024). Conscious sedation in dentistry: narrative review. *Oral & Implantology*. https://doi.org/10.11138/oi.v16i1.19.

Czeizel, A. E., Kazy, Z., & Puhó, E. (2003). A population-based case-control teratological study of oral nystatin treatment during pregnancy. *Scandinavian Journal of Infectious Diseases*, 35(11–12), 830–835. https://doi.org/10.1080/00365540310016844.

Da Silveira, M., Da Conceição Coêlho, O., & Germano, A. (2023). Assessment of cardiovascular alterations and catecholamines serum concentration after oral surgery in patients receiving local anesthetics with epinephrine: A randomized, blind, controlled clinical trial. *Clinical Oral Investigations*, 27, 7651–7662. https://doi.org/10.1007/s00784-023-05354-y.

Dalamagka, M. (2024). Emergence Delirium in children. *International Journal of Science and Research Archive*. https://doi.org/10.30574/ijsra.2024.12.2.1408.

Dallmann, A., Mian, P., den Anker, J. V., & Allegaert, K. (2019). Clinical pharmacokinetic studies in pregnant women and the relevance of pharmacometric tools. *Current Pharmaceutical Design, 25*(5), 483–495.

Damé-Teixeira, N., El-Gendy, R., Silva, I., Holanda, C., De Oliveira, A., Romeiro, L., & Tostes, M. (2022). Sustainable multifunctional phenolic lipids as potential therapeutics in dentistry. *Scientific Reports, 12*, Article 13292. https://doi.org/10.1038/s41598-022-13292-0.

Dancer, S. (2001). The problem with cephalosporins. *The Journal of Antimicrobial Chemotherapy, 48*(4), 463–478. https://doi.org/10.1093/JAC/48.4.463.

Dar-Odeh, N. S., Abu-Hammad, O. A., Al-Omiri, M. K., Khraisat, A. S., & Shehabi, A. A. (2010). Antibiotic prescribing practices by dentists: A review. *Therapeutics and Clinical Risk Management*, 301–306.

Dar-Odeh, N., Elsayed, S., Babkair, H., Abu-Hammad, S., Althagafi, N., Bahabri, R., Eldeen, Y., Aljohani, W., & Abu-Hammad, O. (2020). What the dental practitioner needs to know about pharmaco-therapeutic modalities of COVID-19 treatment: A review. *Journal of Dental Sciences*, 16, 806–816. https://doi.org/10.1016/j.jds.2020.11.007.

Dar-Odeh, N., Fadel, H. T., Abu-Hammad, S., Abdeljawad, R. A., & Abu-Hammad, O. A. (2018). Antibiotic prescribing for oro-facial infections in the paediatric outpatient: A review. *Antibiotics, 7*(2), 38.

Darouiche, R. O. (1998). Oropharyngeal and esophageal candidiasis in immunocompromised patients: Treatment issues. *Clinical Infectious Diseases, 26*(2), 259–274. https://doi.org/10.1086/516315.

Darwish, D., Kumar, P., Urs, K., & Dave, S. (2024). Inhaled Anesthetics: Beyond the Operating Room. *Journal of Clinical Medicine*, 13. https://doi.org/10.3390/jcm13247513.

Dasari, N., Jiang, A., Skochdopole, A., Chung, J., Reece, E., Vorstenbosch, J., & Winocour, S. (2021). Updates in diabetic wound healing, inflammation, and scarring. *Seminars in Plastic Surgery*, 35(3), 153–158. https://doi.org/10.1055/s-0041-1731460.

DaSilva, A., Robinson, M., Shi, W., & McCauley, L. (2022). The forefront of dentistry—Promising tech-innovations and new treatments. *JDR Clinical & Translational Research, 7*(1_suppl), 16S–24S. https://doi.org/10.1177/23800844221116850.

Davari, A., Ataei, E., & Assarzadeh, H. (2013). Dentin hypersensitivity: Etiology, diagnosis and treatment; a literature review. *Journal of Dentistry (Shiraz, Iran), 14*(3), 136–145.

Davis, B. (2010). How are odontogenic infections best managed? *Journal of the Canadian Dental Association, 76*, a37.

Davis, G., Hathway, R., Shipley, D., & Staines, K. (2024). The management of pemphigus vulgaris and mucous membrane pemphigoid in a joint oral medicine and dermatology clinic: A five-year narrative review. *British Dental Journal, 236*(4), 311-316.

Dayer, P., Desmeules, J., Leemann, T., & Striberni, R. (1988). Bioactivation of the narcotic drug codeine in human liver is mediated by the polymorphic monooxygenase catalyzing debrisoquine 4-hydroxylation (cytochrome P-450 dbl/bufI). *Biochemical and Biophysical Research Communications, 152*(1), 411–416.

De Andrade, N., Motta, R., Bergamaschi, C., Oliveira, L., Guimarães, C., De Oliveira Araújo, J., & Lopes, L. (2019). Bleeding risk in patients using oral anticoagulants undergoing surgical procedures in dentistry: A systematic review and meta-analysis. *Frontiers in Pharmacology, 10*, 866. https://doi.org/10.3389/fphar.2019.00866.

De Barros Padilha, D., Veiga, N., Mello-Moura, A., & Correia, P. (2023). Virtual reality and behaviour management in paediatric dentistry: A systematic review. *BMC Oral Health, 23*. https://doi.org/10.1186/s12903-023-03595-7.

de Carvalho Minighini, E., Bragança, K. P., & Anastácio, L. R. (2020). Warfarin drug interaction with vitamin K and other foodstuffs. *Revista Chilena de Nutrición, 47*, 470–477.

De Carvalho, D., De Souza, H., De Assis, P., Alciati, C., & Ortolani, C. (2024). Essential oils from the perspective of dentistry. *Brazilian Journal of Health Aromatherapy and Essential Oil, 2*(2), Article 4. https://doi.org/10.62435/2965-7253.bjhae.2024.iisinaroma4.

De Freitas Rosa Remiro, P., Nagahara, M., Azoubel, R., Franz-Montan, M., D'ávila, M., & Moraes, Â. (2022). Polymeric biomaterials for topical drug delivery in the oral cavity: Advances on devices and manufacturing technologies. Pharmaceutics, 15(1), 12. https://doi.org/10.3390/pharmaceutics15010012.

De Lacerda, D., Honorato, P., De Albuquerque, J., De Araujo, L., Rocha, F., De Macêdo, M., De Freitas Neto, V., Cavalcante, A., De Moura Leite, I., Celeste, H., & Gomes, T. (2024). Pharmacology of general anesthetic agents in cardiac surgery: Pharmacokinetic and pharmacodynamic properties. *III Seven International Medical and Nursing Congress*. https://doi.org/10.56238/iiicongressmedicalnursing-035.

De Oliveira Araújo, J., Bergamaschi, C., Lopes, L., Guimarães, C., De Andrade, N., Ramacciato, J., & Motta, R. (2021). Effectiveness and safety of oral sedation in adult patients undergoing dental procedures: A systematic review. *BMJ Open, 11*, e043363. https://doi.org/10.1136/bmjopen-2020-043363.

De Oliveira, A., Rodrigues, J., De Souza, I., Oliveira, T., Santos, M., Varallo, F., & Pereira, L. (2024). Strategies employed and experiences associated with the implementation of pharmaceutical services and interventions in geriatric wards: A scoping review. *British Journal of Clinical Pharmacology*, 91, 729–739. https://doi.org/10.1111/bcp.16373.

De Oliveira, N., Azevedo, J., Macedo, N., Baggio, G., Cardoso, M., Souza, P., & Couto, S. (2024). Oral pseudomembranous candidiasis in hospitalized patients: A "hidden" cause for concern. *Oral Surgery, Oral Medicine, Oral Pathology and Oral Radiology*. https://doi.org/10.1016/j.oooo.2023.12.063.

Decloux, D., & Ouanounou, A. (2020). Local Anaesthesia in Dentistry: A Review. *International Dental Journal*, 71, 87 - 95. https://doi.org/10.1111/idj.12615.

Dedha, K., Nautiyal, A., Bali, S., Aggarwal, P., Garg, A., & Kumar, V. (2024). Treatment of periodontal abscess. *Santosh University Journal of Health Sciences*. https://doi.org/10.4103/sujhs.sujhs_68_23.

Deepak, T. A., Manjunath, M., & Thakur, H. (2021). Efficacy of curcumin and topical steroids in the treatment for oral submucous fibrosis: A comparative study. *Journal of Pharmacy and Bioallied Sciences, 13*(Suppl 1), S542-S548. https://doi.org/10.4103/jpbs.JPBS_687_20.

Deluke, D., Cannon, D., Carrico, C., Byrne, E., & Laskin, D. (2018). Is Maximal Dosage for Local Anesthetics Taught Consistently Across U.S. Dental Schools? A National Survey. *Journal of Dental Education*, 82 6, 621-624. https://doi.org/10.21815/JDE.018.071.

Demeester, C., Robins, D., Edwina, A., Tournoy, J., Augustijns, P., Ince, I., Lehmann, A., Vertzoni, M., & Schlender, J. (2023). Physiologically based pharmacokinetic (PBPK) modelling of oral drug absorption in older adults—An AGePOP review. *European Journal of Pharmaceutical Sciences*, 106496. https://doi.org/10.1016/j.ejps.2023.106496.

Deng, L., Du, C., Song, P., Chen, T., Rui, S., Armstrong, D., & Deng, W. (2021). The role of oxidative stress and antioxidants in diabetic wound healing. *Oxidative Medicine and Cellular Longevity*, 2021, 8852759. https://doi.org/10.1155/2021/8852759.

Deng, Q., Li, Y., He, W., Chen, T., Liu, N., Qiu, Z., Shang, Z., & Wang, Z. (2025). A polyene macrolide targeting phospholipids in the fungal cell membrane. *Nature, 640*, 743–751. https://doi.org/10.1038/s41586-025-08678-9.

Denisco, R. C., Kenna, G. A., O'Neil, M. G., Kulich, R. J., Moore, P. A., Kane, W. T., Mehta, N. R., Hersh, E. V., & Katz, N. P. (2011). Prevention of prescription opioid abuse: The role of the dentist. *Journal of the American Dental Association (1939), 142*(7), 800–810. https://doi.org/10.14219/jada.archive.2011.0268.

Deniz-Sungur, D., Aksel, H., Karaismailoğlu, E., & Sayin, T. (2020). The prescribing of antibiotics for endodontic infections by dentists in Turkey: A comprehensive survey. *International Endodontic Journal*. https://doi.org/10.1111/iej.13390.

Deray, G., Buti, M., Gane, E., Jia, J., Chan, H., Craxì, A., Piratvisuth, T., & Pol, S. (2015). Hepatitis B virus infection and the kidney: Renal abnormalities in HBV patients, antiviral drugs handling, and specific follow-up. *International Journal of Nephrology*, 2015, 1–11. https://doi.org/10.1155/2015/596829.

Derwich, M., Górski, B., Amm, E., & Pawłowska, E. (2023). Oral glucosamine in the treatment of temporomandibular joint osteoarthritis: A systematic review. *International Journal of Molecular Sciences, 24*, 4925. https://doi.org/10.3390/ijms24054925.

Derwich, M., Mituś-Kenig, M., & Pawłowska, E. (2021). Mechanisms of action and efficacy of hyaluronic acid, corticosteroids and platelet-rich plasma in the treatment of temporomandibular joint osteoarthritis—A systematic review. *International Journal of Molecular Sciences, 22*, 7405. https://doi.org/10.3390/ijms22147405.

Deus, F., & Ouanounou, A. (2022). Chlorhexidine in Dentistry: Pharmacology, Uses, and Adverse Effects. *International Dental Journal*, 72, 269 - 277. https://doi.org/10.1016/j.identj.2022.01.005.

Deus, F., & Ouanounou, A. (2022). Chlorhexidine in dentistry: Pharmacology, uses, and adverse effects. *International Dental Journal, 72*, 269–277. https://doi.org/10.1016/j.identj.2022.01.005.

Dézsi, C., Dézsi, B., & Dézsi, A. (2017). Management of dental patients receiving antiplatelet therapy or chronic oral anticoagulation: A review of the latest evidence. *European Journal of General Practice, 23*, 196–201. https://doi.org/10.1080/13814788.2017.1350645.

Dhar, V., Gosnell, E., Jayaraman, J., Law, C., Majstorović, M., Marghalani, A., Randall, C., Townsend, J., Wells, M., Chen, C., & Wedeward, R. (2023). Nonpharmacological behavior guidance for the pediatric dental patient. Pediatric Dentistry, 45(5), 385–410.

Dhatariya, K., Levy, N., Russon, K., Patel, A., Frank, C., Mustafa, O., Newland-Jones, P., Rayman, G., Tinsley, S., & Dhesi, J. (2024). Perioperative use of glucagon-like peptide-1 receptor agonists and sodium-glucose cotransporter 2 inhibitors for diabetes mellitus. *British Journal of Anaesthesia*. https://doi.org/10.1016/j.bja.2023.12.015.

Dhingra, K., & Vandana, K. (2017). Effectiveness of *Azadirachta indica* (neem) mouthrinse in plaque and gingivitis control: A systematic review. *International Journal of Dental Hygiene, 15*, 4–15. https://doi.org/10.1111/idh.12191.

Dhingra, K., & Vandana, K. L. (2017). Effectiveness of *Azadirachta indica* (neem) mouthrinse in plaque and gingivitis control: A systematic review. *International Journal of Dental Hygiene, 15*(1), 4–15.

Dhivya, S. (2018). Antibacterial efficacy of neem and cinnamon mouth rinse on salivary mutans streptococci and its effect on plaque and gingival health among 15–17 year old students in Madurai city: A double blind, randomized controlled trial.

Didona, D., Caposiena Caro, R. D., Sequeira Santos, A. M., Solimani, F., & Hertl, M. (2022). Therapeutic strategies for oral lichen planus: State of the art and new insights. *Frontiers in Medicine, 9*, 997190. https://doi.org/10.3389/fmed.2022.997190.

Dighriri, I., Mobarki, A., Althomali, N., Alqurashi, K., Daghriri, O., Howimel, B., Alahmad, I., Alsaadi, R., Alsufyani, M., Balobade, M., Altemani, R., Alatawi, B., Sharoufna, W., Almuntashiri, T., & Almushawwah, S. (2021). Detect drug interactions with metronidazole. *Journal of Pharmaceutical Research International*. https://doi.org/10.9734/jpri/2021/v33i47a33049.

Ding, H., Wu, J., Zhao, W., Matinlinna, J., Burrow, M., & Tsoi, J. (2023). Artificial intelligence in dentistry—A review. *Frontiers in Dental Medicine, 4*. https://doi.org/10.3389/fdmed.2023.1085251.

Dinos, G. P. (2017). The macrolide antibiotic renaissance. *British Journal of Pharmacology, 174*(18), 2967–2983. https://doi.org/10.1111/bph.13936.

Dionne, R., & Berthold, C. (2001). Therapeutic uses of non-steroidal anti-inflammatory drugs in dentistry.. *Critical reviews in oral biology and medicine : an official publication of the American Association of Oral Biologists*, 12 4, 315-30. https://doi.org/10.1177/10454411010120040301.

Dios, P. D., Monteiro, L., Pimolbutr, K., Gobbo, M., France, K., Bindakhil, M., ... & Edefonti, V. (2023). World Workshop on Oral Medicine VIII: Dentists' compliance with infective endocarditis prophylaxis guidelines for patients with high-risk cardiac conditions: A systematic review. *Oral Surgery, Oral Medicine, Oral Pathology and Oral Radiology, 135*(6), 757–771.

Dipalma, G., Inchingolo, A. D., Inchingolo, A. M., Piras, F., Carpentiere, V., Garofoli, G., Azzollini, D., Campanelli, M., Paduanelli, G., Palermo, A., et al., (2023). Artificial intelligence and its clinical applications in orthodontics: A systematic review. *Diagnostics, 13*, Article 243677. https://doi.org/10.3390/diagnostics13243677.

Dixon, J. C., Speidel, B. D., & Dixon, J. J. (1998). Neonatal flumazenil therapy reverses maternal diazepam. *Acta Paediatrica*, 87(2), 225–226. https://doi.org/10.1111/j.1651-2227.1998.tb01423.x.

Diz Dios, P., Tomas Carmona, I., Limeres Posse, J., Medina Henriquez, J., Fernandez Feijoo, J., & Alvarez Fernandez, M. (2006). Comparative efficacies of amoxicillin, clindamycin, and moxifloxacin in prevention of bacteremia following dental extractions. *Antimicrobial Agents and Chemotherapy, 50*(9), 2996–3002.

Dogan, G., Polat, Y., & Özüdoğru, S. (2025). Parental awareness and attitudes towards pediatric dentistry and children's oral health. *BMC Oral Health,* 25, 60. https://doi.org/10.1186/s12903-025-06037-8.

Doganay, O., Atalay, B., Karadag, E., Aga, U., & Tuğrul, M. (2018). Bleeding frequency of patients taking ticagrelor, aspirin, clopidogrel, and dual antiplatelet therapy after tooth extraction and minor oral surgery. *Journal of the American Dental Association, 149*(2), 132–138. https://doi.org/10.1016/j.adaj.2017.09.052.

Donaldson, M., & Goodchild, J. H. (2012). Pregnancy, breast-feeding and drugs used in dentistry. *Journal of the American Dental Association*, 143(8), 858–871. https://doi.org/10.14219/jada.archive.2012.0290.

Dong, X. (2018). Current strategies for brain drug delivery. *Theranostics, 8*(6), 1481–1493. https://doi.org/10.7150/thno.21254.

Donker, E., Bakkum, M., Richir, M., & Tichelaar, J. (2024). Bridging the gap between clinical pharmacology and rational drug prescribing 2.0: An up-date after 30 years. *British Journal of Clinical Pharmacology*. https://doi.org/10.1111/bcp.16051.

Doogue, M. P., & Polasek, T. M. (2013). The ABCD of clinical pharmacokinetics. *Therapeutic Advances in Drug Safety, 4*(1), 5–7.

Doshi, M., Shehabi, Z., Liu, S., & Geddis-Regan, A. (2024). General Anaesthesia in Special Care Dentistry. Part 1: Justifying and Planning the Use of General Anaesthesia. *Dental Update*. https://doi.org/10.12968/denu.2024.51.11.780.

Dowdy, R., Forgy, S., Hefnawi, O., & Neimar, T. (2023). A review of current oral sedation agents for pediatric dentistry. *Anesthesia Progress,* 70(2), 68–77. https://doi.org/10.2344/anpr-268717.

Dragovic, S., Schneider, G., García, P., Hinzmann, D., Sleigh, J., Kratzer, S., & Kreuzer, M. (2023). Predictors of Low Risk for Delirium during Anesthesia Emergence. *Anesthesiology*, 139, 757 - 768. https://doi.org/10.1097/ALN.0000000000004754.

Drenth-van Maanen, A. C., Wilting, I., & Jansen, P. A. (2020). Prescribing medicines to older people—How to consider the impact of ageing on human organ and body functions. *British Journal of Clinical Pharmacology, 86*(10), 1921–1930.

Droździk, A., & Droździk, M. (2023). Drug-Induced Gingival Overgrowth—Molecular Aspects of Drug Actions. *International Journal of Molecular Sciences*, 24. https://doi.org/10.3390/ijms24065448.

Duarte, M., Santos, P., Da Silva, M., De Oliveira Antonino, M., Cunha, R., De Queiroz Marques Filho, E., De Melo Júnior, P., De Ataíde Filho, A., Travassos, R., & Silva, L. (2025). Oral manifestations and complications resulting from diabetes: An interdisciplinary analysis in health. *Brazilian Journal of Implantology and Health*

Sciences, 7(2), 2172–2183. https://doi.org/10.36557/2674-8169.2025v7n2p2172-2183.

Ducharme, J., & Farinotti, R. (1996). Clinical pharmacokinetics and metabolism of chloroquine: Focus on recent advancements. *Clinical Pharmacokinetics, 31*, 257–274.

Dudek, B., Tymińska, J., Szymczyk-Ziółkowska, P., Chodaczek, G., Migdał, P., Czajkowska, J., & Junka, A. (2023). In vitro activity of octenidine dihydrochloride-containing lozenges against biofilm-forming pathogens of oral cavity and throat. *Applied Sciences, 13*, Article 52974. https://doi.org/10.3390/app13052974.

Duffy, C., Huang, Y., Andrikopoulou, M., Stern-Ascher, C., Wright, J., Goffman, D., D'Alton, M., & Friedman, A. (2019). Clindamycin, gentamicin, and risk of Clostridium difficile infection and acute kidney injury during delivery hospitalizations. *Obstetrics & Gynecology*. https://doi.org/10.1097/AOG.0000000000003568.

Duggal, S., Chandrika, P., Nasyam, F., Singh, D., Devraj, I., & Anand, C. (2024). Herbal dentistry: Nurturing oral health with natural remedies. *Journal of Pharmacy & Bioallied Sciences, 16*, S1932–S1934. https://doi.org/10.4103/jpbs.jpbs_18_24.

Đukić, L., Soulis, G., Janssens, B., Müller, F., Petrovic, M., & Kossioni, A. (2024). Appropriate use of antibiotics for oral/dental conditions in older adults: A narrative review. *Acta Clinica Belgica*, 79, 193–204. https://doi.org/10.1080/17843286.2024.2359182.

Dumbreck, S., Flynn, A., Nairn, M., Wilson, M., Treweek, S., Mercer, S. W., ... & Guthrie, B. (2015). Drug-disease and drug-drug interactions: Systematic examination of recommendations in 12 UK national clinical guidelines. *BMJ, 350*.

Dundee, J., Halliday, N., Harper, K., & Brogden, R. (2012). Midazolam. *Drugs*, 28, 519-543. https://doi.org/10.2165/00003495-198428060-00002.

Duvaldestin, P. (1981). Pharmacokinetics in Intravenous Anaesthetic Practice. *Clinical Pharmacokinetics*, 6, 61-82. https://doi.org/10.2165/00003088-198106010-00003.

Ebert, N., Jakob, O., Gaedeke, J., Van Der Giet, M., Kuhlmann, M. K., Martus, P., ... & Schaeffner, E. S. (2017). Prevalence of reduced kidney function and albuminuria in older adults: The Berlin Initiative Study. *Nephrology Dialysis Transplantation, 32*(6), 997–1005.

Edelstein, B., Basch, C., Zybert, P., Wolf, R., Custodio-Lumsden, C., Levine, J., Trent, R., Estrada, I., Koch, P., Andrews, H., & Kunzel, C. (2025). Chronic disease management of early childhood dental caries: Practices of US pediatric dentists. *Preventing Chronic Disease*, 22, 240151. https://doi.org/10.5888/pcd22.240151.

Edwards, D., Bowles, S., Svensson, C., & Rybak, M. (1988). Inhibition of drug metabolism by quinolone antibiotics. *Clinical Pharmacokinetics, 15*, 194–204. https://doi.org/10.2165/00003088-198815030-00004.

Edwards, I. R., & Aronson, J. K. (2000). Adverse drug reactions: Definitions, diagnosis, and management. *The Lancet, 356*(9237), 1255–1259.

Elhassy, G., & El-Naihoum, N. (2024). Trends in prescribing systemic antibiotics by Libyan dentists and periodontists. *AlQalam Journal of Medical and Applied Sciences*, 1043–1053.

Elhusseiny, G., & Saleh, W. (2024). Oral health in children with chronic kidney disease, hemodialysis, and renal transplantation: A comprehensive narrative review of the oral manifestations and dental implications. *Clinical Medicine Insights: Pediatrics*, 18, 11795565241271689. https://doi.org/10.1177/11795565241271689.

Elion, G. (1982). Mechanism of action and selectivity of acyclovir. *The American Journal of Medicine*, 73(1A), 7–13. https://doi.org/10.1016/0002-9343(82)90055-9.

Elmaghraby, D., Alsalman, G., Alawadh, L., Al-Abdulqader, S., Alaithan, M., & Alnuwaysir, B. (2023). Integrated traditional herbal medicine in the treatment of gastrointestinal disorder: The pattern of use and the knowledge of safety among the Eastern Region Saudi population. *BMC Complementary Medicine and Therapies, 23*. https://doi.org/10.1186/s12906-023-04197-0.

Elmarakeby, A., Alrashed, A., Zahr, A., Alanazi, F., Alazmi, G., Abulsaud, H., Alsulami, R., Jafar, S., Albalawi, S., Alrosini, S., & Alenazi, S. (2025). The transformative impact of digital technologies on modern dentistry: A narrative review of the applications and benefits. *Journal of Healthcare Sciences*. https://doi.org/10.52533/johs.2025.50103.

Elzagallaai, A., Greff, M., & Rieder, M. (2017). Adverse drug reactions in children: The double-edged sword of therapeutics. *Clinical Pharmacology & Therapeutics*, 101(6), 725–735. https://doi.org/10.1002/cpt.677.

Emmett, S., Hill, N., & Dajas-Bailador, F. (2019). Principles of clinical pharmacology. In *Clinical Pharmacology for Prescribing*. https://doi.org/10.1093/oso/9780199694938.003.0009.

Encinosa, W., Bernard, D., & Selden, T. (2021). Opioid and non-opioid analgesic prescribing before and after the CDC's 2016 opioid guideline. *International Journal of Health Economics and Management, 22*, 1-52. https://doi.org/10.1007/s10754-021-09307-4.

Engelen, E., Schutgens, R., Mauser-Bunschoten, E., Van Es, R., & Van Galen, K. (2018). Antifibrinolytic therapy for preventing oral bleeding in people on anticoagulants undergoing minor oral surgery or dental extractions. *Cochrane Database of Systematic Reviews, 7*, CD012293. https://doi.org/10.1002/14651858.CD012293.pub2.

Erdmann, A., RehmannSutter, C., & Bozzaro, C. (2021). Patients' and professionals' views related to ethical issues in precision medicine: A mixed research synthesis. *BMC Medical Ethics, 22*. https://doi.org/10.1186/s12910-021-00682-8.

Erdő, F., Bors, L., Farkas, D., Bajza, Á., & Gizurarson, S. (2018). Evaluation of intranasal delivery route of drug administration for brain targeting. *Brain Research Bulletin, 143*, 155–170. https://doi.org/10.1016/j.brainresbull.2018.10.009.

Ericson, J., Benjamin, D., Boakye-Agyeman, F., Balevic, S., Cotten, C., Adler-Shohet, F., Laughon, M., Poindexter, B., Harper, B., Payne, E., Kaneshige, K., & Smith, P. (2022). Exposure-safety relationship for acyclovir in the treatment of neonatal herpes simplex virus disease. *Early Human Development*, 170, 105616. https://doi.org/10.1016/j.earlhumdev.2022.105616.

Ernst, E. (2002). Toxic heavy metals and undeclared drugs in Asian herbal medicines. *Trends in Pharmacological Sciences, 23*(3), 136–139.

Escribano, M., Figuero, E., Martín, C., Tobías, A., Serrano, J., Roldán, S., & Herrera, D. (2016). Efficacy of adjunctive anti-plaque chemical agents: A systematic review and network meta-analyses of the Turesky modification of the Quigley and Hein plaque index. *Journal of Clinical Periodontology, 43*(12), 1059–1073. https://doi.org/10.1111/jcpe.12616.

Estrela, C., Guedes, O. A., Silva, J. A., Leles, C. R., Estrela, C. R., & Pécora, J. D. (2011). Diagnostic and clinical factors associated with pulpal and periapical pain. *Brazilian Dental Journal, 22*(4), 306–311. https://doi.org/10.1590/s0103-64402011000400008.

Etwel, F., Faught, L., Rieder, M., & Koren, G. (2017). The risk of adverse pregnancy outcome after first trimester exposure to H1 antihistamines: A systematic review and meta-analysis. *Drug Safety*, 40, 121–132. https://doi.org/10.1007/s40264-016-0479-9.

Evans, S. W., & McCahon, R. A. (2019). Management of postoperative pain in maxillofacial surgery. *British Journal of Oral and Maxillofacial Surgery, 57*(1), 4-11.

Falagas, M., Rafailidis, P., & Rosmarakis, E. (2007). Arrhythmias associated with fluoroquinolone therapy. *International Journal of Antimicrobial Agents, 29*(4), 374–379. https://doi.org/10.1016/J.IJANTIMICAG.2006.11.011.

Falatah, A., Almalki, R., Al-Qahtani, A., Aljumaah, B., Almihdar, W., & Almutairi, A. (2023). Comprehensive strategies in endodontic pain management: An integrative narrative review. *Cureus, 15*. https://doi.org/10.7759/cureus.50371.

Fatima, F., Kamal, A., Fida, M., Ahmed, M., & Mahmood, H. (2019). Adjunctive surgical procedures enhancing treatment outcome - A literature review. *JPMA. The Journal of the Pakistan Medical Association, 69*(5), 705–710.

Fayans, E. P., Stuart, H. R., Carsten, D., et al., (2010). Local anesthetic use in the pregnant and postpartum patient. *Dental Clinics of North America*, 54(4), 697–713. https://doi.org/10.1016/j.cden.2010.06.002

Feldman, C., Fredericks-Younger, J., Lu, S., Desjardins, P., Malmstrom, H., Miloro, M., Warburton, G., Ward, B., Ziccardi, V., & Fine, D. (2022). The Opioid Analgesic Reduction Study (OARS)—A comparison of opioid vs. non-opioid combination analgesics for management of post-surgical pain: A double-blind randomized clinical trial. *Trials, 23*. https://doi.org/10.1186/s13063-022-06064-8.

Fernandez, C., & Angeles, B. (2025). Comparison of Analgesic Efficiency between Local Infiltration of a Long-Acting Analgesic and Regional Nerve Block among Patients Undergoing Arthroscopic Anterior Cruciate Ligament Reconstruction: Meta-Analysis of Randomized Controlled Trials. *Clinics in Orthopedic Surgery*, 17, 228 - 237. https://doi.org/10.4055/cios23149.

Ferrante, L., Trilli, I., Di Noia, A., Sabatelli, F., Memè, L., Bambini, F., Sampalmieri, F., Bordea, I., Qorri, E., Almasri, L., Alkassab, M., Almasri, M., & Palermo, A. (2024). Pharmacological approaches to sedation in pediatric dentistry: A narrative review. *Oral & Implantology*. https://doi.org/10.11138/oi163.1suppl476-491.

Ferrillo, M., Giudice, A., Marotta, N., Fortunato, F., Di Venere, D., Ammendolia, A., Fiore, P., & De Sire, A. (2022). Pain management and rehabilitation for central sensitization in temporomandibular disorders: A comprehensive review. *International Journal of Molecular Sciences, 23*, 12164. https://doi.org/10.3390/ijms232012164.

Feucht, C., & Patel, D. R. (2011). Principles of pharmacology. *Pediatric Clinics of North America, 58*(1), 11–ix. https://doi.org/10.1016/j.pcl.2010.10.005.

Fichtenbaum, C. J., Zackin, R., Rajicic, N., et al., (2000). Amphotericin B oral suspension for fluconazole-refractory oral candidiasis in persons with HIV infection. Adult AIDS

Clinical Trials Group Study Team 295. *AIDS, 14*(6), 845–852. https://doi.org/10.1097/00002030-200004140-00010.

Figuero, E., Roldán, S., Serrano, J., Escribano, M., Martín, C., & Preshaw, P. (2019). Efficacy of adjunctive therapies in patients with gingival inflammation: A systematic review and meta-analysis. *Journal of Clinical Periodontology*. https://doi.org/10.1111/jcpe.13244.

Fine, D., Furgang, D., Barnett, M., Drew, C., Steinberg, L., Charles, C., & Vincent, J. (2000). Effect of an essential oil-containing antiseptic mouthrinse on plaque and salivary Streptococcus mutans levels. *Journal of Clinical Periodontology, 27*(3), 157–161. https://doi.org/10.1034/J.1600-051X.2000.027003157.X.

Finegold, S. M. (1980). Metronidazole. *Annals of Internal Medicine, 93*(4), 585–587. https://doi.org/10.7326/0003-4819-93-4-585.

Fiorillo, L., D'amico, C., Meto, A., Mehta, V., Lo Giudice, G., & Cervino, G. (2024). Sodium hypochlorite accidents in endodontic practice: Clinical evidence and state of the art. *The Journal of Craniofacial Surgery, 35*, e636–e645. https://doi.org/10.1097/SCS.0000000000010407.

Fisher, C., Janda, A. M., Zhao, X., Deng, Y., Bardia, A., Yanez, N. D., ... & Schonberger, R. B. (2025). Opioid dose variation in cardiac surgery: a multicenter study of practice. *Anesthesia & Analgesia, 140*(5), 1016-1027. https://doi.org/10.1213/ANE.0000000000007128.

Folly, P. (2024). Artificial intelligence in dentistry. *BDJ Student*. https://doi.org/10.1038/s41406-024-1432-5.

Foster, H., & Fitzgerald, J. (2005). Dental disease in children with chronic illness. Archives of Disease in Childhood, 90(7), 703–705. https://doi.org/10.1136/adc.2004.058065.

Fouad, A. F. (2012). Management of postoperative pain and swelling in endodontics. *Oral Surgery, Oral Medicine, Oral Pathology and Oral Radiology, 113*(6), 721-728. https://doi.org/10.1016/j.oooo.2012.03.011.

Fozzard, H., Lee, P., & Lipkind, G. (2005). Mechanism of local anesthetic drug action on voltage-gated sodium channels. Current Pharmaceutical Design, 11 21, 2671-86. https://doi.org/10.2174/1381612054546833.

Frank, A., Singh, P., Singh, K., Arora, S., Sharma, R., & Bajwa, N. (2023). Advanced oral drug delivery systems for combating and preventing paediatric periodontal disease. *Letters in Drug Design & Discovery*, 20(8), 836–844. https://doi.org/10.2174/1570180820666230823093604.

Frasca, L., Sarubbi, A., Longo, F., Costa, F., Sarubbi, D., Strumia, A., Marziali, V., & Crucitti, P. (2025). Remifentanil-Propofol-Ketamine- Based Total Intravenous Anesthesia with Spontaneous Breathing for Adult Rigid Bronchoscopy. *Journal of Clinical Medicine*, 14. https://doi.org/10.3390/jcm14020377.

Freo, U., Ruocco, C., Valerio, A., Scagnol, I., & Nisoli, E. (2021). Paracetamol: A review of guideline recommendations. *Journal of Clinical Medicine*, 10(15), 3420. https://doi.org/10.3390/jcm10153420.

Fuchi, I., & Noda, K. (2010). Labor control under epidural anesthesia: placental transfer and newborn metabolism of local anesthetics. Asia-Oceania Journal of Obstetrics and Gynaecology, 13 4, 427-32. https://doi.org/10.1111/J.1447-0756.1987.TB00286.X.

Fujimoto, T., Iizuka, S., Enomoto, M., Abe, K., Yamashita, K., Hanaoka, N., Okabe, N., Yoshida, H., Yasui, Y., Kobayashi, M., Fujii, Y., Tanaka, H., Yamamoto, M., & Shimizu, H. (2012). Hand, foot, and mouth disease caused by Coxsackievirus A6, Japan, 2011. *Emerging Infectious Diseases*, 18(2), 337–339. https://doi.org/10.3201/eid1802.111147.

Funck-Brentano, C. (1993). Pharmacokinetic and pharmacodynamic profiles of d-sotalol and d, l-sotalol. *European Heart Journal, 14*(suppl_H), 30–35.

Fung, S. (2024). Corticosteroids are still first-line therapies for bullous pemphigoid, with biologics finding use in difficult-to-treat disease. *Drugs & Therapy Perspectives, 40*(8), 310-314. https://doi.org/10.1007/s40267-024-01085-6.

Gallagher, P., & O'Mahony, D. (2008). STOPP (Screening Tool of Older Persons' potentially inappropriate prescriptions): Application to acutely ill elderly patients and comparison with Beers' criteria. *Age and Ageing*, 37(6), 673–679. https://doi.org/10.1093/ageing/afn197.

Galpin, J., Shinaberger, J., Stanley, T., Blumenkrantz, M., Bayer, A., Friedman, G., Montgomerie, J., Guze, L., Coburn, J., & Glassock, R. (1978). Acute interstitial nephritis due to methicillin. *The American Journal of Medicine, 65*(5), 756–765. https://doi.org/10.1016/0002-9343(78)90793-3.

Gambeta, E., Chichorro, J. G., & Zamponi, G. W. (2020). Trigeminal neuralgia: An overview from pathophysiology to pharmacological treatments. *Molecular Pain, 16*, 1744806920901890.

Gambhir, R. (2016). Herbal formulations: The next level in oral care. *International Journal of Green Pharmacy, 10*. https://doi.org/10.22377/ijgp.v10i3.697.

Gan, T., Belani, K., Bergese, S., Chung, F., Diemunsch, P., Habib, A., Jin, Z., Kovac, A., Meyer, T., Urman, R., Apfel, C., Ayad, S., Beagley, L., Candiotti, K., Englesakis, M., Hedrick, T., Kranke, P., Lee, S., Lipman, D., Minkowitz, H., Morton, J., & Philip, B. (2020). Fourth Consensus Guidelines for the Management of Postoperative Nausea and Vomiting. *Anesthesia & Analgesia*, 131, 411 - 448. https://doi.org/10.1213/ANE.0000000000004833.

Gao, C., Dong, X., Zhang, J., Mao, L., Guo, C., Qin, X., & Zou, Z. (2024). Recommendations for the selection of nucleoside analogues as antihuman herpesvirus drugs: A real-world analysis of reported cases from the FDA adverse event reporting system. *Expert Opinion on Drug Safety*, 24(6), 695–709. https://doi.org/10.1080/14740338.2024.2374919.

Gao, F., & Wu, Y. (2023). Procedural sedation in pediatric dentistry: A narrative review. *Frontiers in Medicine, 10*, 1186823. https://doi.org/10.3389/fmed.2023.1186823.

Gao, S., Zhang, S., Mei, M., Lo, E., & Chu, C. (2016). Caries remineralisation and arresting effect in children by professionally applied fluoride treatment: A systematic review. BMC Oral Health, 16, 12. https://doi.org/10.1186/s12903-016-0171-6.

Garcia, I., Kuska, R., & Somerman, M. (2013). Expanding the foundation for personalized medicine. *Journal of Dental Research, 92*(1_suppl), S10–S13. https://doi.org/10.1177/0022034513487209.

Garg, A., Sharma, G., Goyal, A., Ghosh, G., Si, S., & Rath, G. (2020). Recent advances in topical carriers of anti-fungal agents. *Heliyon*, 6. https://doi.org/10.1016/j.heliyon.2020.e04663.

Garstka, A., Kozowska, L., Kijak, K., Brzózka, M., Gronwald, H., Skomro, P., & Lietz-Kijak, D. (2023). Accurate diagnosis and treatment of painful temporomandibular disorders: A literature review supplemented by own clinical experience. *Pain Research & Management, 2023*, 1002235. https://doi.org/10.1155/2023/1002235.

Geng, S., Wang, J., Bai, X., Hou, Y., Li, J., & Ban, J. (2023). Comparison of nerve block anesthesia and local infiltration anesthesia with lidocaine hydrochloride in primary root canal treatment of mandibular molars. *Tropical Journal of Pharmaceutical Research*. https://doi.org/10.4314/tjpr.v22i4.21.

George, M. K. (2010). Pharmacokinetics. In G. M. Kapalka (Ed.), *Nutritional and Herbal Therapies for Children and Adolescents* (pp. 13–46). Academic Press. https://doi.org/10.1016/B978-0-12-374927-7.00002-9.

Geziry, A., Toble, Y., Kadhi, F., Pervaiz, M., & Nobani, M. (2018). Non-pharmacological pain management. In Pain Management in Special Circumstances. *IntechOpen*. https://doi.org/10.5772/intechopen.79689.

Ghafoor, H., Haroon, S., Atique, S., Huda, A., Ahmed, O., Khair, A., & Samad, A. (2023). Neurological Complications of Local Anesthesia in Dentistry: A Review. *Cureus*, 15. https://doi.org/10.7759/cureus.50790.

Ghasemi, S., & Vahidi, F. (2021). Medications used in oral surgery. In *Innovative Perspectives in Oral and Maxillofacial Surgery* (pp. 1–20). https://doi.org/10.1007/978-3-030-75750-2_51.

Gheorghe, D., Niculescu, A., Bîrcă, A., & Grumezescu, A. (2021). Biomaterials for the prevention of oral candidiasis development. *Pharmaceutics*, 13(6), 803. https://doi.org/10.3390/pharmaceutics13060803.

Ghorbani, H., Minasyan, A., Ansari, D., Ghorbani, P., Wood, D., Yeremyan, R., Ghorbani, S., & Minasian, N. (2024). Anti-diabetic therapies on dental implant success in diabetes mellitus: A comprehensive review. *Frontiers in Pharmacology, 15*, 1506437. https://doi.org/10.3389/fphar.2024.1506437.

Gidley, M., & Sanders, J. (1983). Mechanisms of antibacterial formaldehyde delivery from noxythiolin and other 'masked-formaldehyde' compounds. *Journal of Pharmacy and Pharmacology, 35*, 257–261. https://doi.org/10.1111/j.2042-7158.1983.tb02876.x.

Gilson, A., Chladek, J., Stone, J., Watterson, T., Lehnbom, E., Hoffins, E., Berbakov, M., Moon, J., Jacobson, N., Holden, R., Gangnon, R., Pigarelli, D., Welch, L., Portillo, E., Shiyanbola, O., Gollhardt, J., Walker, K., & Chui, M. (2024). Older adult misuse of over-the-counter medications: Effectiveness of a novel pharmacy-based intervention to improve patient safety. *Journal of Patient Safety*, 21, 38–47. https://doi.org/10.1097/PTS.0000000000001288.

Gizani, S., Seremidi, K., Katsouli, K., Markouli, A., & Kloukos, D. (2022). Basic behavioral management techniques in paediatric dentistry: A systematic review and meta-analysis. *Journal of Dentistry*, 104303. https://doi.org/10.1016/j.jdent.2022.104303

Glaser, R. J., Dankner, A., Mathes, S. B., & Harford, C. G. (1948). Effect of penicillin on the bacteremia following dental extraction. *The American Journal of Medicine, 4*(1), 55–65.

Glück, T., Kiefmann, B., Grohmann, M., Falk, W., Straub, R., & Schölmerich, J. (2005). Immune status and risk for infection in patients receiving chronic immunosuppressive therapy. *The Journal of Rheumatology*, 32(8), 1473–1480.

Goel, D., Chaudhary, S., Manuja, N., & Goel, G. (2024). Clinical perspective of antimicrobial drugs in pediatric dentistry: An update. *Indian Journal of Dental Sciences*, 16(1), 88–93. https://doi.org/10.4103/ijds.ijds_88_23.

Goel, D., Goel, G., Chaudhary, S., & Jain, D. (2020). Antibiotic prescriptions in pediatric dentistry: A review. *Journal of Family Medicine and Primary Care*, 9(1), 473–480. https://doi.org/10.4103/jfmpc.jfmpc_1097_19.

Golub, L., Suomalainen, K., & Sorsa, T. (1992). Host modulation with tetracyclines and their chemically modified analogues. *Current Opinion in Dentistry, 2*, 80–90.

Gong, C., Duong, A., & Zangwill, K. (2024). Response to "Estimating the cost of inappropriate antibiotic prophylaxis prior to dental procedures." *Infection Control & Hospital Epidemiology*, 45, 556. https://doi.org/10.1017/ice.2023.235.

González-Martínez, R., Cortell-Ballester, I., Herráez-Vilas, J. M., Arnau-de Bolós, J. M., & Gay-Escoda, C. (2012). Antibiotic prescription in the treatment of odontogenic infection by health professionals: A factor to consensus. *Medicina Oral, Patologia Oral y Cirugia Bucal, 17*(3), e452–e456. https://doi.org/10.4317/medoral.17504.

Gonzalez, D., Delmore, P., Bloom, B. T., et al., (2016). Clindamycin pharmacokinetics and safety in preterm and term infants. *Antimicrobial Agents and Chemotherapy, 60*(5), 2888–2894.

Goodchild, J. H., & Donaldson, M. (2017). New sedation and general anesthesia guidelines: Why the changes? *Journal of the American Dental Association, 148*(3), 138–142.

Gordon Arbuthnott, & Garcia-Muñoz. (2010). Neuropharmacology. In E. C. Johnstone, D. C. Owens, S. M. Lawrie, A. M. McIntosh, & M. Sharpe (Eds.), *Companion to Psychiatric Studies* (8th ed., pp. 45–76). Churchill Livingstone. https://doi.org/10.1016/B978-0-7020-3137-3.00003-6.

Gordon, J., Walker, C., Lamster, I., West, T., Socransky, S., Seiger, M., & Fasciano, R. (1985). Efficacy of clindamycin hydrochloride in refractory periodontitis: 12-month results. *Journal of Periodontology, 56*(Suppl 11S), 75–80. https://doi.org/10.1902/jop.1985.56.11s.75.

Gordon, J., Walker, C., Murphy, J., Goodson, J., & Socransky, S. (1981). Concentration of tetracycline in human gingival fluid after single doses. *Journal of Clinical Periodontology, 8*(2), 117–121. https://doi.org/10.1111/J.1600-051X.1981.TB02351.X.

Gordon, S., Riedy, C., Stohler, C., & Vujicic, M. (2022). Trends in scope of practice for oral health care: Future transformative effects. *JDR Clinical & Translational Research, 7*(1_suppl), 31S–39S. https://doi.org/10.1177/23800844221116845.

Gorle, A., & Khairnar, D. (2018). An approach to improve therapeutic efficacy of doxycycline hyclate in treatment of periodontitis. *Iranian Journal of Pharmaceutical Research (IJPR), 17*, 1550–1562. https://doi.org/10.22037/ijpr.2018.2279.

Goswami, M., Johar, S., & Khokhar, A. (2023). Oral health considerations and dental management for epileptic children in pediatric dental care. *International Journal of Clinical Pediatric Dentistry*, 16, 170–176. https://doi.org/10.5005/jp-journals-10005-2516.

Graziani, F., Izzetti, R., Perić, M., Marhl, U., Nisi, M., & Gennai, S. (2024). Early periodontal wound healing after chlorhexidine rinsing: a randomized clinical trial. *Clinical Oral Investigations*, 28. https://doi.org/10.1007/s00784-024-05643-0.

Greco, M., Caruso, P., Angelotti, G., Aceto, R., Coppalini, G., Martinetti, N., Albini, M., Bash, L., Carvello, M., Piccioni, F., Monzani, R., Montorsi, M., & Cecconi, M. (2023). REVersal of nEuromusculAr bLocking Agents in Patients Undergoing General Anaesthesia (REVEAL Study). *Journal of Clinical Medicine*, 12. https://doi.org/10.3390/jcm12020563.

Griffith, A., Mateen, A., Markowitz, K., Singer, S., Cugini, C., Shimizu, E., Wiedman, G., & Kumar, V. (2022). Alternative antibiotics in dentistry: Antimicrobial peptides. *Pharmaceutics, 14*. https://doi.org/10.3390/pharmaceutics14081679.

Gronich, N. (2024). Central nervous system medications: Pharmacokinetic and pharmacodynamic considerations for older adults. *Drugs & Aging*, 41, 507–519. https://doi.org/10.1007/s40266-024-01117-w.

Gronich, N., Stein, N., & Muszkat, M. (2021). Association between use of pharmacokinetic-interacting drugs and effectiveness and safety of direct acting oral anticoagulants: Nested case-control study. *Clinical Pharmacology & Therapeutics, 110*(6), 1526–1536.

Gross, A., Hanna, D., Rowan, S., Bleasdale, S., & Suda, K. (2019). Successful implementation of an antibiotic stewardship program in an academic dental practice. *Open Forum Infectious Diseases, 6*, ofz067. https://doi.org/10.1093/ofid/ofz067.

Gu, Y., Walker, C., Ryan, M., Payne, J., & Golub, L. (2012). Non-antibacterial tetracycline formulations: Clinical applications in dentistry and medicine. *Journal of Oral Microbiology, 4*, Article 19227. https://doi.org/10.3402/jom.v4i0.19227.

Guentsch, A., Jentsch, H., Pfister, W., Hoffmann, T., & Eick, S. (2008). Moxifloxacin as an adjunctive antibiotic in the treatment of severe chronic periodontitis. *Journal of Periodontology, 79*(10), 1894–1903.

Guggenheimer, J., & Moore, P. A. (2011). The therapeutic applications of and risks associated with acetaminophen use: A review and update. *Journal of the American Dental Association*, 142(1), 38–44. https://doi.org/10.14219/jada.archive.2011.0021.

Gülcan, H., & Gülşen, U. (2021). The use of corticosteroid in the treatment of central giant cell granuloma. *Düzce Üniversitesi Sağlık Bilimleri Enstitüsü Dergisi, 11*(2), 257-260.

Güner, M. D., & Ekmekci, P. E. (2019). Healthcare professionals' pharmacovigilance knowledge and adverse drug reaction reporting behavior and factors determining the reporting rates. *Journal of Drug Assessment, 8*(1), 13–20.

Guo, Z., Zhou, Y., Fu, M., Zheng, L., & Shi, L. (2024). Trends and patterns of antibiotic using from 2014 to 2018 in stomatology hospitals of China. *Oral Diseases*. https://doi.org/10.1111/odi.15042.

Gupta, C., Kumari, A., Garg, A. P., Catanzaro, R., & Marotta, F. (2011). Comparative study of cinnamon oil and clove oil on some oral microbiota. *Acta Bio-Medica: Atenei Parmensis, 82*(3), 197–199.

Gupta, M., Gupta, M., & , A. (2015). Oral conditions in renal disorders and treatment considerations – A review for pediatric dentist. *The Saudi Dental Journal*, 27(3), 113–119. https://doi.org/10.1016/j.sdentj.2014.11.014.

Gupta, Y. K. (2010). Pharmacovigilance programme for India. *RMLH Report*.

Gurzawska-Comis, K., Becker, K., Brunello, G., Gurzawska, A., & Schwarz, F. (2020). Recommendations for dental care during COVID-19 pandemic. *Journal of Clinical Medicine, 9*. https://doi.org/10.3390/jcm9061833.

Gussow, L. (2023). The myth that metronidazole and alcohol cause a disulfiram-like reaction. *Emergency Medicine News*. https://doi.org/10.1097/01.eem.0000990104.46586.c8.

Guzzi, R., & Bartucci, R. (2022). Interactive multiple binding of oleic acid, warfarin and ibuprofen with human serum albumin revealed by thermal and fluorescence studies. *European Biophysics Journal*, 51, 41 - 49. https://doi.org/10.1007/s00249-021-01582-w.

Haas, D. M., Marsh, D. J., Dang, D. T., Parker, C. B., Wing, D. A., Simhan, H. N., ... & Reddy, U. M. (2018). Prescription and other medication use in pregnancy. *Obstetrics & Gynecology*, 131(5), 789–798. https://doi.org/10.1097/AOG.0000000000002582.

Hacker, K. (2024). The burden of chronic disease. *Mayo Clinic Proceedings: Innovations, Quality & Outcomes*, 8, 112–119. https://doi.org/10.1016/j.mayocpiqo.2023.08.005.

Hackett, N., De Oliveira, G., Jain, U., & Kim, J. (2015). ASA class is a reliable independent predictor of medical complications and mortality following surgery.. *International journal of surgery*, 18, 184-90 . https://doi.org/10.1016/j.ijsu.2015.04.079.

Hadaya, D., Soundia, A., Gkouveris, I., Bezouglaia, O., Dry, S., Pirih, F., Aghaloo, T., & Tetradis, S. (2021). Antiresorptive-type and discontinuation-timing affect ONJ burden. *Journal of Dental Research, 100*, 746–753. https://doi.org/10.1177/0022034520986804.

Hagai, A., Diav-Citrin, O., Shechtman, S., & Ornoy, A. (2015). Pregnancy outcome after in utero exposure to local anesthetics as part of dental treatment: A prospective comparative cohort study. *Journal of the American Dental Association*, 146 8, 572-580 . https://doi.org/10.1016/j.adaj.2015.04.002.

Hagenbuch, B. (2010). Drug uptake systems in liver and kidney: A historic perspective. *Clinical Pharmacology & Therapeutics, 87*. https://doi.org/10.1038/clpt.2009.235.

Hakim, L., Yari, A., Nikparto, N., Mehraban, S., Cheperli, S., Asadi, A., Darehdor, A., Nezaminia, S., Dortaj, D., Nazari, Y., Dehghan, M., Hojjat, P., Mohajeri, M., & Jebelli, M. (2024). The current applications of nano and biomaterials in drug delivery of dental implant. *BMC Oral Health, 24*. https://doi.org/10.1186/s12903-024-03911-9.

Hakim, L., Yazdanian, M., Alam, M., Abbasi, K., Tebyaniyan, H., Tahmasebi, E., Khayatan, D., Seifalian, A., Ranjbar, R., & Yazdanian, A. (2021). Biocompatible and biomaterials application in drug delivery system in oral cavity. *Evidence-based Complementary and Alternative Medicine: eCAM, 2021*. https://doi.org/10.1155/2021/9011226.

Hale, T. W. (2010). Medications and mother's milk: A manual of lactational pharmacology (14th ed.). Hale Publishing.

Hanberg, P., Rasmussen, H. C., Bue, M., Stilling, M., Jørgensen, A. R., Petersen, E. K., ... & Klug, T. E. (2024). Penicillin concentrations in oropharyngeal and frontal sinus tissue following enteral and intravenous administration measured by microdialysis in a porcine model. *European Journal of Pharmaceutical Sciences, 201*, 106859.

Hapala, I., Klobučníková, V., Mazáňová, K., & Kohút, P. (2005). Two mutants selectively resistant to polyenes reveal distinct mechanisms of antifungal activity by nystatin and amphotericin B. *Biochemical Society Transactions, 33*(Pt 5), 1206–1209. https://doi.org/10.1042/BST20051206.

Hara, T., Ozawa, A., Shibutani, K., Tsujino, K., Miyauchi, Y., Kawano, T., Ito, K., Sakai, H., & Yokota, M. (2023). Practical guide for safe sedation. *Journal of Anesthesia*, 1–17. https://doi.org/10.1007/s00540-023-03177-5.

Harbaugh, C. M., Lee, J. S., Hu, H. M., McCabe, S. E., Voepel-Lewis, T., Englesbe, M. J., ... & Waljee, J. F. (2018). Persistent opioid use among pediatric patients after surgery. *Pediatrics, 141*(1).

Harbaugh, C. M., Nalliah, R. P., Hu, H. M., Englesbe, M. J., Waljee, J. F., & Brummett, C. M. (2018). Persistent opioid use after wisdom tooth extraction. *JAMA, 320*(5), 504-506.

Harding, A. (1994). Pharmacologic considerations in pediatric dentistry. *Dental Clinics of North America*, 38(4), 733–753. https://doi.org/10.1016/s0011-8532(22)00187-2

Hargreaves, K. M., & Cohen, S. (2011). *Cohen's pathways of the pulp* (10th ed.). Mosby.

Hargreaves, K., & Abbott, P. V. (2005). Drugs for pain management in dentistry. *Australian Dental Journal, 50*, S14-S22.

Harman, K. E., Brown, D., Exton, L. S., Groves, R. W., Hampton, P. J., Mohd Mustapa, M. F., Setterfield, J. F., & Yesudian, P. D. (2017). British Association of Dermatologists' guidelines for the management of pemphigus vulgaris 2017. *The British Journal of Dermatology, 177*(5), 1170–1201. https://doi.org/10.1111/bjd.15930.

Harnoss, J., Elrub, Q., Jung, J., Koburger, T., Assadian, O., Dissemond, J., Baguhl, R., Papke, R., & Kramer, A. (2018). Irritative potency of selected wound antiseptics in the hen's egg test on chorioallantoic membrane to predict their compatibility to wounds. *Wound Repair and Regeneration, 27*, 126–134. https://doi.org/10.1111/wrr.12689.

Harrison, C., & Bratcher, D. (2008). Cephalosporins: A review. *Pediatrics in Review, 29*(8), 264–267; quiz 273. https://doi.org/10.1542/pir.29-8-264.

Hartigan-Go, K. Y., & Wong, J. Q. (2000). Inclusion of therapeutic failures as adverse drug reactions. *Side Effects of Drugs Annual, 23*, 27–33. http://www.sciencedirect.com/science/article/pii/S0378608000800069.

Hashim, N., Babiker, R., Chaitanya, N., Mohammed, R., Priya, S., Padmanabhan, V., Ahmed, A., Dasnadi, S., Islam, M., Gismalla, B., & Rahman, M. (2025). New insights in natural bioactive compounds for periodontal disease: Advanced molecular mechanisms and therapeutic potential. *Molecules, 30*, 40807. https://doi.org/10.3390/molecules30040807.

Hashim, N., Babiker, R., Rahman, M., Mohamed, R., Priya, S., Chaitanya, N., Islam, M., & Gobara, B. (2024). Natural bioactive compounds in the management of periodontal diseases: A comprehensive review. *Molecules, 29*, 33044. https://doi.org/10.3390/molecules29133044.

Hauser, A., Attwood, M., Rask-Andersen, M., Schiöth, H., & Gloriam, D. (2017). Trends in GPCR drug discovery: New agents, targets and indications. *Nature Reviews Drug Discovery, 16*, 829–842. https://doi.org/10.1038/nrd.2017.178.

Havers-Borgersen, E., Engelund, A. P., Butt, J. H., Østergaard, L., Køber, L., & Fosbøl, E. L. (2023). Prescription practices of antibiotic prophylaxis among patients at high risk of infective endocarditis. *American Heart Journal Plus: Cardiology Research and Practice, 26*, 100254.

He, X., Wang, X., Wang, B., & Zhu, A. (2023). The association between mild cognitive impairment and medication non-adherence among elderly patients with chronic diseases. *Cureus*, 15, e47756. https://doi.org/10.7759/cureus.47756.

Heavner, J. (2007). Local anesthetics. *Current Opinion in Anaesthesiology*, 20, 336–342. https://doi.org/10.1097/ACO.0b013e3281c10a08.

Hedaya, M. A. (2024). Routes of drug administration. In *Pharmaceutics* (pp. 537-554). Academic Press.

Heinonen, O. P., Slone, D., & Shapiro, S. (1977). *Birth defects and drugs in pregnancy*. Publishing Sciences Group.

Helander, E., Kaye, A., Eng, M., Emelife, P., Motejunas, M., Bonneval, L., Terracciano, J., Cornett, E., & Kaye, A. (2019). Regional Nerve Blocks—Best Practice Strategies for Reduction in Complications and Comprehensive Review. *Current Pain and Headache Reports*, 23, 1-9. https://doi.org/10.1007/s11916-019-0782-0.

Hendrickson, R. G., & McKeown, N. J. (2012). Is maternal opioid use hazardous to breast-fed infants? *Clinical Toxicology*, 50(1), 1–14. https://doi.org/10.3109/15563650.2011.635147.

Herkenne, C., Alberti, I., Naik, A., Kalia, Y. N., Mathy, F. X., Préat, V., & Guy, R. H. (2008). In vivo methods for the assessment of topical drug bioavailability. *Pharmaceutical Research, 25*(1), 87–103. https://doi.org/10.1007/s11095-007-9429-7.

Hernández Ceruelos, A., Romero-Quezada, L. C., Ruvalcaba Ledezma, J. C., & López Contreras, L. (2019). Therapeutic uses of metronidazole and its side effects: An update. *European Review for Medical and Pharmacological Sciences, 23*(1), 397–401. https://doi.org/10.26355/eurrev_201901_16788.

Herrera, D., Matesanz, P., Martín, C., Oud, V., Feres, M., & Teughels, W. (2020). Adjunctive effect of locally delivered antimicrobials in periodontitis therapy: A systematic review and meta-analysis. *Journal of Clinical Periodontology*. https://doi.org/10.1111/jcpe.13230.

Herrera, D., Roldán, S., & Sanz, M. (2000). The periodontal abscess: A review. *Journal of Clinical Periodontology, 27*(6), 377–386.

Hersh, E. V., Moore, P. A., Grosser, T., Polomano, R. C., Farrar, J. T., Saraghi, M., Juska, S. A., Mitchell, C. H., & Theken, K. N. (2020). Nonsteroidal anti-inflammatory drugs and opioids in postsurgical dental pain. *Journal of Dental Research, 99*(7), 777–786. https://doi.org/10.1177/0022034520914254.

Hilgers, K. K., Douglass, J., & Mathieu, G. P. (2003). Adolescent pregnancy: A review of dental treatment guidelines. *Pediatric Dentistry*, 25(5), 459–467.

Hillman, D., Platt, P., & Eastwood, P. (2003). The upper airway during anaesthesia.. *British journal of anaesthesia*, 91 1, 31-9 . https://doi.org/10.1093/BJA/AEG126.

Hintjens, J., Daems, L., & Bossuyt, M. (1994). Melkersson Rosenthal syndrome. Review of the literature. *Acta Stomatologica Belgica, 91*(3), 143–154.

Hirayama, K., Kanda, N., Hashimoto, H., Yoshimoto, H., Goda, K., Mitsutake, N., & Hatakeyama, S. (2025). Antibiotic prescription trends in dentistry: A descriptive study using Japan's national database. *Journal of Public Health Dentistry, 85*, 153–159. https://doi.org/10.1111/jphd.12663.

Ho, J., Van Riet, T., Afrian, Y., Sem, K., Spijker, R., De Lange, J., & Lindeboom, J. (2021). Adverse effects following dental local anesthesia: a literature review. *Journal of Dental Anesthesia and Pain Medicine*, 21, 507 - 525. https://doi.org/10.17245/jdapm.2021.21.6.507.

Hodge, R. (1993). Famciclovir and penciclovir: The mode of action of famciclovir including its conversion to penciclovir. *Antiviral Chemistry & Chemotherapy*, 4(2), 67–84. https://doi.org/10.1177/095632029300400201.

Hodgens, A., & Sharman, T. (2024). Corticosteroids. In *StatPearls*. StatPearls Publishing. https://www.ncbi.nlm.nih.gov/books/NBK554612/.

Hof, H. (2006). A new, broad-spectrum azole antifungal: Posaconazole – mechanisms of action and resistance, spectrum of activity. *Mycoses, 49*(Suppl 1), 2–6. https://doi.org/10.1111/j.1439-0507.2006.01295.x.

Holford, N. H. (1986). Clinical pharmacokinetics and pharmacodynamics of warfarin: Understanding the dose-effect relationship. *Clinical Pharmacokinetics, 11*, 483–504.

Holt, A., Strange, J., Nouhravesh, N., Nielsen, S., Malik, M., Schjerning, A., Køber, L., Torp-Pedersen, C., Gislason, G., McGettigan, P., Schou, M., & Lamberts, M. (2023). Heart failure following anti-inflammatory medications in patients with type 2 diabetes mellitus. *Journal of the American College of Cardiology*, 81(15), 1459–1470. https://doi.org/10.1016/j.jacc.2023.02.027.

Holt, S., Schmiedl, S., & Thürmann, P. (2010). Potentially inappropriate medications in the elderly: The PRISCUS list. *Deutsches Ärzteblatt International*, 107(31–32), 543–551. https://doi.org/10.3238/arztebl.2010.0543.

Hooper, D. C. (2001). Emerging mechanisms of fluoroquinolone resistance. *Emerging Infectious Diseases, 7*(2), 337.

Horváth, B., Kloesel, B., Todd, M., Cole, D., & Prielipp, R. (2021). The Evolution, Current Value, and Future of the American Society of Anesthesiologists Physical Status Classification System. *Anesthesiology*. https://doi.org/10.1097/ALN.0000000000003947.

Houghton, I., Aun, C., & Leung, D. (1993). Minimum Alveolar Concentration of Halothane: An Ethnic Comparison. *Journal of the Royal Army Medical Corps*, 139, 117 - 119. https://doi.org/10.1136/jramc-139-03-10.

Howard, C. B., Griffin, W. C., & Lopez, M. F. (2013). Neuroadaptive changes that result from chronic drug exposure. In P. M. Miller (Ed.), *Biological Research on Addiction* (pp. 169–178). Academic Press. https://doi.org/10.1016/B978-0-12-398335-0.00018-2

Howie, W. O., & McMullen, P. C. (2006). Breastfeeding problems following anesthetic administration. *Journal of Perinatal Education*, 15(3), 50–57. https://doi.org/10.1624/105812406X118877.

Hoyert, D. L., & Xu, J. Q. (2012). Deaths: Preliminary data for 2011. *National Vital Statistics Reports,* 61, 1–52.

Hsu, S. H., Cheng, A., Chang, T., Pao, L., Hsiong, C., & Wang, H. (2021). Precisely adjusting the hepatic clearance of highly extracted drugs using the modified well-stirred model. *Biomedicine & Pharmacotherapy, 141*, 111855. https://doi.org/10.1016/j.biopha.2021.111855.

Hubbard, C. C., Evans, C. T., Calip, G. S., Rowan, S. A., Gellad, W. F., Campbell, A., Gross, A. E., Hershow, R. C., McGregor, J. C., Sharp, L. K., & Suda, K. J. (2021). Characteristics associated with opioid and antibiotic prescribing by dentists. *American Journal of Preventive Medicine, 60*(5), 648–657. https://doi.org/10.1016/j.amepre.2020.11.017.

Hung, K., Yeung, A., Bornstein, M., & Schwendicke, F. (2022). Personalized dental medicine, artificial intelligence, and their relevance for dentomaxillofacial imaging. *Dentomaxillofacial Radiology, 52*(1), 20220335. https://doi.org/10.1259/dmfr.20220335.

Hussain, H., & Al-Drobie, B. (2022). Clinicopathological assessment of chronic hyperplastic candidiasis. *Journal of Baghdad College of Dentistry, 34*(4). https://doi.org/10.26477/jbcd.v34i4.3274.

Hussain, U., Alam, S., Rehman, K., Antonoglou, G., & Papageorgiou, S. (2022). Effects of chlorhexidine use on periodontal health during fixed appliance orthodontic treatment: A systematic review and meta-analysis. *European Journal of Orthodontics, 44*(2), 123–134. https://doi.org/10.1093/ejo/cjac044.

Hutchison, R., Chon, E., Tucker, W., Gilder, R., Moss, J., & Daniel, P. (2006). A Comparison of a Fentanyl, Morphine, and Hydromorphone Patient-Controlled Intravenous Delivery for Acute Postoperative Analgesia: A Multicenter Study of Opioid-Induced Adverse Reactions. *Hospital Pharmacy*, 41, 659 - 663. https://doi.org/10.1310/hpj4107-659.

Hyllested, M., Jones, S., Pedersen, J., & Kehlet, H. (2002). Comparative effect of paracetamol, NSAIDs or their combination in postoperative pain management: A qualitative review. *British Journal of Anaesthesia*, 88(2), 199–214. https://doi.org/10.1093/bja/88.2.199.

Ibrahim, M. (2023). Acute oral toxicity, haematobiochemical parameters and histopathological evaluation of povidone iodine in mice. *Arid Zone Journal of Basic and Applied Research, 10*(7), 898–887. https://doi.org/10.55639/607.898887.

Ibrahim, N., Edis, Z., & Al-Owais, K. (2020). Adherence of geriatric patients and their beliefs toward their medicines in the United Arab Emirates. *Journal of Pharmacy & Bioallied Sciences,* 12, 22–30. https://doi.org/10.4103/jpbs.JPBS_93_19.

Ibrahim, N., Wong, Y., Lean, Q., Ramasamy, K., Lim, S., Tan, M., & Majeed, A. (2023). Medication self-management among older adults with cognitive frailty. *Research in Social & Administrative Pharmacy.* https://doi.org/10.1016/j.sapharm.2023.11.001.

Ilett, K., & Kristensen, J. (2005). Drug use and breastfeeding. *Expert Opinion on Drug Safety*, 4(4), 745–768. https://doi.org/10.1517/14740338.4.4.745.

Ilyes, I., Boariu, M., Rusu, D., Iorio-Siciliano, V., Vela, O., Boia, S., Kardaras, G., Surlin, P., Calniceanu, H., Jentsch, H., Lodin, A., & Stratul, S. (2024). A single dose of piperacillin plus tazobactam gel as an adjunct to professional mechanical plaque removal (PMPR) in patients with peri-implant mucositis: A 6-month double-blind randomized clinical trial. *Antibiotics, 13*, 30269. https://doi.org/10.3390/antibiotics 13030269.

Inchingolo, A. M., Inchingolo, A. D., Carpentiere, V., Del Vecchio, G., Ferrante, L., Di Noia, A., Palermo, A., Di Venere, D., Dipalma, G., Inchingolo, F. (2023). Predictability of dental distalization with clear aligners: A systematic review. *Bioengineering, 10*, 1390. https://doi.org/10.3390/bioengineering10121390.

Inchingolo, F., Inchingolo, A. M., Malcangi, G., Ferrante, L., Trilli, I., Di Noia, A., Piras, F., Mancini, A., Palermo, A., Inchingolo, A. D., et al., (2024). The interaction of cytokines in orthodontics: A systematic review. *Applied Sciences, 14*, 5133. https://doi.org/10.3390/app14125133.

Inchingolo, F., Inchingolo, A., Ferrante, L., Ruvo, E., Noia, A., Palermo, A., , A., & Dipalma, G. (2024). Pharmacological Sedation in Paediatric Dentistry. *European journal of paediatric dentistry*, 1 . https://doi.org/10.23804/ejpd.2024.2204.

Ing, J. W. (2017). Head and neck cancer pain. *Otolaryngologic Clinics of North America, 50*(4), 793-806.

Iqbal, M., & Aneja, E. (2024). Safety profile of benzodiazepines during pregnancy. *Psychiatry and Psychological Disorders*, 4(1), 1–7. https://doi.org/10.58489/2836-3558/024

Ishikane, M., Tanaka, C., Ono, S., Kusama, Y., Tsuzuki, S., Muraki, Y., Yamasaki, D., Tanabe, M., & Ohmagari, N. (2019). 773. First national survey of antibiotic use prescribed by all dentists in Japan from 2015 to 2017 using the National Database of Health Insurance Claims and Specific Health Checkups of Japan (NDB). *Open Forum Infectious Diseases, 6*, S343–S344. https://doi.org/10.1093/ofid/ofz360.841.

Ismail, J. (2018). Low-Dose Epinephrine Boluses: No Risk of Arrhythmias?. *Pediatric Critical Care Medicine*. https://doi.org/10.1097/PCC.0000000000001517.

Ito, S. (2011). Pharmacokinetics 101. *Paediatrics & Child Health, 16*(9), 535–536. https://doi.org/10.1093/pch/16.9.535.

Ito, S., Blajchman, A., Stephenson, M., Eliopoulos, C., & Koren, G. (1993). Prospective follow-up of adverse reactions in breast-fed infants exposed to maternal medication. *American Journal of Obstetrics and Gynecology,* 168(5), 1393–1399. https://doi.org/ 10.1016/0002-9378(93)90385-7.

Iwasawa, A., Niwano, Y., Kohno, M., & Ayaki, M. (2011). Bactericidal effects and cytotoxicity of new aromatic dialdehyde disinfectants (ortho-phthalaldehyde). *Biocontrol Science, 16*(4), 165–170. https://doi.org/10.4265/BIO.16.165.

Jackson, M. A., Schutze, G. E., & Committee on Infectious Diseases. (2016). The use of systemic and topical fluoroquinolones. *Pediatrics, 138*(5).

Jafarzadeh, M., Ghasemi, R., Asnaashari, E., Ponnet, K., & Moeeni, M. (2025). Your right to choose: Parents' preferences toward a pediatric dental center. *BMC Oral Health,* 25, 57. https://doi.org/10.1186/s12903-025-05707-x.

Jaffal, K., Chevillard, L., & Mégarbane, B. (2023). Lipid Emulsion to Treat Acute Poisonings: Mechanisms of Action, Indications, and Controversies. *Pharmaceutics,* 15. https://doi.org/10.3390/pharmaceutics15051396.

Jain, M., Prakash, A., & Medhi, B. (2021). Narrow therapeutic index drugs and role of therapeutic drug monitoring. *Drug Bulletin, 46*(1), 1–5.

Jain, N., Gupta, A., & N, M. (2013). An insight into neurophysiology of pulpal pain: Facts and hypotheses. *The Korean Journal of Pain, 26*(4), 347–355. https://doi.org/10.3344/kjp.2013.26.4.347.

Jakubovics, N., Goodman, S., Mashburn-Warren, L., Stafford, G., & Cieplik, F. (2021). The dental plaque biofilm matrix. *Periodontology 2000, 86*, 32–56. https://doi.org/10.1111/prd.12361.

Jamaldini, S. (2020). Personalized medicine approach in dental management, abilities and challenges: A review article. *Journal of Dental Medicine, 32*(4), 247–254.

James, P., Worthington, H., Parnell, C., Harding, M., Lamont, T., Cheung, A., Whelton, H., & Riley, P. (2017). Chlorhexidine mouthrinse as an adjunctive treatment for gingival health. *Cochrane Database of Systematic Reviews, 3*, CD008676. https://doi.org/10.1002/14651858.CD008676.pub2.

Janakiram, C., Nayar, S., Varma, B., Ramanarayanan, V., Mathew, A., Suresh, R., & Puttaiah, R. (2020). Dental care implications in coronavirus disease-19 scenario: Perspectives. *The Journal of Contemporary Dental Practice, 21*(8), 935–941. https://doi.org/10.5005/jp-journals-10024-2896.

Janev, N., & Ouanounou, A. (2023). Local anesthetics in oral and maxillofacial medicine: pharmacology, adverse effects, drug interactions and clinical manifestations. *Journal of Oral and Maxillofacial Anesthesia*. https://doi.org/10.21037/joma-23-27.

Janev, N., & Ouanounou, A. (2023). Local anesthetics in oral and maxillofacial medicine: pharmacology, adverse effects, drug interactions and clinical manifestations. *Journal of Oral and Maxillofacial Anesthesia*. https://doi.org/10.21037/joma-23-27.

Jauro, S., Ndumnego, O., Ellis, C., Buys, A., Beyer, W., & Van Heerden, H. (2020). Immunogenicity and protective efficacy of a non-living anthrax vaccine versus a live spore vaccine with simultaneous penicillin-G treatment in cattle. *Vaccines, 8*, Article 595. https://doi.org/10.3390/vaccines8040595.

Jedlicka, J., Groene, P., Linhart, J., Raith, E., Mustapha, D., & Conzen, P. (2021). Inhalational Anaesthetics: An Update on Mechanisms of Action and Toxicity. . https://doi.org/10.33696/neurol.2.037.

Jedlička, J., Groene, P., Linhart, J., Raith, E., Mustapha, D., & Conzen, P. (2021). Inhalationsanästhetika. *Der Anaesthesist*, 70, 343-355. https://doi.org/10.1007/s00101-020-00908-1.

Jeffcoat, M. K., Williams, R. C., Reddy, M. S., English, R., & Goldhaber, P. (1988). Flurbiprofen treatment of human periodontitis: Effect on alveolar bone height and metabolism. *Journal of Periodontal Research, 23*(6), 381–385. https://doi.org/10.1111/j.1600-0765.1988.tb01617.x.

Jeffres, M., Porter, M., Ricco, M., Norvell, M., Koonce, R., Bassler, E., & Hogan, C. (2022). 988. Risk of surgical site infection and Clostridioides difficile infection after perioperative clindamycin in patients labeled penicillin and/or cephalosporin allergic. *Open Forum Infectious Diseases*. https://doi.org/10.1093/ofid/ofac492.830.

Jiang, W. X., Zhang, Y., Yang, K. S., Zhang, H., Lu, K., & Sun, L. G. (2013). Efficacy of salvianolic acid B combined with triamcinolone acetonide in the treatment of oral submucous fibrosis. *Oral Surgery, Oral Medicine, Oral Pathology and Oral Radiology, 115*(3), 339-344. https://doi.org/10.1016/j.oooo.2012.10.006.

Jiang, X., Li, Y., Chen, N., Zhou, M., & He, L. (2023). Corticosteroids for preventing postherpetic neuralgia. *Cochrane Database of Systematic Reviews, 12*, CD005582. https://doi.org/10.1002/14651858.CD005582.pub5.

Jiao, Y., Tay, F., Niu, L., & Chen, J. (2019). Advancing antimicrobial strategies for managing oral biofilm infections. *International Journal of Oral Science, 11*. https://doi.org/10.1038/s41368-019-0062-1.

Joda, T., Bornstein, M., Jung, R., Ferrari, M., Waltimo, T., & Zitzmann, N. (2020). Recent trends and future direction of dental research in the digital era. *International Journal of Environmental Research and Public Health, 17*(6), 1987. https://doi.org/10.3390/ijerph17061987.

John, G., Schwarz, F., & Becker, J. (2015). Taurolidine as an effective and biocompatible additive for plaque-removing techniques on implant surfaces. *Clinical Oral Investigations, 19*, 1069–1077. https://doi.org/10.1007/s00784-014-1337-8.

Johnston, S. (2016). An evidence summary of the management of patients taking direct oral anticoagulants (DOACs) undergoing dental surgery. *International Journal of Oral and Maxillofacial Surgery, 45*(5), 618–630. https://doi.org/10.1016/j.ijom.2015.12.010.

Joly, P., & Tedbirt, B. (2022). Topical corticosteroids in bullous pemphigoid: What we have learned after two decades. *Annales de Dermatologie et de Vénéréologie, 149*(2), 79-80. https://doi.org/10.1016/j.annder.2022.01.009.

Joseph, J. M., & Raphael, K. G. (2000). Phantom tooth pain: A new look at an old dilemma. *Pain Medicine, 1*(1), 68–77. https://doi.org/10.1046/j.1526-4637.2000.00012.x.

Joshi, D., Garg, T., Goyal, A., & Rath, G. (2016). Advanced drug delivery approaches against periodontitis. *Drug Delivery, 23*, 363–377. https://doi.org/10.3109/10717544.2014.935531.

Joshi, G. (2020). General anesthetic techniques for enhanced recovery after surgery: Current controversies.. *Best practice & research. Clinical anaesthesiology*, 35 4, 531-541 . https://doi.org/10.1016/j.bpa.2020.08.009.

Jovanović, M., & Vučićević, K. (2022). Pediatric pharmacokinetic considerations and implications for drug dosing. *Arhiv za farmaciju,* 72(2), 105–112. https://doi.org/10.5937/arhfarm72-37605.

Jovanović, Ž., & Vulić, P. (2025). Self-medication and knowledge of pregnant women about the use of medication during pregnancy in the cities of Rijeka and Zadar, Croatia. *Frontiers in Pharmacology*, 16, 1536050. https://doi.org/10.3389/fphar.2025.1536050.

Jung, D., Mayersohn, M., Perrier, D., Calkins, J., & Saunders, R. (1982). Thiopental disposition in lean and obese patients undergoing surgery. *Anesthesiology, 56*(4), 269–274.

Jurić, S., Newport, D., Ritchie, J., Galanti, M., & Stowe, Z. (2009). Zolpidem (Ambien®) in pregnancy: Placental passage and outcome. *Archives of Women's Mental Health,* 12, 441–446. https://doi.org/10.1007/s00737-009-0100-7.

Juszczuk-Kubiak, E. (2024). Molecular aspects of the functioning of pathogenic bacteria biofilm based on quorum sensing (QS) signal-response system and innovative non-antibiotic strategies for their elimination. *International Journal of Molecular Sciences, 25*. https://doi.org/10.3390/ijms25052655.

Kadirovna, M., Tillaevna, S., & Otabekovich, T. (2024). Clinical protocols of dental treatment of patients with cardiovascular diseases (review of scientific research). *European International Journal of Multidisciplinary Research and Management Studies*, 4(4), 62–68. https://doi.org/10.55640/eijmrms-04-04-09.

Kadu, N., Khan, T., Khan, S., & Adling, Y. S. (2024). Identifying barriers to the rational use of antibiotics in dental practice: A questionnaire based study. *International Journal of All Research Education and Scientific Methods, 12*(12), 1548–1554.

Kalita, S., Goyal, R., Kumar, H., Yadav, D., Talreja, L., & Jaiswal, P. (2024). Efficacy of dexamethasone in reducing postoperative symptoms of the surgical extraction of impacted third molars. *Cureus, 16*(10), e72035. https://doi.org/10.7759/cureus.72035.

Kallali, B., Singh, K., & Thaker, V. (2011). Corticosteroids in dentistry. *Journal of Indian Academy of Oral Medicine and Radiology, 23*(2), 128-131.

Kamath, S., & Jawdekar, A. (2023). A comparison of innovative app-based prescriptions with conventional prescriptions for children by general dentists: A mixed methods study. Cureus, 15(6), e33583. https://doi.org/10.7759/cureus.33583.

Kanan, M., Atif, S., Mohammed, F., Balahmar, Y., Adawi, Y., AlSaleem, R., Farhan, A., Alghoribi, M., Mohammed, S., Alshanbari, R., Fahad, M., Kallab, R., Mohammed, R., Alassaf, D., & Hazza, A. (2023). A systematic review on the clinical pharmacokinetics of cephalexin in healthy and diseased populations. *Antibiotics, 12*. https://doi.org/10.3390/antibiotics12091402.

Kapoor, D., Garg, R., Gaur, M., Patel, M., Minglani, V., Prajapati, B., Huanbutta, K., Sangnim, T., & Sriamornsak, P. (2024). Pediatric drug delivery challenges: Enhancing compliance through age-appropriate formulations and safety measures. *Journal of Drug Delivery Science and Technology*, 85, 105720. https://doi.org/10.1016/j.jddst.2024.105720.

Katsarov, P., Shindova, M., Lukova, P., Belcheva, A., Delattre, C., & Pilicheva, B. (2021). Polysaccharide-based micro- and nanosized drug delivery systems for potential application in the pediatric dentistry. *Polymers, 13*. https://doi.org/10.3390/polym13193342.

Kaufmann, C. P., Tremp, R., Hersberger, K. E., & Lampert, M. L. (2014). Inappropriate prescribing: A systematic overview of published assessment tools. *European Journal of Clinical Pharmacology, 70*(1), 1–11. https://doi.org/10.1007/s00228-013-1575-8.

Kaur, G., Arora, M., & Majeti, R. (2019). Oral drug delivery technologies—A decade of developments. *The Journal of Pharmacology and Experimental Therapeutics, 370*(3), 529–543. https://doi.org/10.1124/jpet.118.

Kaye, A., Jeha, G., Renschler, J., Fuller, M., Pham, A., & Cornett, E. (2020). Anesthetic Agents in Pediatric Patients, A Comprehensive Review of Pharmacological Considerations in Clinical Practice. *Medical research archives*, 8. https://doi.org/10.18103/mra.v8i4.2057.

Keller, F., & Hann, A. (2018). Clinical pharmacodynamics: Principles of drug response and alterations in kidney disease. *Clinical Journal of the American Society of Nephrology, 13*(9), 1413–1420.

Kende, P., Wadewale, M., Mathai, P., Landge, J., Desai, H., & Nimma, V. (2021). Role of Superficial Cervical Plexus Nerve Block as an Adjuvant to Local Anesthesia in the Maxillofacial Surgical Practice. *Journal Of Oral And Maxillofacial Surgery: Official*

Journal Of The American Association Of Oral And Maxillofacial Surgeons. https://doi.org/10.1016/j.joms.2021.05.005.

Kern, J. (2023). Ramsay Hunt syndrome in an immunocompromised patient. *Journal of Clinical and Medical Images, Case Reports*. https://doi.org/10.55920/2771-019x/1506.

Kesado, T., Watanabe, K., Asahi, Y., Isono, M., & Ueno, K. (1984). Comparative antibacterial activities of 7 alpha-methoxy cephalosporins and 7 beta-methoxyiminoacetamido cephalosporins against *Bacteroides fragilis*. *Antimicrobial Agents and Chemotherapy, 25*, 131–133. https://doi.org/10.1128/AAC.25.1.131.

Khan, D. A., & Solensky, R. (2010). Drug allergy. *Journal of Allergy and Clinical Immunology, 125*(3), S126–S137. https://doi.org/10.1016/j.jaci.2009.10.028.

Khan, S., Stannard, N., & Greijn, J. (2011). Precipitation of thiopental with muscle relaxants: a potential hazard. *JRSM short reports*, *2*(7), 58. https://doi.org/10.1258/shorts.2011.011031

Kharouf, N., Haikel, Y., & Ball, V. (2020). Polyphenols in dental applications. *Bioengineering, 7*(3), Article 72. https://doi.org/10.3390/bioengineering7030072.

Khattab, A., & Malik, T. (2020). Temporomandibular joint dysfunction. In *Practical Chronic Pain Management* (pp. 1–20). https://doi.org/10.1007/978-3-030-46675-6_12.

Khbrani, A., Al-Shahrani, A., Alzahrani, H., Almalki, A., Alhawsaw, F., Almalki, W., Almutairi, K., & Zahrani, A. (2022). Role and common types of herbal medicine used for oral health in the Middle-East. *International Journal of Community Medicine and Public Health*. https://doi.org/10.18203/2394-6040.ijcmph20223322.

Kheshti, R., Aalipour, M., & Namazi, S. (2016). A comparison of five common drug–drug interaction software programs regarding accuracy and comprehensiveness. *Journal of Research in Pharmacy Practice, 5*(4), 257–263.

Khurshid, Z. (2023). Digital dentistry: Transformation of oral health and dental education with technology. *European Journal of Dentistry, 17*, 943–944. https://doi.org/10.1055/s-0043-1772674.

Kilgore, D. (2019). Integrative approaches to managing pain in geriatric patients. *Innovation in Aging, 3*, S402. https://doi.org/10.1093/geroni/igz038.1493.

Kim, H., Jung, J., Kim, S., Byun, J., Park, M., & Yeo, S. (2017). Comparison of acyclovir and famciclovir for Ramsay Hunt syndrome. *Otology & Neurotology*. https://doi.org/10.1097/MAO.0000000000001367.

Kim, J., Gharpure, A., Teng, J., Zhuang, Y., Howard, R., Zhu, S., Noviello, C., Walsh, R., Lindahl, E., & Hibbs, R. (2020). Shared structural mechanisms of general anesthetics and benzodiazepines. *Nature*, 585, 303 - 308. https://doi.org/10.1038/s41586-020-2654-5.

Kim, S., & Fechner, J. (2022). Remimazolam – current knowledge on a new intravenous benzodiazepine anesthetic agent. *Korean Journal of Anesthesiology*, 75, 307 - 315. https://doi.org/10.4097/kja.22297.

Kim, S., Hahn, S., Jang, M., Choi, Y., Hong, H., Lee, J., & Kim, H. (2019). Evaluation of the safety of using propofol for paediatric procedural sedation: A systematic review and meta-analysis. *Scientific Reports*, 9. https://doi.org/10.1038/s41598-019-48724-x.

Kim, T., Heo, S., Chandika, P., Kim, Y., Kim, H., Kang, H., Je, J., Qian, Z., Kim, N., & Jung, W. (2024). A literature review of bioactive substances for the treatment of periodontitis: In vitro, in vivo and clinical studies. *Heliyon, 10*, e24216. https://doi.org/10.1016/j.heliyon.2024.e24216.

Kimberlin, D., Weller, S., Whitley, R., Andrews, W., Hauth, J., Lakeman, F., & Miller, G. (1998). Pharmacokinetics of oral valacyclovir and acyclovir in late pregnancy. *American Journal of Obstetrics and Gynecology*, 179(4), 846–851. https://doi.org/10.1016/S0002-9378(98)70176-0.

Kimura, T. (2021). Stability and safety of inhibitor cystine knot peptide, GTx115, from the tarantula spider Grammostola rosea. *Toxins, 13*. https://doi.org/10.3390/toxins13090621.

Kinariwala, N., Samaranayake, L., Oberoi, G., & Agis, H. (2020). Future trends of 3D guidance in dentistry. In *3D Printing in Medicine* (pp. 203–215). https://doi.org/10.1007/978-3-030-55281-7_10.

King, A., Bathgate, T., & Phillips, I. (2002). Erythromycin susceptibility of viridans streptococci from the normal throat flora of patients treated with azithromycin or clarithromycin. *Clinical Microbiology and Infection, 8*(2), 85–92. https://doi.org/10.1046/J.1469-0691.2002.00347.X.

King, C., Rogers, P., Cleary, J., & Chapman, S. (1998). Antifungal therapy during pregnancy. *Clinical Infectious Diseases*, 27(5), 1151–1160. https://doi.org/10.1086/514977.

Kitson, K., Ormond, K., & Pergament, E. (2000). Surgery and pregnancy. *ITIS Newsletter,* 7(5), 1–5.

Klebanoff, M. A. (2009). The Collaborative Perinatal Project: A 50-year retrospective. *Paediatric and Perinatal Epidemiology*, 23(1), 2–8. https://doi.org/10.1111/j.1365-3016.2008.00980.x.

Kligman, S., Ren, Z., Chung, C., Perillo, M., Chang, Y., Koo, H., Zheng, Z., & Li, C. (2021). The impact of dental implant surface modifications on osseointegration and biofilm formation. Journal of Clinical Medicine, 10. https://doi.org/10.3390/jcm10081641.

Klingberg, G., Ridell, K., Brogårdh-Roth, S., Vall, M., & Berlin, H. (2017). Local analgesia in paediatric dentistry: A systematic review of techniques and pharmacologic agents. *European Archives of Paediatric Dentistry*, 18(5), 323–329. https://doi.org/10.1007/s40368-017-0302-z.

Klysik, K., Pietraszek, A., Karewicz, A., & Nowakowska, M. (2018). Acyclovir in the treatment of herpes viruses: A review. *Current Medicinal Chemistry*. https://doi.org/10.2174/0929867325666180309105519.

Knuf, K., & Maani, C. V. (2025). Nitrous oxide. In *StatPearls*. StatPearls Publishing. https://www.ncbi.nlm.nih.gov/books/NBK532922/.

Koch, G., & Brave, D. (2013). Intralesional corticosteroid injection for the management of chronic periapical lesions. *Journal of Endodontics, 39*(10), 1251-1255. https://doi.org/10.1016/j.joen.2013.06.012.

Koen, B., & Belpaire, F. M. (2008). Physiological aspects determining the pharmacokinetic properties of drugs. In C. G. Wermuth, D. Aldous, P. Raboisson, & D. Rognan (Eds.),

The Practice of Medicinal Chemistry (4th ed., pp. 539–559). Academic Press. https://doi.org/10.1016/B978-0-12-417205-0.00023-7.

Kolokotronis, A., Louloudiadis, K., Fotiou, G., & Matiais, A. (2001). Oral manifestations of infections due to varicella zoster virus in otherwise healthy children. *The Journal of Clinical Pediatric Dentistry*, 25(2), 107–112. https://doi.org/10.17796/jcpd.25.2.p255673211764073.

Kommu, S., Carter, C., & Whitfield, P. (2024). Adverse drug reactions. In *StatPearls [Internet]*. StatPearls Publishing.

Kondreddy, K., Mohanty, A., Desai, V., Surekha, G., Khader, A., Mathur, S., & Shetty, S. (2025). The effect of adjunctive antimicrobial therapy on the clinical outcomes of non-surgical periodontal treatment: A systematic review. *Journal of Pharmacy & Bioallied Sciences, 17*, S463–S466. https://doi.org/10.4103/jpbs.jpbs_1426_24.

Koolivand, H., Shooreshi, M., Safari-Faramani, R., Borji, M., Mansoory, M., Moradpoor, H., Bahrami, M., & Azizi, S. (2024). Comparison of the effectiveness of virtual reality-based education and conventional teaching methods in dental education: A systematic review. *BMC Medical Education*, 24. https://doi.org/10.1186/s12909-023-04954-2.

Koren, G., Nordon, G., Radinsky, K., & Shalev, V. (2019). Clinical pharmacology of old age. *Expert Review of Clinical Pharmacology*, 12, 749–755. https://doi.org/10.1080/17512433.2019.1632188.

Koren, G., Pastuszak, A., & Ito, S. (1998). Drugs in pregnancy. *New England Journal of Medicine*, 338(16), 1128–1137. https://doi.org/10.1056/NEJM199804163381607.

Kornman, K., & Duff, G. (2012). Personalized medicine. *Journal of Dental Research*, 91(1_suppl), S11–S18. https://doi.org/10.1177/0022034512449171.

Kotowska-Rodziewicz, A., Zalewska, A., & Maciejczyk, M. (2023). A review of preclinical and clinical studies in support of the role of non-steroidal anti-inflammatory drugs in dentistry. *Medical Science Monitor, 29*, e940635. https://doi.org/10.12659/MSM.940635.

Kounatidis, D., Dalamaga, M., Grivakou, E., Karampela, I., Koufopoulos, P., Dalopoulos, V., Adamidis, N., Mylona, E., Kaziani, A., & Vallianou, N. (2024). Third-generation tetracyclines: Current knowledge and therapeutic potential. *Biomolecules, 14*. https://doi.org/10.3390/biom14070783.

Kovesdy, C. (2022). Epidemiology of chronic kidney disease: An update 2022. *Kidney International Supplements*, 12(1), 7–11. https://doi.org/10.1016/j.kisu.2021.11.003

Kramer, K. J., Riley, C. J., & Brady, J. W. (2020). Overview of local anesthesia. In *Applied Head and Neck Anatomy for the Facial Cosmetic Surgeon* (pp. 3-15). Cham: Springer International Publishing. https://doi.org/10.1007/978-3-030-57931-9_1.

Krogman, W., Woodard, T., & McKay, R. (2023). Anesthetic Mechanisms: Synergistic Interactions With Lipid Rafts and Voltage-Gated Sodium Channels. *Anesthesia & Analgesia*, 139, 92 - 106. https://doi.org/10.1213/ANE.0000000000006738.

Kuang, W., Luo, X., Wang, J., & Zeng, X. (2021). Research progress on Melkersson-Rosenthal syndrome. *Zhejiang Da Xue Xue Bao Yi Xue Ban, 50*(2), 148-154. https://doi.org/10.3724/zdxbyxb-2021-0103.

Kudiyirickal, M. G., & Hollinshead, F. (2012). Clinical profile of orofacial infections: An experience from two primary care dental practices. *Medicina Oral, Patologia Oral y Cirugia Bucal, 17*(4), e533.

Kumar, A. (2016). The effect of corticosteroids on orthodontic tooth movement – A review. *IOSR Journal of Dental and Medical Sciences, 15*, 56-61. https://doi.org/10.9790/0853-1509015661

Kumar, A., Khrime, D., Bansal, N., Pandey, A. N., & Varma, A. (2016). Evaluation of antibiotic dose adjustment in patients with renal insufficiency in a tertiary care center. *International Journal of Contemporary Medical Research, 3*(5), 1383–1385.

Kumar, A., Nagpal, A., & Vohra, P. (2015). Personalized medicine: A step forward in dental treatment. *Journal of Indian Academy of Oral Medicine and Radiology*, 27(1), 76–80. https://doi.org/10.4103/0972-1363.167089.

Kumar, A., Singh, M., & Gupta, A. (2014). Prophylactic use of antibiotics in dentistry–a review. *International Journal of Contemporary Research, 2*(5), 36–40.

Kumar, D., Goyal, R., Arora, S., & Kusum, K. (2022). Assessment of efficacy of local anesthesia with 2 different concentrations of adrenaline in patients undergoing mandibular third molar extraction. *International Journal of Applied Dental Sciences*, 8(1), 142–145. https://doi.org/10.22271/oral.2022.v8.i1c.1420.

Kumar, N., Khare, V. V., Jamdade, A., Aggarwal, A., Rathore, N. S., & Yadav, S. (2022). Antibiotic susceptibility of the bacteria causing odontogenic infections: An observational study. *Journal of Indian Academy of Oral Medicine and Radiology, 34*(4), 442–446.

Kunrath, M., Shah, F., & Dahlin, C. (2022). Bench-to-bedside: Feasibility of nano-engineered and drug-delivery biomaterials for bone-anchored implants and periodontal applications. *Materials Today Bio,* 18, 100540. https://doi.org/10.1016/j.mtbio.2022.100540.

Kuriyama, T., Karasawa, T., Nakagawa, K., Nakamura, S., & Yamamoto, E. (2002a). Antimicrobial susceptibility of major pathogens of orofacial odontogenic infections to 11 β-lactam antibiotics. *Oral Microbiology and Immunology, 17*(5), 285–289.

Kuriyama, T., Karasawa, T., Nakagawa, K., Yamamoto, E., & Nakamura, S. (2002b). Bacteriology and antimicrobial susceptibility of gram-positive cocci isolated from pus specimens of orofacial odontogenic infections. *Oral Microbiology and Immunology, 17*(2), 132–135.

Kussainova, Z., Kulmaganbetov, M., Abiltayev, A., Bulegenov, T., & Salikhanov, I. (2025). Risk of infective endocarditis following invasive dental procedures: A systematic review and meta-analysis. *Public Health Reviews, 45*, 1607684.

Kuswandani, F., Balafif, F. F., Najmi, N., & Rafisa, A. (2023). Analgesic efficacy of etoricoxib on acute dental pain due to dental extraction and periodontal surgery: Rapid review. *European Journal of Theoretical and Applied Sciences, 1*(4), 1006-1014.

Kuzulugil, D., Papeix, G., Luu, J., & Kerridge, R. (2019). Recent advances in diabetes treatments and their perioperative implications. *Current Opinion in Anaesthesiology, 32*, 398–404. https://doi.org/10.1097/ACO.0000000000000735.

La Torre, G., Vitello, T., Cocchiara, R., & Della Rocca, C. (2023). Relationship between formaldehyde exposure, respiratory irritant effects and cancers: A review of reviews. *Public Health, 218*, 186–196. https://doi.org/10.1016/j.puhe.2023.03.009.

Labanca, M., Gianò, M., Franco, C., & Rezzani, R. (2023). Orofacial pain and dentistry management: Guidelines for a more comprehensive evidence-based approach. *Diagnostics, 13*. https://doi.org/10.3390/diagnostics13172854.

Lacroix, I., Damase-Michel, C., Lapeyre-Mestre, M., & Montastruc, J. L. (2000). Prescription of drugs during pregnancy in France. *The Lancet*, 356(9243), 1735–1736. https://doi.org/10.1016/S0140-6736(00)03208-0.

Lagerin, A., Lundh, L., Törnkvist, L., & Fastbom, J. (2020). District nurses' use of a decision support and assessment tool to improve the quality and safety of medication use in older adults: A feasibility study. *Primary Health Care Research & Development,* 21, e9. https://doi.org/10.1017/S1463423620000092.

Lammert, C., Bjornsson, E., Niklasson, A., & Chalasani, N. (2010). Oral medications with significant hepatic metabolism at higher risk for hepatic adverse events. *Hepatology*, 51(2), 615–626. https://doi.org/10.1002/hep.23317.

Lamy, P. P. (1991). Physiological changes due to age: Pharmacodynamic changes of drug action and implications for therapy. *Drugs & Aging, 1*, 385–404.

LaPlante, K., Dhand, A., Wright, K., & Lauterio, M. (2022). Re-establishing the utility of tetracycline-class antibiotics for current challenges with antibiotic resistance. *Annals of Medicine, 54*, 1686–1700. https://doi.org/10.1080/07853890.2022.2085881.

Larrey, D., Vial, T., Micaleff, A., Babany, G., Morichau-Beauchant, M., Michel, H., & Benhamou, J. (1992). Hepatitis associated with amoxycillin-clavulanic acid combination: Report of 15 cases. *Gut, 33*, 368–371. https://doi.org/10.1136/gut.33.3.368.

Larsen, M. K., Kofod, T., Christiansen, A. E., & Starch-Jensen, T. (2018). Different dosages of corticosteroid and routes of administration in mandibular third molar surgery: A systematic review. *Journal of Oral & Maxillofacial Research, 9*(2), e1. https://doi.org/10.5037/jomr.2018.9201.

Larsen, T., & Fiehn, N. (2017). Dental biofilm infections – an update. *APMIS, 125*, 376–384. https://doi.org/10.1111/apm.12688.

Lau, A. H., Evans, R., Chang, C. W., & Seligsohn, R. (1987). Pharmacokinetics of metronidazole in patients with alcoholic liver disease. *Antimicrobial Agents and Chemotherapy, 31*(11), 1662–1664. https://doi.org/10.1128/AAC.31.11.1662.

Lau, C., & Smith, G. (2022). Recurrent aphthous stomatitis: A comprehensive review and recommendations on therapeutic options. *Dermatologic Therapy*, 35. https://doi.org/10.1111/dth.15500.

Laudenbach, J., & Epstein, J. (2009). Treatment strategies for oropharyngeal candidiasis. *Expert Opinion on Pharmacotherapy, 10*(9), 1413–1421. https://doi.org/10.1517/14656560902952854.

Laursen, C., Lunn, T., Hägi-Pedersen, D., Brorson, S., Lindberg-Larsen, M., Overgaard, S., Jakobsen, J., & Mathiesen, O. (2025). Recommended use of non-steroidal anti-inflammatory drugs for pain treatment following primary total hip and knee arthroplasties in Denmark: A national survey. *Acta Anaesthesiologica Scandinavica, 69*(6), e70055. https://doi.org/10.1111/aas.70055.

Lavelle, E., & Kurra, S. (2018). *Pharmacology of Inhaled Anesthetics*, 177-193. https://doi.org/10.1007/978-3-319-62067-1_10.

Lee, H., Ciancio, S., Tüter, G., Ryan, M., Komaroff, E., & Golub, L. (2004). Subantimicrobial dose doxycycline efficacy as a matrix metalloproteinase inhibitor in chronic periodontitis patients is enhanced when combined with a non-steroidal anti-inflammatory drug. *Journal of Periodontology, 75*(3), 453–463. https://doi.org/10.1902/JOP.2004.75.3.453.

Lei, Z. N., Tian, Q., Teng, Q. X., Wurpel, J. N., Zeng, L., Pan, Y., & Chen, Z. S. (2023). Understanding and targeting resistance mechanisms in cancer. *MedComm, 4*(3), e265.

Leresche, L. (2022). Commentary: The changing face of dentistry. *JDR Clinical & Translational Research*, 7(1_suppl), 40S–46S. https://doi.org/10.1177/23800844221116840.

Lerman, J. (2022). Induction of anesthesia with sevoflurane in children: Curiosities and controversies. *Pediatric Anesthesia*, 32, 1100 - 1103. https://doi.org/10.1111/pan.14537.

Lerman, J., & Jöhr, M. (2009). Inhalational anesthesia vs total intravenous anesthesia (TIVA) for pediatric anesthesia. *Pediatric Anesthesia*, 19. https://doi.org/10.1111/j.1460-9592.2009.02962.x.

Leszczyńska, A., Buczko, P., Buczko, W., & Pietruska, M. (2011). Periodontal pharmacotherapy—An updated review. *Advances in Medical Sciences, 56*(2), 123–131. https://doi.org/10.2478/v10039-011-0044-9.

Levine, E., Rabii, K., Thampi, S., Pasha, K., & Coplan, N. (2020). Abstract 16229: Nonsteroidal anti-inflammatory drug use and heart failure hospitalizations: Are patients being screened? *Circulation*, 142(Suppl_3), A16229. https://doi.org/10.1161/circ.142.suppl_3.16229.

Levison, M. E., & Levison, J. H. (2009). Pharmacokinetics and pharmacodynamics of antibacterial agents. *Infectious Disease Clinics of North America, 23*(4), 791–815, vii. https://doi.org/10.1016/j.idc.2009.06.008

Li, H., Sun, J., Wang, X., & Shi, J. (2021). Oral microbial diversity analysis among atrophic glossitis patients and healthy individuals. *Journal of Oral Microbiology, 13*(1), 1984063. https://doi.org/10.1080/20002297.2021.1984063.

Li, L., Wang, Y., & Wang, S. (2021). Efficacy comparison of chlorhexidine and iodine preparation in reduction of surgical site infection: A systemic review and meta-analysis. *International Journal of Nursing Studies, 127*, 104059. https://doi.org/10.1016/j.ijnurstu.2021.104059.

Li, L., Zhang, W., Yang, Y., Zhao, L., Zhou, X., & Zhang, J. (2018). Dental management of patient with dual antiplatelet therapy: A meta-analysis. *Clinical Oral Investigations, 23*, 1615–1623. https://doi.org/10.1007/s00784-018-2591-y.

Li, M., & Ramos, L. G. (2017). Drug-induced QT prolongation and torsades de pointes. *Pharmacy and Therapeutics, 42*(7), 473–477.

Li, X., Gu, J., Xiao, Q., Liu, Y., Zhou, P., Fan, L., Zhang, X., Lu, X., Wu, J., Liu, Z., & He, W. (2022). Liposomal codelivery of inflammation inhibitor and collagen protector to the plaque for effective anti-atherosclerosis. *Chinese Chemical Letters*. https://doi.org/10.1016/j.cclet.2022.04.081.

Li, Y., Jiang, Y., & Zhang, L. (2024). The effect of different dosage of intranasal dexmedetomidine on preventing emergence delirium or agitation in children: A network meta-analysis of randomized controlled trials. *PLOS ONE*, 19. https://doi.org/10.1371/journal.pone.0304796.

Li, Z., Tangadanchu, V., Battini, N., Bheemanaboina, R., Zang, Z., Zhang, S., & Zhou, C. (2019). Indole-nitroimidazole conjugates as efficient manipulators to decrease the genes expression of methicillin-resistant Staphylococcus aureus. *European Journal of Medicinal Chemistry, 179*, 723–735. https://doi.org/10.1016/j.ejmech.2019.06.093

Li, Z., Yang, M., Liao, T., Zhou, Y., Yue, H., Piao, Z., & Zhou, L. (2020). Combined inferior alveolar nerve block anaesthesia and local infiltration anaesthesia in extraction of impacted mandibular third molars: a randomised controlled trial. *British Dental Journal.* https://doi.org/10.1038/s41415-020-2002-z.

Liang, G., Qian, H., Sun, C., Zhang, H., Li, Z., Li, S., Jing, K., Zhao, C., Wang, Y., Xiang, R., Li, X., & Feng, S. (2024). Dupilumab, corticosteroids and their combination for the treatment of bullous pemphigoid. *Anais Brasileiros de Dermatologia.* https://doi.org/10.1016/j.abd.2024.04.012.

Liao, Y., Parajuli, J., Jao, Y., Kitko, L., & Berish, D. (2021). Non-pharmacological interventions for pain in people with dementia: A systematic review. *International Journal of Nursing Studies*, 124, 104082. https://doi.org/10.1016/j.ijnurstu.2021.104082.

Lillis, T., Ziakas, A., Koskinas, K., Tsirlis, A., & Giannoglou, G. (2011). Safety of dental extractions during uninterrupted single or dual antiplatelet treatment. *American Journal of Cardiology, 108*(7), 964–967. https://doi.org/10.1016/j.amjcard.2011.05.029.

Lim, S., & Pettit, R. (2019). Pharmacokinetic considerations in pediatric pharmacotherapy. *American Journal of Health-System Pharmacy*, 76(19), 1472–1480. https://doi.org/10.1093/ajhp/zxz161.

Lin, C. P., Wang, Y. L., Shen, L. J., & Lin, C. P. (2019). The dentin permeability of anti-inflammatory and antibacterial drugs: In vitro study. *Journal of the Formosan Medical Association, 118*(4), 828–832. https://doi.org/10.1016/j.jfma.2018.09.009.

Lin, S., Hoffman, R., Nabriski, O., Moreinos, D., & Dummer, P. (2021). Management of patients receiving novel antithrombotic treatment in endodontic practice: Review and clinical recommendations. *International Endodontic Journal.* https://doi.org/10.1111/iej.13533.

Lin, Y., Wan, L., & Jamison, R. (2017). Using integrative medicine in pain management: An evaluation of current evidence. *Anesthesia & Analgesia, 125*, 2081–2093. https://doi.org/10.1213/ANE.0000000000002579.

Lindberg, C., Boreus, L. O., de Chateau, P., Lindstrom, B., Lonnerholm, G., & Nyberg, L. (1984). Transfer ofterbutaline into breast milk. European Journal of Respiratory Diseases, 134, 87–91.

Lipp, K., Casamassimo, P., Griffen, A., Smiley, M., Bryant, J., Draper, J., & Kumar, A. (2021). Effect of Intrapapillary Local Anesthetic on Postoperative Pain Following Dental Treatment Under General Anesthesia in Pediatric Patients. *Anesthesia progress*, 68 4, 206-213 . https://doi.org/10.2344/anpr-68-02-06.

Liu, C., Xiong, Y., Zhu, T., Liu, W., Tang, W., & Zeng, W. (2022). Management of tooth extraction in patients taking antiresorptive drugs: An evidence mapping review and meta-analysis. *Journal of Clinical Medicine, 12*, 10239. https://doi.org/10.3390/jcm12010239.

Liu, Y., Ren, Z., Hwang, G., & Koo, H. (2018). Therapeutic strategies targeting cariogenic biofilm microenvironment. *Advances in Dental Research, 29*, 86–92. https://doi.org/10.1177/0022034517736497.

Lobo, S., Argolinha, I., Machado, V., Botelho, J., Rua, J., Li, J., & Mendes, J. (2025). Advances in digital technologies in dental medicine: Enhancing precision in virtual articulators. *Journal of Clinical Medicine, 14*. https://doi.org/10.3390/jcm14051495.

Lodi, G., Manfredi, M., Mercadante, V., Murphy, R., & Carrozzo, M. (2020). Interventions for treating oral lichen planus: Corticosteroid therapies. *Cochrane Database of Systematic Reviews, 2020*(2), CD001168. https://doi.org/10.1002/14651858.CD001168.pub3.

Löffler, C., & Böhmer, F. (2017). The effect of interventions aiming to optimise the prescription of antibiotics in dental care—A systematic review. *PLoS ONE, 12*, e0188061. https://doi.org/10.1371/journal.pone.0188061.

Lone, P., Wani, N., Ain, Q., Heer, A., Devi, R., & Mahajan, S. (2021). Common postoperative complications after general anesthesia in oral and maxillofacial surgery. *National Journal of Maxillofacial Surgery*, 12, 206 - 210. https://doi.org/10.4103/njms.NJMS_66_20.

López-Valverde, A., Montero, J., Albaladejo, A., & De Diego, G. (2011). The Discovery of Surgical Anesthesia. *Journal of Dental Research*, 90, 31 - 34. https://doi.org/10.1177/0022034510385239.

López-Velasco, A., Puche-Torres, M., Carrera-Hueso, F., & Silvestre, F. (2021). General anesthesia for oral and dental care in paediatric patients with special needs: A systematic review. *Journal of Clinical and Experimental Dentistry*, 13, e303 - e312. https://doi.org/10.4317/jced.57852.

Lottinger, C. (2019). Local anesthetics in dentistry. *Clinical Dentistry Reviewed*, 3. https://doi.org/10.1007/s41894-019-0055-7.

Lou, J., Duan, H., Qin, Q., Teng, Z., Gan, F., Zhou, X., & Zhou, X. (2023). *Advances in oral drug delivery systems: Challenges and opportunities. Pharmaceutics*, 15(2), 484. https://doi.org/10.3390/pharmaceutics15020484.

Louizos, C., Yáñez, J. A., Forrest, M. L., & Davies, N. M. (2014). Understanding the hysteresis loop conundrum in pharmacokinetic/pharmacodynamic relationships. *Journal of Pharmacy & Pharmaceutical Sciences, 17*(1), 34–91.

Loyola-Rodriguez, J. P., Franco-Miranda, A., Loyola-Leyva, A., Perez-Elizalde, B., Contreras-Palma, G., & Sanchez-Adame, O. (2019). Prevention of infective endocarditis and bacterial resistance to antibiotics: A brief review. *Special Care in Dentistry, 39*(6), 603–609.

Lu, H., & Rosenbaum, S. (2014). Developmental pharmacokinetics in pediatric populations. *Journal of PediatricPharmacology and Therapeutics*, 19(4), 262–276. https://doi.org/10.5863/1551-6776-19.4.262.

Luchian, I., Goriuc, A., Martu, M. A., & Covasa, M. (2021). Clindamycin as an alternative option in optimizing periodontal therapy. *Antibiotics, 10*(7), 814. https://doi.org/10.3390/antibiotics10070814.

Luchian, I., Goriuc, A., Mârțu, M., & Covașă, M. (2021). Clindamycin as an alternative option in optimizing periodontal therapy. *Antibiotics, 10*, Article 814. https://doi.org/10.3390/antibiotics10070814.

Luckey, A. E., & Parsa, C. J. (2003). Fluid and electrolytes in the aged. *Archives of Surgery, 138*(10), 1055–1060.

Lusk, R., Fekety, F., Silva, J., Bodendorfer, T., Devine, B., Kawanishi, H., Korff, L., Nakauchi, D., Rogers, S., & Siskin, S. (1977). Gastrointestinal side effects of clindamycin and ampicillin therapy. *The Journal of Infectious Diseases, 135*(Suppl), S111–S119. https://doi.org/10.1093/INFDIS/135.SUPPLEMENT.S111.

MacCarthy, E. P., & Bloomfield, S. S. (1983). Labetalol: A review of its pharmacology, pharmacokinetics, clinical uses and adverse effects. *Pharmacotherapy: The Journal of Human Pharmacology and Drug Therapy, 3*(4), 193–217.

Machion, L., Andia, D., Lecio, G., Nociti, F., Casati, M., Sallum, A., & Sallum, E. (2006). Locally delivered doxycycline as an adjunctive therapy to scaling and root planing in the treatment of smokers: A 2-year follow-up. *Journal of Periodontology, 77*(4), 606–613. https://doi.org/10.1902/JOP.2006.050087.

Maciag, M., Ward, S., O'Connell, A., & Broyles, A. (2020). Hypersensitivity to tetracyclines: Skin testing, graded challenge, and desensitization regimens. *Annals of Allergy, Asthma & Immunology*. https://doi.org/10.1016/j.anai.2020.02.007.

Macpherson, L., & Binnie, V. (1996). A survey of general anaesthesia, sedation and resuscitation in general dental practice. *British Dental Journal*, 181, 199-203. https://doi.org/10.1038/sj.bdj.4809212.

Madadi, P., Moretti, M., Djokanovic, N., et al., (2009). Guidelines for maternal codeine use during breastfeeding. *Canadian Family Physician*, 55(11), 1077–1078. https://www.cfp.ca/content/55/11/1077.

Maggiolo, F., Caprioli, S., & Suter, F. (1990). Risk/benefit analysis of quinolone use in children: The effect on diarthrodial joints. *Journal of Antimicrobial Chemotherapy, 26*(4), 469–471.

Mahalingam, N. (2025). Preparation of Neem and Stevia mouthwash and its antimicrobial activity against oral pathogens. *Cuestiones de Fisioterapia.* https://doi.org/10.48047/8ceb1j15.

Mahmoud, R., Arbel, S., Ianculovici, C., Peleg, O., Kleinman, S., & Shuster, A. (2023). Antimicrobial therapy in the management of odontogenic infections: The penicillin-allergic patient. *International Journal of Oral and Maxillofacial Surgery*. https://doi.org/10.1016/j.ijom.2023.09.001.

Mai, S., Mauger, M., Niu, L., Barnes, J., Kao, S., Bergeron, B., Ling, J., & Tay, F. (2017). Potential applications of antimicrobial peptides and their mimics in combating caries and pulpal infections. *Acta Biomaterialia, 49*, 16–35. https://doi.org/10.1016/j.actbio.2016.11.026.

Maji, A., Soutar, C., Zhang, J., Lewandowska, A., Uno, B., Yan, S., Shelke, Y., Murhade, G., Nimerovsky, E., Borcik, C., Arango, A., Lange, J., Marin-Toledo, J., Lyu, Y., Bailey, K., Roady, P., Holler, J., Khandelwal, A., SantaMaria, A., Sanchez, H., Juvvadi, P., Johns, G., Hageman, M., Krise, J., Gebremariam, T., Youssef, E., Bartizal, K., Marr, K., Steinbach, W., Ibrahim, A., Patterson, T., Wiederhold, N., Andes, D., Pogorelov, T., Schwieters, C., Fan, T., Rienstra, C., & Burke, M. (2023). Tuning sterol extraction kinetics yields a renal-sparing polyene antifungal. *Nature, 623*, 1079–1085. https://doi.org/10.1038/s41586-023-06710-4.

Malamed, S. F. (2017). *Sedation: A guide to patient management* (6th ed.). Elsevier.

Malcangi, G., Patano, A., Guglielmo, M., Sardano, R., Palmieri, G., Di Pede, C., De Ruvo, E., Inchingolo, A., Mancini, A., Inchingolo, F., Bordea, I., Dipalma, G., & Inchingolo,

A. (2023). Precision medicine in oral health and diseases: A systematic review. *Journal of Personalized Medicine, 13*. https://doi.org/10.3390/jpm13050725.

Malsagova, K. A., Butkova, T. V., Kopylov, A. T., Izotov, A. A., Potoldykova, N. V., Enikeev, D. V., ... & Kaysheva, A. L. (2020). Pharmacogenetic testing: A tool for personalized drug therapy optimization. *Pharmaceutics, 12*(12), 1240.

Managutti, A., Prakasam, M., Puthanakar, N., Menat, S., Shah, D., & Patel, H. (2015). Comparative analysis of local anesthesia with 2 different concentrations of adrenaline: A randomized and single blind study. *Journal of International Oral Health*, 7, 24–27. https://www.ncbi.nlm.nih.gov/pmc/articles/PMC4382572/.

Manak, T., & Metelitsa, C. (2021). Oral health status of patients due to immunosuppressive therapy after organ transplantation operations. *Clinical Review for General Practice*, 2(10), 1–7. https://doi.org/10.47407/kr2021.2.10.00116.

Manchikanti, L., Kaye, A., Knezevic, N., McAnally, H., Slavin, K., Trescot, A., Blank, S., Pampati, V., Abdi, S., Grider, J., Kaye, A., Manchikanti, K., Cordner, H., Gharibo, C., Harned, M., Albers, S., Atluri, S., Aydin, S., Bakshi, S., Barkin, R., Benyamin, R., Boswell, M., Buenaventura, R., Calodney, A., Cedeño, D., Datta, S., Deer, T., Fellows, B., Galan, V., Grami, V., Hansen, H., Helm, S., Justiz, R., Koyyalagunta, D., Malla, Y., Navani, A., Nouri, K., Pasupuleti, R., Sehgal, N., Silverman, S., Simopoulos, T., Singh, V., Solanki, D., Staats, P., Vallejo, R., Wargo, B., Watanabe, A., & Hirsch, J. (2017). Responsible, safe, and effective prescription of opioids for chronic non-cancer pain: American Society of Interventional Pain Physicians (ASIPP) guidelines. *Pain Physician, 20*(2S), S3-S92. https://doi.org/10.36076/ppj.2017.s92.

Manfredi, M., Dave, B., Percudani, D., Christoforou, J., Karasneh, J., Diz Dios, P., ... & Patton, L. L. (2019). World workshop on oral medicine VII: Direct anticoagulant agents management for invasive oral procedures: A systematic review and meta-analysis. *Oral Diseases, 25*, 157–173. https://doi.org/10.1111/odi.13086.

Manfredini, M., Poli, P. P., Creminelli, L., Porro, A., Maiorana, C., & Beretta, M. (2021). Comparative risk of bleeding of anticoagulant therapy with vitamin K antagonists (VKAs) and with non-vitamin K antagonists in patients undergoing dental surgery. *Journal of Clinical Medicine, 10*(23), 5526. https://doi.org/10.3390/jcm10235526.

Mangoni, A., Woodman, R., & Jarmuzewska, E. (2025). Pharmacokinetic and pharmacodynamic alterations in older people: What we know so far. *Expert Opinion* on *Drug Metabolism & Toxicology*. https://doi.org/10.1080/17425255.2025.2503848.

Manihani, A. (2020). Dental management in medically compromised patients: An overview. *International Journal of Contemporary Research and Review*, 11(8), 20741–20746. https://doi.org/10.15520/ijcrr.v11i08.832.

Mann, N., Mathes, T., Sönnichsen, A., Pieper, D., Klager, E., Moussa, M., & Thürmann, P. (2023). Potentially inadequate medications in the elderly: PRISCUS 2.0—First update of the PRISCUS list. *Deutsches Ärzteblatt International*. https://doi.org/10.3238/arztebl.m2022.0377.

Manoharan, P., & Rajesh, P. (2019). Bacterial infections of the oral cavity. In *Pocket Guide to Bacterial Infections*. https://doi.org/10.1201/B22196-7.

Mansour, G., Ouda, S., Shaker, A., & Abdallah, H. (2014). Clinical efficacy of new aloe vera- and myrrh-based oral mucoadhesive gels in the management of minor recurrent aphthous stomatitis: A randomized, double-blind, vehicle-controlled study. *Journal of Oral Pathology & Medicine, 43*(6), 405–409. https://doi.org/10.1111/jop.12130.

Mansour, O., Russo, R., Straub, L., Bateman, B., Gray, K., Huybrechts, K., & Hernández-Díaz, S. (2023). Prescription medication use during pregnancy in the United States 2011–2020: Trends and safety evidence. *American Journal of Obstetrics and Gynecology*. https://doi.org/10.1016/j.ajog.2023.12.020.

Mao, X., Auer, D., Buchalla, W., Hiller, K., Maisch, T., Hellwig, E., Al-Ahmad, A., & Cieplik, F. (2020). Cetylpyridinium chloride: Mechanism of action, antimicrobial efficacy in biofilms, and potential risks of resistance. *Antimicrobial Agents and Chemotherapy, 64*(7), e00576-20. https://doi.org/10.1128/AAC.00576-20.

Marbach, J. J., & Raphael, K. G. (2000). Phantom tooth pain: A new look at an old dilemma. *Pain Medicine, 1*(1), 68–77. https://doi.org/10.1046/j.1526-4637.2000.00012.x.

Marek, C., & Timmons, S. (2019). Antimicrobials in pediatric dentistry. In A. Nowak, J. Christensen, & P. Townsend (Eds.), *Pediatric Dentistry* (7th ed., pp. 325–334). Elsevier. https://doi.org/10.1016/B978-0-323-60826-8.00009-2.

Marik, P. (2004). Propofol: therapeutic indications and side-effects. *Current pharmaceutical design*, 10 29, 3639-49 . https://doi.org/10.2174/1381612043382846.

Marinelli, G., Inchingolo, A., Balestriere, L., Fiore, A., Ciocia, C., Inchingolo, F., Corsalini, M., Minervini, G., Palermo, A., Vinjolli, F., Farronato, M., Maspero, C., Guerra, F., De Paula Guerra, A., Inchingolo, A., & Dipalma, G. (2024). Personalized approaches to oral health and disease management. *Oral & Implantology*. https://doi.org/10.11138/oi.v16i3.2suppl.136.

Marinho, V., Higgins, J., Sheiham, A., & Logan, S. (2004). One topical fluoride (toothpastes, or mouthrinses, or gels, or varnishes) versus another for preventing dental caries in children and adolescents.. The Cochrane database of systematic reviews, 1, CD002780. https://doi.org/10.1002/14651858.CD002780.PUB2.

Marinho, V., Worthington, H., Walsh, T., & Clarkson, J. (2013). Fluoride varnishes for preventing dental caries in children and adolescents.. The Cochrane database of systematic reviews, 7, CD002279. https://doi.org/10.1002/14651858.CD002279.pub2.

Mariño, Y. B., Cristo, H. G. G., Vidal, M. D., Marrero, Y. P., Labrada, S. M., & Díaz, L. E. R. (2023). Behavior of stomatological emergencies of dental origin. Mario Pozo Ochoa Stomatology Clinic. 2022–2023. *Odontologia (Montevideo), 1*, 06–06.

Marshall, J. G. (2002). Consideration of steroids for endodontic pain. *Endodontic Topics, 3*, 41-51.

Martínez, C., Gómez, D., & Oh, M. (2017). Use of traditional herbal medicine as an alternative in dental treatment in Mexican dentistry: A review. *Pharmaceutical Biology, 55*, 1992–1998. https://doi.org/10.1080/13880209.2017.1347188.

Martinez, M. N., & Amidon, G. L. (2002). A mechanistic approach to understanding the factors affecting drug absorption: A review of fundamentals. *The Journal of Clinical Pharmacology, 42*(6), 620–643.

Marwa, K., Goldin, J., & Kondamudi, N. P. (2025). Type IV Hypersensitivity Reaction. In *StatPearls*. StatPearls Publishing.

Masereeuw, R., & Russel, F. (2001). Mechanisms and clinical implications of renal drug excretion. *Drug Metabolism Reviews, 33*, 299–351. https://doi.org/10.1081/DMR-120000654.

Maslamani, M., & Sedeqi, F. (2018). Antibiotic and analgesic prescription patterns among dentists or management of dental pain and infection during endodontic treatment. *Medical Principles and Practice, 27*(1), 66–72. https://doi.org/10.1159/000486416.

Mason, D., & Young, E. (1989). Oral sedation in dentistry. *University of Toronto dental journal*, 2 2, 25-30.

Matheson, I., Lunde, P. K., & Notarianni, L. (1985). Infant rash caused by paracetamol in breast milk? Pediatrics, 76(4), 651–652. https://doi.org/10.1542/peds.76.4.651.

Mathew, M., Verma, A., Gigi, G., Patil, H., & Shaikh, A. (2024). Cephalosporins in pediatrics: Navigating antimicrobial resistance impact and adverse effects – A comprehensive review. *IP Indian Journal of Clinical and Experimental Dermatology*. https://doi.org/10.18231/j.ijced.2024.023.

Mathews, B., Thalody, A., Miraj, S., Kunhikatta, V., Rao, M., & Saravu, K. (2019). Adverse effects of fluoroquinolones: A retrospective cohort study in a South Indian tertiary healthcare facility. *Antibiotics, 8*, Article 104. https://doi.org/10.3390/antibiotics8030104.

Mathias, N., & Hussain, M. (2010). Non-invasive systemic drug delivery: Developability considerations for alternate routes of administration. *Journal of Pharmaceutical Sciences, 99*(1), 1–20. https://doi.org/10.1002/jps.21793.

Matsuda, Y., Mizuno, R., Miyajima, S., Arakawa, S., & Kabasawa, Y. (2022). A case of oral health management for a patient with extensive ulceration of the oral mucosa due to herpes zoster. *Healthcare*, 10(11), 2249. https://doi.org/10.3390/healthcare10112249.

Matsuki, A., & Zsigmond, E. (1973). The first three days in the history of surgical anaesthesia in England. *Anaesthesia*, 28. https://doi.org/10.1111/J.1365-2044.1973.TB00311.X.

Matthews, T., & Boehme, R. (1988). Antiviral activity and mechanism of action of ganciclovir. *Reviews of Infectious Diseases*, 10(Suppl 3), S490–S494. https://doi.org/10.1093/clinids/10.supplement_3.s490.

Maxwell, S. (2009). Rational prescribing: The principles of drug selection. *Clinical Medicine, 16*(5), 459–464. https://doi.org/10.7861/clinmedicine.16-5-459.

Mazaleuskaya, L. L., Sangkuhl, K., Thorn, C. F., FitzGerald, G. A., Altman, R. B., & Klein, T. E. (2015). PharmGKB summary: Pathways of acetaminophen metabolism at the therapeutic versus toxic doses. *Pharmacogenetics and Genomics, 25*(8), 416–426.

Maze, M., & Fujinaga, M. (2000). Recent advances in understanding the actions and toxicity of nitrous oxide. *Anaesthesia*, 55. https://doi.org/10.1046/j.1365-2044.2000.01463.x.

Mazoit, J., & Dalens, B. (2004). Pharmacokinetics of Local Anaesthetics in Infants and Children. *Clinical Pharmacokinetics*, 43, 17-32. https://doi.org/10.2165/00003088-200443010-00002.

Mazze, R. I., Wilson, A. I., Rice, S. A., & Baden, J. M. (1984). Reproduction and fetal development in rats exposed to nitrous oxide. *Teratology*, 30(2), 259–265. https://doi.org/10.1002/tera.1420300215.

Mburia-Mwalili, A., & Yang, W. (2014). Birth defects surveillance in the United States: Challenges and implications of International Classification of Diseases, Tenth Revision, Clinical Modification implementation. *International Scholarly Research Notices*, 2014, 212874. https://doi.org/10.1155/2014/212874.

McCormack, W. M., George, H., Donner, A., et al., (1977). Hepatotoxicity of erythromycin estolate during pregnancy. Antimicrobial Agents and Chemotherapy, 12(5), 630–635. https://doi.org/10.1128/aac.12.5.630.

McCullough, M., & Savage, N. (2005). Oral viral infections and the therapeutic use of antiviral agents in dentistry. *Australian Dental Journal*, 50(Suppl 2), S31–S35. https://doi.org/10.1111/j.1834-7819.2005.tb00382.x.

Mcdonnell, G., & Russell, A. (2001). Antiseptics and disinfectants: Activity, action, and resistance. *Clinical Microbiology Reviews, 14*, 227–264. https://doi.org/10.1128/cmr.14.1.227-227.2001.

McGowan, K., McGowan, T., & Ivanovski, S. (2018). Optimal dose and duration of amoxicillin-plus-metronidazole as an adjunct to non-surgical periodontal therapy: A systematic review and meta-analysis of randomized, placebo-controlled trials. *Journal of Clinical Periodontology, 45*(1), 56–67. https://doi.org/10.1111/jcpe.12830.

McGrath, C., Chau, C., & Molina, G. (2025). Monitoring oral health remotely: Ethical considerations when using AI among vulnerable populations. *Frontiers in Oral Health,* 6. https://doi.org/10.3389/froh.2025.1587630.

McKendrick, M. W., & Geddes, A. M. (1979). Neutropenia associated with metronidazole. *British Medical Journal, 2*(6193), 795. https://doi.org/10.1136/bmj.2.6193.795-b.

Mclennan, F., & Ward, P. (2023). General anaesthesia for dentistry. *Anaesthesia & Intensive Care Medicine*. https://doi.org/10.1016/j.mpaic.2023.05.002.

Medeiros, F. B., de Rezende, N. P. M., Franco, J. B., de Andrade, A. P., Timerman, L., Gallottini, M., ... & Ortega, K. L. (2017). Quantification of bleeding during dental extraction in patients on dual antiplatelet therapy. *International Journal of Oral and Maxillofacial Surgery, 46*(9), 1151–1157. https://doi.org/10.1016/j.ijom.2017.05.013.

Media, E., Visual, A., Berlubang, G., Meningkatkan, D., Anak, P., Harto, T., Afriani, B., & Adelia, S. (2025). Effectiveness of audio visual media for dental cavities in enhancing children's knowledge. *Cendekia Medika: Jurnal Stikes Al-Ma`arif Baturaja*, 10(1), 1–8. https://doi.org/10.52235/cendekiamedika.v10i1.468.

Meesters, K., Balbas-Martinez, V., Allegaert, K., Downes, K., & Michelet, R. (2024). Personalized dosing of medicines for children: A primer on pediatric pharmacometrics for clinicians. *Paediatric Drugs*, 26(2), 133–146. https://doi.org/10.1007/s40272-024-00633-x.

Mehran, M., Ansari, G., Golpayegani, V., Shayeghi, S., & Shafiei, L. (2018). Comparison of sedative effects of oral midazolam/chloral hydrate and midazolam/promethazine in pediatric dentistry. *Journal of Dental Research, Dental Clinics, Dental Prospects*, 12, 221 - 226. https://doi.org/10.15171/joddd.2018.034.

Mehrotra, D., & Manju, R. (2023). Herbal dentistry: A narrative review. *Journal of Clinical and Diagnostic Research*. https://doi.org/10.7860/jcdr/2023/63457.18045.

Mendia, J., Cuddy, M. A., & Moore, P. A. (2012). Drug therapy for the pregnant dental patient. Compendium of Continuing Education in Dentistry, 33(8), 568–596.

Meng, X. N., Ma, J. F., Liu, Y. H., Li, S. Q., Wang, X., Zhu, J., ... & Fu, S. B. (2024). Dynamic genomic changes in methotrexate-resistant human cancer cell lines beyond DHFR amplification suggest potential new targets for preventing drug resistance. *British Journal of Cancer*, 1–9.

Mezzour, M., Elharti, K., & Elwady, W. (2018). Focus on oral pemphigus vulgaris's management. *International Journal of Applied Dental Sciences, 4*(2), 289-292.

Michel-Levy, J. (2020). Pharmacokinetics and Pharmacodynamics of Local Anesthetics. Topics in Local Anesthetics. https://doi.org/10.5772/intechopen.91700.

Michelogiannakis, D., Al-Shammery, D., Rossouw, P. E., Ahmed, H. B., Akram, Z., Romanos, G. E., & Javed, F. (2018). Influence of corticosteroid therapy on orthodontic tooth movement: A narrative review of studies in animal models. *Orthodontics & Craniofacial Research, 21*(4), 216-224. https://doi.org/10.1111/ocr.12243.

Michenfelder, J., Sundt, T., Fode, N., & Sharbrough, F. (1987). Isoflurane When Compared to Enflurane and Halothane Decreases the Frequency of Cerebral Ischemia During Carotid Endarterectomy. *Anesthesiology*, 67, 336–340. https://doi.org/10.1097/00000542-198709000-00010.

Micó-Llorens, J. M., Satorres-Nieto, M., Gargallo-Albiol, J., Arnabat-Domínguez, J., Berini-Aytés, L., & Gay-Escoda, C. (2006). Efficacy of methylprednisolone in controlling complications after impacted lower third molar surgical extraction. *European Journal of Clinical Pharmacology, 62*(9), 693–698. https://doi.org/10.1007/s00228-006-0164-5.

Milia, E., Sotgiu, M., Spano, G., Filigheddu, E., Gallusi, G., & Campanella, V. (2022). Recurrent aphthous stomatitis (RAS): guideline for differential diagnosis and management. *European journal of paediatric dentistry*, 23 1, 73-78. https://doi.org/10.23804/ejpd.2022.23.01.14.

Milky, G., & Thomas, J. (2020). Shared decision making, satisfaction with care and medication adherence among patients with diabetes. *Patient Education and Counseling,* 103(2), 324–330. https://doi.org/10.1016/j.pec.2019.10.008.

Ming, Y., Wu, Z., Wu, Z., & Chu, S. (2021). Effects of different anesthesia methods on maternal and neonatal outcomes in pregnant patients with pulmonary arterial hypertension: a meta-analysis. *Archives of Gynecology and Obstetrics*, 306, 7 - 15. https://doi.org/10.1007/s00404-021-06274-6.

Miniaci, A., & Gupta, V. (2023). Loading dose. In *StatPearls*. StatPearls Publishing.

Mishra, A., Amalakara, J., Avula, H., & Reddy, K. (2017). Effect of diclofenac mouthwash on postoperative pain after periodontal surgery. *Journal of Clinical and Diagnostic Research, 11*(4), ZC24–ZC26. https://doi.org/10.7860/JCDR/2017/22165.9658.

Misra, S., Kaur, M., Deb, T., Kaushik, A., Vohra, A., Sindhwani, K., & Saranjhna, A. (2025). Agreement and correlation between WHO-UMC Causality scale and the Naranjo algorithm for causality assessment of adverse drug reactions at tertiary care center in Northern India. *Journal of Family Medicine and Primary Care*, 14, 1252 - 1258. https://doi.org/10.4103/jfmpc.jfmpc_1148_24.

Mitchell, D., Kuljanin, M., Li, J., Van Vranken, J., Bulloch, N., Schweppe, D., Huttlin, E., & Gygi, S. (2023). A proteome-wide atlas of drug mechanism of action. *Nature Biotechnology*, 1–13. https://doi.org/10.1038/s41587-022-01539-0.

Mittal, M., Gupta, N., Parashar, P., Mehra, V., & Khatri, M. (2014). Phytochemical evaluation and pharmacological activity of *Syzygium aromaticum*: A comprehensive review. *International Journal of Pharmacy and Pharmaceutical Sciences, 6*, 67–72.

Mo, Y., Zhang, H., Shen, J., Chen, J., Hong, J., Xu, Y., & Qian, C. (2022). Prophylactic and therapeutic HPV vaccines: Current scenario and perspectives. *Frontiers in Cellular and Infection Microbiology*, 12, 909223. https://doi.org/10.3389/fcimb.2022.909223.

Modell, W., & Garrett, M. (1960). Interactions between pharmacodynamic and placebo effects in drug evaluations in man. *Nature, 185*(4712), 538–539.

Moghadam, E., Yazdanian, M., Tahmasebi, E., Tebyanian, H., Ranjbar, R., Yazdanian, A., Seifalian, A., & Tafazoli, A. (2020). Current herbal medicine as an alternative treatment in dentistry: *In vitro, in vivo* and clinical studies. *European Journal of Pharmacology*, Article 173665. https://doi.org/10.1016/j.ejphar.2020.173665.

Mohammadi, Z., & Abbott, P. V. (2009). On the local applications of antibiotics and antibiotic-based agents in endodontics and dental traumatology. *International Endodontic Journal, 42*(7), 555–567. https://doi.org/10.1111/j.1365-2591.2009.01564.x.

Mokrzecki, S. M., Mallett, A., Sen Gupta, T., Perks, S., & Pain, T. (2023). Do educational interventions improve prescribing skills of medical students compared to no additional learning? A systematic review. *Medical Education Online, 28*(1), 2259166. https://doi.org/10.1080/10872981.2023.2259166.

Mombelli, A., & Samaranayake, L. (2004). Topical and systemic antibiotics in the management of periodontal diseases. *International dental journal*, 54 1, 3-14 . https://doi.org/10.1111/J.1875-595X.2004.TB00246.X.

Monette, P., & Schwartz, A. (2023). Optimizing medications with the Geriatrics 5Ms: An age-friendly approach. *Drugs & Aging*, 40, 391–396. https://doi.org/10.1007/s40266-023-01016-6.

Monteiro, C., Duarte, A., & Alves, G. (2020). Adverse drug reactions in elderly: A five-year review of spontaneous reports to the Portuguese pharmacovigilance system. *Expert Opinion on Drug Safety*, 20, 109–118. https://doi.org/10.1080/14740338.2020.1849137.

Monteiro, M., Tonelli, H., Reis, A., Casati, M., Silvério, K., Júnior, F., Sallum, E., & Casarin, R. (2020). Triclosan toothpaste as an adjunct therapy to plaque control in children from periodontitis families: A crossover clinical trial. *Clinical Oral Investigations, 24*, 1421–1430. https://doi.org/10.1007/s00784-019-03121-6.

Moore, P. A. (1999). Dental therapeutic indications for the newer long-acting macrolide antibiotics. *Journal of the American Dental Association, 130*(9), 1341–1343. https://doi.org/10.14219/jada.archive.1999.0404.

Moore, P. A., & Hersh, E. V. (2010). Local anesthetics: Pharmacology and toxicology. *Dental Clinics of North America*, 54(4), 587–599. https://doi.org/10.1016/j.cden.2010.06.001.

Moore, P. A., Ziegler, K. M., Lipman, R. D., Aminoshariae, A., Carrasco-Labra, A., & Mariotti, A. (2018). Benefits and harms associated with analgesic medications used in the management of acute dental pain: An overview of systematic reviews. *The Journal of the American Dental Association, 149*(4), 256-265.

Moore, R. (2022). Trusting the dentist—Expecting a leap of faith vs. a well-defined strategy for anxious patients. Dentistry Journal, 10(4), 66. https://doi.org/10.3390/dj10040066.

Mörch, C., Atsu, S., Cai, W., Li, X., Madathil, S., Liu, X., Mai, V., Tamimi, F., Dilhac, M., & Ducret, M. (2021). Artificial intelligence and ethics in dentistry: A scoping review. *Journal of Dental Research*, 100, 1452–1460. https://doi.org/10.1177/00220345211013808.

Moreno-Ligero, M., Moral-Munoz, J., Salazar, A., & Failde, I. (2023). Health intervention for improving pain, quality of life, and functional disability in patients with chronic pain: Systematic review. *JMIR mHealth and uHealth, 11*. https://doi.org/10.2196/40844.

Morgado-Sevillano, D., Rodríguez-Molinero, J., García-Bravo, C., Peña-Cardelles, J. F., Ruiz-Roca, J. A., García-Guerrero, I., & Gómez-de Diego, R. (2024). Oral surgery considerations in patients at high-risk of complications related to drug intake: A systematic review. *The Saudi Dental Journal, 36*(12), 1503–1508. https://doi.org/10.1016/j.sdentj.2024.12.004.

Morishita, K., Soutome, S., Otsuru, M., Hayashida, S., Murata, M., Sasaki, M., ... & Umeda, M. (2022). Relationship between drug holiday of the antiresorptive agents and surgical outcome of medication-related osteonecrosis of the jaw in osteoporosis patients. *Scientific Reports, 12*(1), 11545. https://doi.org/10.1038/s41598-022-15720-7.

Motov, S., Masoudi, A., Drapkin, J., Sotomayor, C., Kim, S., Butt, M., Likourezos, A., Fassassi, C., Hossain, R., Brady, J., Rothberger, N., Flom, P., & Marshall, J. (2019). Comparison of oral ibuprofen at three single-dose regimens for treating acute pain in the emergency department: A randomized controlled trial. *Annals of Emergency Medicine*. https://doi.org/10.1016/j.annemergmed.2019.05.037.

Moudgal, V., & Sobel, J. (2003). Antifungal drugs in pregnancy: A review. *Expert Opinion on Drug Safety*, 2(5), 475–483. https://doi.org/10.1517/14740338.2.5.475.

Mountziaris, P. M., Kramer, P. R., & Mikos, A. G. (2009). Emerging intra-articular drug delivery systems for the temporomandibular joint. *Methods, 47*(2), 134–140. https://doi.org/10.1016/j.ymeth.2008.09.001.

Moussa, R., Alghazaly, A., Althagafi, N., Eshky, R., & Borzangy, S. (2021). Effectiveness of virtual reality and interactive simulators on dental education outcomes: Systematic review. *European Journal of Dentistry*, 16, 14–31. https://doi.org/10.1055/s-0041-1731837.

Muanda, F., Sheehy, O., & Bérard, A. (2017). Use of antibiotics during pregnancy and the risk of major congenital malformations: A population based cohort study. *British Journal of Clinical Pharmacology, 83*, 2557–2571. https://doi.org/10.1111/bcp.13364.

Muanda, F., Sheehy, O., & Bérard, A. (2017). Use of antibiotics during pregnancy and the risk of major congenital malformations: A population based cohort study. *British Journal of Clinical Pharmacology*, 83, 2557–2571. https://doi.org/10.1111/bcp.13364.

Muhammad, H., Khan, B., Idrees, O., Irfan, S., Chishti, H., Tayyab, R., Alam, N., Bin, H., & Khan, T. (2025). Impact of Oral Hygiene Products on the Oral Microbiome and

Susceptibility to Thrush: A Narrative Review. *Journal of Medical & Health Sciences Review*. https://doi.org/10.62019/2n6bbp62.

Muhson, Z., & Al-Obaidi, W. (2024). Knowledge and behavior of a group of dentists towards antibiotic prescription to pediatric patients in Baghdad. *Mustansiria Dental Journal*, 19(1), 1–8. https://doi.org/10.32828/mdj.v19i1.990.

Muller, A. E., Mouton, J. W., Oostvogel, P. M., et al., (2010). Pharmacokinetics of clindamycin in pregnant women in the peripartum period. *Antimicrobial Agents and Chemotherapy, 54*(5), 2175–2181. https://doi.org/10.1128/AAC.01017-09.

Müller, M. (1983). Mode of action of metronidazole on anaerobic bacteria and protozoa. *Surgery, 93*(1 Pt 2), 165–171.

Munteanu, A., Holban, A., Pauna, M., Imre, M., Farcaşiu, A., & Farcaşiu, C. (2022). Review of Professionally Applied Fluorides for Preventing Dental Caries in Children and Adolescents. *Applied Sciences*. https://doi.org/10.3390/app12031054.

Murphy, A., Patel, U., Wilson, G., & Suda, K. (2024). Prevalence of unnecessary antibiotic prescriptions among dental visits, 2019. *Infection Control & Hospital Epidemiology*, 45, 890–899. https://doi.org/10.1017/ice.2024.13.

Musaimi, O., Lombardi, L., Williams, D., & Albericio, F. (2022). Strategies for improving peptide stability and delivery. *Pharmaceuticals, 15*. https://doi.org/10.3390/ph15101283.

Musale, G., & Naveriya, A. (2024). Overview of Ketamine Activity in General Anaesthesia. *International Journal of Advanced Research in Science, Communication and Technology*. https://doi.org/10.48175/ijarsct-22736.

Mustilwar, R., Shetti, A., Bhadange, S., Mani, A., Padmawar, D., & Vadvadgi, V. (2018). Management of medically compromised patients in dentistry – A review. International Journal of Scientific Research, 7(8), 1–3.

Muthu, K., Saravanan, D., Rethinam, S., Madeswaran, S., & Suresh, N. (2021). Appraising the Clinical Efficacy of Herbal Topical Medications in the Treatment of Recurrent Aphthous Stomatitis - A Review. *Journal of Young Pharmacists*. https://doi.org/10.5530/jyp.2021.13.87.

Nadig, K., & Taylor, N. G. (2018). Management of odontogenic infection at a district general hospital. *British Dental Journal, 224*(12), 962–966. https://doi.org/10.1038/sj.bdj.2018.445.

Naeem, F., & Naeem, S. (2025). Non-pharmacological behavior management techniques in pediatric dentistry: A narrative review. *Indus Journal of Bioscience Research*, 3(3), 905. https://doi.org/10.70749/ijbr.v3i3.905.

Naik, B., Kuck, K., Saager, L., Kheterpal, S., Domino, K., Posner, K., Sinha, A., Stuart, A., Brummett, C., Durieux, M., Vaughn, M., & Pace, N. (2021). Practice Patterns and Variability in Intraoperative Opioid Utilization: A Report From the Multicenter Perioperative Outcomes Group. *Anesthesia & Analgesia*, 134, 8 - 17. https://doi.org/10.1213/ANE.0000000000005663.

Nakajima, M., Tanner, E., Nakajima, N., Ibsen, K., & Mitragotri, S. (2021). Topical treatment of periodontitis using an iongel. *Biomaterials*, 276, 121069. https://doi.org/10.1016/j.biomaterials.2021.121069.

Naranjo, C. A., Busto, U., Sellers, E. M., Sandor, P., Ruiz, I., Roberts, E. A., ... & Greenblatt, D. J. (1981). A method for estimating the probability of adverse drug reactions. *Clinical Pharmacology & Therapeutics, 30*(2), 239–245.

Nashkova, S., Atanasova, S., & Toneva, V. (2017). Prevention and dental treatment of patients with epilepsy. *Journal of IMAB*, 20(3), 1945–1950. https://doi.org/10.5272/jimab.2017203.1945.

Naso, M. F., Tomkowicz, B., Perry, W. L., III, & Strohl, W. R. (2017). Adeno-associated virus (AAV) as a vector for gene therapy. *BioDrugs, 31*(4), 317–334.

Nateghi, M. R., Saremi, A., Abbasi, B., & Karimi, E. (2021). *Balancing Blood Pressure: Understanding Hemodynamic Fluctuations in Spinal Anesthesia.*

Naud, J., Michaud, J., Beauchemin, S., Hébert, M., Roger, M., Lefrancois, S., Leblond, F., & Pichette, V. (2011). Effects of chronic renal failure on kidney drug transporters and cytochrome P450 in rats. *Drug Metabolism and Disposition*, 39, 1363–1369. https://doi.org/10.1124/dmd.111.039115.

Navabi, N., Afshari, Z., Kamyabi, H., & Mohammadi, M. (2023). Side effects and short effects of using three common mouthwashes on oral health and quality of life: A quasi-experimental study. *International Journal of Dental Hygiene, 21*(2), 123–134. https://doi.org/10.1111/idh.12761

Navarro, J., & Monsan, P. (1976). Studies on the mechanism of interaction of glutaraldehyde with microorganisms (author's transl). *Annales de Microbiologie, 127B*(3), 295–307.

Nayak-Rao, S. (2010). Aminoglycoside use in renal failure. *Indian Journal of Nephrology*, 20(3), 121–124. https://doi.org/10.4103/0971-4065.70839.

Nazar, S., Dave, M., & Barry, S. (2023). Antibiotic prescription practices among dentists treating children in the UK. *Faculty Dental Journal*, 14(2), 22–27. https://doi.org/10.1308/rcsfdj.2023.22.

Needleman, I., Nibali, L., & Di Iorio, A. (2015). Professional mechanical plaque removal for prevention of periodontal diseases in adults–systematic review update. *Journal of Clinical Periodontology, 42*, S12–S35. https://doi.org/10.1111/jcpe.12341.

Needleman, I., Suvan, J., Moles, D. R., & Pimlott, J. (2005). A systematic review of professional mechanical plaque removal for prevention of periodontal diseases. *Journal of Clinical Periodontology, 32*, 229–282. https://doi.org/10.1111/J.1600-051X.2005.00804.X.

Neininger, M., Jeschke, S., Kiesel, L., Bertsche, T., & Bertsche, A. (2021). Physicians' perspectives on adverse drug reactions in pediatric routine care: A survey. *World Journal of Pediatrics*, 18, 50–58. https://doi.org/10.1007/s12519-021-00478-1.

Neves, J., Notario-Pérez, F., & Sarmento, B. (2021). Women-specific routes of administration for drugs: A critical overview. *Advanced Drug Delivery Reviews*, 113865. https://doi.org/10.1016/j.addr.2021.113865.

Neville, B. W., Damm, D. D., Allen, C. M., & Bouquot, J. E. (2002). *Oral and maxillofacial pathology* (2nd ed.). W. B. Saunders.

Newman, H. N. (1998). The rationale for chemical adjuncts in plaque control. *International Dental Journal, 48*(S3), 298–304. https://doi.org/10.1111/J.1875-595X.1998.TB00720.X.

Ngcobo, N. (2025). Influence of ageing on the pharmacodynamics and pharmacokinetics of chronically administered medicines in geriatric patients: A review. Clinical Pharmacokinetics, 64, 335–367. https://doi.org/10.1007/s40262-024-01466-0.

Ngeow, W. C., & Lim, D. (2016). Do corticosteroids still have a role in the management of third molar surgery? *Advances in Therapy, 33*(7), 1105–1139. https://doi.org/10.1007/s12325-016-0357-y.

Nguyen, F., Starosta, A., Arenz, S., Sohmen, D., Dönhöfer, A., & Wilson, D. (2014). Tetracycline antibiotics and resistance mechanisms. *Biological Chemistry, 395*, 559–575. https://doi.org/10.1515/hsz-2013-0292.

Niebyl, J. (2003). Antibiotics and Other Anti-infective Agents in Pregnancy and Lactation. *American Journal of Perinatology*, 20, 405 - 414. https://doi.org/10.1055/s-2003-45391.

Nielsen, K., Jakobsen, K., Jensen, J., Grønhøj, C., & Von Buchwald, C. (2021). The effect of prophylactic HPV vaccines on oral and oropharyngeal HPV infection—A systematic review. *Viruses*, 13(7), 1339. https://doi.org/10.3390/v13071339.

Nielsen, R. P., Nikolajsen, L., Paltved, C., & Aagaard, R. (2021). Effect of simulation-based team training in airway management: A systematic review. *Anaesthesia, 76*(10), 1404–1415.

Nikolishyna, E., Marchenko, A., Ilenko, N., & Lytovchenko, I. (2020). Local treatment of chronic candidiasis stomatitis. *Ukrainian Journal of Medicine, Biology and Sports*, 5(2), 121–125. https://doi.org/10.26693/jmbs05.02.121.

Niu, J., Straubinger, R. M., & Mager, D. E. (2019). Pharmacodynamic drug–drug interactions. *Clinical Pharmacology & Therapeutics, 105*(6), 1395–1406.

Niu, J., Yin, I., Mei, M., Wu, W., Li, Q., & Chu, C. (2021). The multifaceted roles of antimicrobial peptides in oral diseases. *Molecular Oral Microbiology*. https://doi.org/10.1111/omi.12333.

Niu, J., Yin, I., Wu, W., Li, Q., Mei, M., & Chu, C. (2020). Antimicrobial peptides for the prevention and treatment of dental caries: A concise review. *Archives of Oral Biology, 122*, 105022. https://doi.org/10.1016/j.archoralbio.2020.105022.

Noor, N., Legendre, R., Cloutet, A., Chitneni, A., Varrassi, G., & Kaye, A. (2021). A comprehensive review of remimazolam for sedation. *Health psychology research*, 9 1, 24514 . https://doi.org/10.52965/001c.24514.

Nørgaard, M., Pedersen, L., Gislum, M., et al., (2008). Maternal use of fluconazole and risk of congenital malformations: A Danish population-based cohort study. *Journal of Antimicrobial Chemotherapy*, 62(1), 172–176. https://doi.org/10.1093/jac/dkn157.

Nunge, R., Kendle, A., & Alwan, S. (2025). Pain medication use during pregnancy. *Seminars in Perinatology*, 49, 152074. https://doi.org/10.1016/j.semperi.2025.152074.

O'Mahony, D., Cherubini, A., Guiteras, A., Denkinger, M., Beuscart, J., Onder, G., Gudmundsson, A., Cruz-Jentoft, A., Knol, W., Bahat, G., Van Der Velde, N., Petrovic, M., & Curtin, D. (2023). STOPP/START criteria for potentially inappropriate prescribing in older people: Version 3. *European Geriatric Medicine*, 14, 625–632. https://doi.org/10.1007/s41999-023-00777-y.

Oberoi, S. S., Dhingra, C., Sharma, G., & Sardana, D. (2015). Antibiotics in dental practice: How justified are we? *International Dental Journal, 65*, 4–10.

Odubanjo, O., Tipping, B., & Greenstein, L. (2024). Medication adherence in geriatric patients attending medical outpatient department. *South African Family Practice,* 66(1), e6011. https://doi.org/10.4102/safp.v66i1.6011.

Ofori, B., Oraichi, D., Blais, L., et al., (2006). Risk of congenital anomalies in pregnant users of nonsteroidal anti-inflammatory drugs: A nested case-control study. Birth Defects Research Part B: Developmental and Reproductive Toxicology, 77(4), 268–279. https://doi.org/10.1002/bdrb.20090.

Ogunbona, F. A., Smith, I. F., & Olawoye, O. S. (1985). Fat contents of meals and bioavailability of griseofulvin in man. *Journal of Pharmacy and Pharmacology, 37*(4), 283–284.

Okumus, M., Elcim, O., Surmelioglu, O., Ceceli, E., Tuncay, F., & Borman, P. (2012). AB1227 The comparative efficacy of physiotherapy, injection and pharmacotherapy in patients with temporomandibular joint dysfunction. *Annals of the Rheumatic Diseases, 71*, 708. https://doi.org/10.1136/ANNRHEUMDIS-2012-EULAR.1225.

Okunev, I., Frantsve-Hawley, J., & Tranby, E. (2021). *Trends in national opioid prescribing for dental procedures among Medicaid patients.* https://doi.org/10.1101/2021.04.12.21255158.

Olivares-Morales, A., Hatley, O. J., Turner, D., Galetin, A., Aarons, L., & Rostami-Hodjegan, A. (2014). The use of ROC analysis for the qualitative prediction of human oral bioavailability from animal data. *Pharmaceutical Research, 31*, 720–730.

Omori, K., Otsuru, M., Morishita, K., Hayashida, S., Suyama, K., Naruse, T., ... & Umeda, M. (2022). Ineffectiveness of antiresorptive agent drug holidays in osteoporosis patients for treatment of medication-related osteonecrosis of the jaw: Consideration from immunohistological observation of osteoclast suppression and treatment outcomes. *International Journal of Environmental Research and Public Health, 19*(17), 10898. https://doi.org/10.3390/ijerph191710898.

Onemu, S., Odeyemi, O., Adu, M., & Obeagu, M. (2023). Efficacy assessment of some commonly used disinfectants against multidrug resistant bacterial isolates from a tertiary healthcare facility in Benin City, Nigeria. *Newport International Journal of Scientific and Experimental Sciences, 10*(7), 1000. https://doi.org/10.59298/nijses/2023/10.7.1000.

Oo, M., Oo, P., & Saddki, N. (2022). The efficacy of 0.05% cetylpyridinium chloride mouthwash as an adjunct to toothbrushing compared with 0.12% chlorhexidine gluconate mouthwash in reducing dental plaque and gingival inflammation: A randomized control trial. *International Journal of Dental Hygiene, 20*(2), 123–130. https://doi.org/10.1111/idh.12614.

Osborne, L., Leistikow, N., & Rocha, R. (2020). FDA rules for pregnancy and lactation labeling and their clinical implications. In Principles and Practice of Pharmaceutical Medicine (pp. 397–404). https://doi.org/10.1007/978-3-030-29081-8_26.

Ottesen, C., Schiodt, M., & Gotfredsen, K. (2020). Efficacy of a high-dose antiresorptive drug holiday to reduce the risk of medication-related osteonecrosis of the jaw (MRONJ): A systematic review. *Heliyon, 6*(4), e03795.

Ottesen, C., Schiodt, M., Jensen, S. S., Kofod, T., & Gotfredsen, K. (2022). Tooth extractions in patients with cancer receiving high-dose antiresorptive medication: A randomized clinical feasibility trial of drug holiday versus drug continuation. *Oral*

Surgery, Oral Medicine, Oral Pathology and Oral Radiology, 133(2), 165–173. https://doi.org/10.1016/j.oooo.2021.06.003.

Ouanounou, A., Goldberg, M., & Haas, D. A. (2017). Pharmacotherapy in temporomandibular disorders: A review. *Journal of the Canadian Dental Association, 83*(7), 1–8.

Ouanounou, A., Ng, K., & Chaban, P. (2020). Adverse drug reactions in dentistry. *International Dental Journal*, 70(6), 385–393. https://doi.org/10.1111/idj.12540.

Owens, R., & Ambrose, P. (2002). Torsades de pointes associated with fluoroquinolones. *Pharmacotherapy: The Journal of Human Pharmacology and Drug Therapy, 22*, 663–668. https://doi.org/10.1592/phco.22.8.663.33201.

Ozcan, G., Aykac, E., Kasap, Y., Nemutlu, N. T., Sen, E., & Aydinkarahaliloglu, N. D. (2016). Adverse drug reaction reporting pattern in Turkey: Analysis of the national database in the context of the first pharmacovigilance legislation. *Drugs-Real World Outcomes, 3*, 33–43.

Özdemir Kabalak, M., Aytac, E. N., Tarhan, N., Karabulut, E., & Keceli, H. G. (2024). Potential barriers to the rational antibiotic use in dental and periodontal practice: A questionnaire-based online survey. *Dental and Medical Problems, 61*(3), 373–383.

Page, A., Clifford, R., Potter, K., Schwartz, D., & Etherton-Beer, C. (2016). The feasibility and effect of deprescribing in older adults on mortality and health: A systematic review and meta-analysis. *British Journal of Clinical Pharmacology*, 82(3), 583–623. https://doi.org/10.1111/bcp.12975.

Painter, W., Robertson, A., Trost, L., Godkin, S., Lampert, B., & Painter, G. (2012). First pharmacokinetic and safety study in humans of the novel lipid antiviral conjugate CMX001, a broad-spectrum oral drug active against double-stranded DNA viruses. *Antimicrobial Agents and Chemotherapy*, 56(5), 2726–2734. https://doi.org/10.1128/AAC.05983-11.

Pais, G., Chang, J., Barreto, E., Stitt, G., Downes, K., Alshaer, M., Lesnicki, E., Panchal, V., Bruzzone, M., Bumanglag, A., Burke, S., & Scheetz, M. (2022). Clinical pharmacokinetics and pharmacodynamics of cefepime. *Clinical Pharmacokinetics, 61*, 929–953. https://doi.org/10.1007/s40262-022-01137-y.

Palmer, S., Tendal, B., Mustafa, R., Vandvik, P., Li, S., Hao, Q., Tunnicliffe, D., Ruospo, M., Natale, P., Saglimbene, V., Nicolucci, A., Johnson, D., Tonelli, M., Rossi, M., Badve, S., Cho, Y., Nadeau-Fredette, A., Burke, M., Faruque, L., Lloyd, A., Ahmad, N., Liu, Y., Tiv, S., Millard, T., Gagliardi, L., Kolanu, N., Barmanray, R., McMorrow, R., Cortez, A., White, H., Chen, X., Zhou, X., Liu, J., Rodríguez, A., González-Colmenero, A., Wang, Y., Li, L., Sutanto, S., Solis, R., González-Colmenero, F., Rodríguez-Gutiérrez, R., Walsh, M., Guyatt, G., & Strippoli, G. (2021). Sodium-glucose cotransporter protein-2 (SGLT-2) inhibitors and glucagon-like peptide-1 (GLP-1) receptor agonists for type 2 diabetes: Systematic review and network meta-analysis of randomised controlled trials. *BMJ*, 372, m4573. https://doi.org/10.1136/bmj.m4573.

Pan, J., Wang, Y., Qian, Y., Zou, J., & Zhang, Q. (2023). Comparison of dental anesthetic efficacy between the periodontal intraligamentary anesthesia and other infiltration anesthesia: a systematic review and meta-analysis. *PeerJ*, 11. https://doi.org/10.7717/peerj.15734.

Panat, S. R., Upadhyay, N., Khan, M., & Iqubal, M. A. (2014). Corticosteroids used in dentistry: An update. *Journal of Dental Sciences and Oral Rehabilitation, 5*, 8992.

Panchal, N., & Sabina, E. (2023). Non-steroidal anti-inflammatory drugs (NSAIDs): A current insight into its molecular mechanism eliciting organ toxicities. *Food and Chemical Toxicology, 172*, 113598. https://doi.org/10.1016/j.fct.2022.113598.

Parekh, S., Gardener, C., Ashley, P., & Walsh, T. (2014). Intraoperative local anaesthesia for reduction of postoperative pain following general anaesthesia for dental treatment in children and adolescents.. *The Cochrane database of systematic reviews*, 12, CD009742 . https://doi.org/10.1002/14651858.CD009742.pub2.

Parhizkar, P., Schmidlin, P., Bornstein, M., & Fakheran, O. (2022). Can adjunctive corticosteroid therapy improve patient-centered outcomes following third molar surgery? A systematic review. *Medicina Oral, Patología Oral y Cirugía Bucal, 27*, e410–e418. https://doi.org/10.4317/medoral.25177.

Parirokh, M., Saffarzadeh, A., Nakhaei, N., & Abbott, P. (2023). The outcome of prescribing antibiotics for the management of patients with endodontic infections. *European Endodontic Journal, 8*(3), 194. https://doi.org/10.14744/eej.2023.39306.

Patel, M. (2022). Oral cavity and *Candida albicans*: Colonisation to the development of infection. *Pathogens, 11*(3), 335. https://doi.org/10.3390/pathogens11030335.

Pathan, H., & Williams, J. (2012). Basic opioid pharmacology: An update. *British Journal of Pain, 6*(1), 11–16. https://doi.org/10.1177/2049463712438493.

Patini, R. (2020). Personalized dentistry: Approaching a new way for diagnosis and treatment of oral diseases. *Journal of Personalized Medicine*, 10(2), 35. https://doi.org/10.3390/jpm10020035.

Patočka, J., Wu, W., Olekšák, P., Jelinkova, R., Nepovimova, E., Spicanova, L., Springerová, P., Alomar, S., Long, M., & Kuča, K. (2024). Fentanyl and its derivatives: Pain-killers or man-killers?. *Heliyon*, 10. https://doi.org/10.1016/j.heliyon.2024.e28795.

Pattyn, J., Hendrickx, G., Vorsters, A., & Van Damme, P. (2021). Hepatitis B vaccines. *The Journal of Infectious Diseases*, 224(Suppl 5), S343–S351. https://doi.org/10.1093/infdis/jiaa668.

Paulraj, S., & Lakshmanan, M. (2021). General Anesthetics. *Introduction to Basics of Pharmacology and Toxicology*. https://doi.org/10.1007/978-981-33-6009-9_8.

Pazan, F., Weiss, C., Wehling, M., & FORTA Group. (2019). The FORTA (Fit fOR The Aged) List 2018: Third version of a validated clinical tool for improved drug treatment in older people. Drugs & Aging, 36, 481–484. https://doi.org/10.1007/s40266-019-00669-6

Peedikayil, F. C. (2016). Antibiotics in odontogenic infections—an update. *J Antimicro, 2*(117), 2472–1212.

Pei, J., Gao, X., Pan, D., Hua, Y., He, J., Liu, Z., & Dang, Y. (2022). Advances in the stability challenges of bioactive peptides and improvement strategies. *Current Research in Food Science, 5*, 2162–2170. https://doi.org/10.1016/j.crfs.2022.10.031.

Penlington, C., Bowes, C., Taylor, G., Otemade, A., Waterhouse, P., Durham, J., & Ohrbach, R. (2022). Psychological therapies for temporomandibular disorders (TMDs). *The Cochrane Database of Systematic Reviews, 8*, CD013515. https://doi.org/10.1002/14651858.CD013515.pub2.

Peppa, M., Krania, M., & Raptis, S. A. (2011). Hypertension and other morbidities with Cushing's syndrome associated with corticosteroids: A review. *Integrated Blood Pressure Control, 4*, 7–16. https://doi.org/10.2147/IBPC.S9486.

Perazella, M. (2009). Renal vulnerability to drug toxicity. *Clinical Journal of the American Society of Nephrology*, 4(7), 1275–1283. https://doi.org/10.2215/CJN.02050309.

Pergolizzi, J. V., Magnusson, P., LeQuang, J. A., Gharibo, C., & Varrassi, G. (2020). The pharmacological management of dental pain. *Expert Opinion on Pharmacotherapy, 21*(5), 591-601.

Perrin, S., Bull, C., Rowe, R., & Black, S. (2022). Local anaesthetic drugs. Anaesthesia & Intensive Care Medicine. https://doi.org/10.1016/j.mpaic.2022.10.012.

Petricas, A., Medvedev, D., & Olkhovskaya, E. (2016). [Classification of local anesthesia methods]. Stomatologiia, 95 4, 4-8. https://doi.org/10.17116/stomat20169544-9.

Petrovic, M., Cammen, T., & Onder, G. (2012). Adverse drug reactions in older people. *Drugs & Aging*, 29, 453–462. https://doi.org/10.2165/11631760-000000000-00000.

Pfizer. (2007). Vibramycin (prescribing information). New York, NY: Pfizer.

Pfizer. (2011). Zithromax (prescribing information). New York, NY: Pfizer.

Pichai, E., & Lakshmanan, M. (2019). Drug Elimination. *Introduction to Basics of Pharmacology and Toxicology*. https://doi.org/10.1007/978-981-32-9779-1_8.

Piekoszewska-Ziętek, P. (2022). The use of antibiotics in paediatric dentistry: A revision of current recommendations. *The Journal of Dentists*. https://doi.org/10.12974/2311-8695.2022.10.2.

Pieper, P. (2015). Use of medication for cardiovascular disease during pregnancy. Nature Reviews Cardiology, 12, 718–729. https://doi.org/10.1038/nrcardio.2015.172

Pierce, R. C., & Kalivas, P. W. (1997). A circuitry model of the expression of behavioral sensitization to amphetamine-like psychostimulants. *Brain Research Reviews, 25*(2), 192–216.

Pieri, M., Ursoleo, D., Di Prima, A., Bugo, S., Barucco, G., Licheri, M., Losiggio, R., Frau, G., & Monaco, F. (2024). Remimazolam for anesthesia and sedation in pediatric patients: a scoping review. *Journal of anesthesia*. https://doi.org/10.1007/s00540-024-03358-w.

Pigò, F., Gottin, M., & Conigliaro, R. (2025). The Incidence of Adverse Events in Adults Undergoing Procedural Sedation with Propofol Administered by Non-Anesthetists: A Systematic Review and Meta-Analysis. *Diagnostics*, 15. https://doi.org/10.3390/diagnostics15101234.

Pilgrim, R., Kwok, M., May, A., Chapman, S., & Jones, M. (2025). The effect of medication use on breastfeeding continuation: A systematic review with narrative synthesis. *International Breastfeeding Journal*, 20, 756. https://doi.org/10.1186/s13006-025-00756-y.

Pillai, S., Johnson, L., & Bagde, H. (2023). Chlorhexidine mouthwash in dentistry. *Journal of Nursing Research, Patient Safety and Practise, 33*(24), 29. https://doi.org/10.55529/jnrpsp.33.24.29.

Pilmis, B., Jullien, V., Sobel, J., Lecuit, M., Lortholary, O., & Charlier, C. (2015). Antifungal drugs during pregnancy: An updated review. *Journal of Antimicrobial Chemotherapy*, 70(1), 14–22. https://doi.org/10.1093/jac/dku355.

Pinto, N., & Dolan, M. E. (2011). Clinically relevant genetic variations in drug metabolizing enzymes. *Current Drug Metabolism, 12*(5), 487–497.

Pintye, A., Bacsó, R., & Kovács, G. (2024). Trans-kingdom fungal pathogens infecting both plants and humans, and the problem of azole fungicide resistance. *Frontiers in Microbiology, 15*, 1354757. https://doi.org/10.3389/fmicb.2024.1354757.

Piper, J. M., Baum, C., & Kennedy, D. L. (1987). Prescription drug use before and during pregnancy in a Medicaid population. *American Journal of Obstetrics and Gynecology*, 157(1), 148–156. https://doi.org/10.1016/S0002-9378(87)80097-1.

Pitman, S., Hoang, U., Wi, C., Alsheikh, M., Hiner, D., & Percival, K. (2019). Revisiting oral fluoroquinolone and multivalent cation drug-drug interactions: Are they still relevant? *Antibiotics, 8*, Article 108. https://doi.org/10.3390/antibiotics8030108.

Pitoy, A., Wowor, V., & Leman, M. (2021). Efektivitas dental health education menggunakan media audio visual dalam meningkatkan pengetahuan siswa sekolah dasar. e-GiGi, 9(2), 49–54. https://doi.org/10.35790/EG.V9I2.34903.

Polizzi, A., Donzella, M., Nicolosi, G., Santonocito, S., Pesce, P., & Isola, G. (2022). Drugs for the quorum sensing inhibition of oral biofilm: New frontiers and insights in the treatment of periodontitis. Pharmaceutics, 14. https://doi.org/10.3390/pharmaceutics14122740.

Polk, R. (1989). Drug-drug interactions with ciprofloxacin and other fluoroquinolones. *The American Journal of Medicine, 87*(5A), 76S–81S. https://doi.org/10.1016/0002-9343(89)90028-4.

Porreca, F., & Navratilova, E. (2017). Reward, motivation, and emotion of pain and its relief. *Pain, 158*, S43-S49.

Porter, R. S. (n.d.). *The Merck Manual Home Health Handbook for Patients and Caregivers: Drug use during pregnancy*. Retrieved June 8, 2012, from www.merck manuals.com/home/womens_health_issues/drug_use_during_pregnancy/drug_use_d uring_pregnancy.html#v810071.

Powell, K., Baltimore, R., Bernstein, H., Bocchini, J., Bradley, J., Brady, M., Dennehy, P., Frenck, R., Kimberlin, D., Long, S., Mcmillan, J., Rubin, L., Baker, C., Hall, C., Meissner, H., Rennels, M., & Saari, T. (2006). The use of systemic fluoroquinolones. *Pediatrics, 118*, 1287–1292. https://doi.org/10.1542/peds.2006-1722.

Practice Guidelines for Moderate Procedural Sedation and Analgesia 2018: A report by the American Society of Anesthesiologists Task Force on Moderate Procedural Sedation and Analgesia, the American Association of Oral and Maxillofacial Surgeons, American College of Radiology, American Dental Association, American Society of Dentist Anesthesiologists, and Society of Interventional Radiology. (2018). *Anesthesiology, 128*(3), 437–479. https://doi.org/10.1097/ALN.0000000000002043.

Prashar, A., Locke, I. C., & Evans, C. S. (2006). Cytotoxicity of clove (*Syzygium aromaticum*) oil and its major components to human skin cells. *Cell Proliferation, 39*(4), 241–248.

Prathoshini, M., Kumar, J., & Ramanathan, V. (2020). Management of recurrent apthous ulcer using Corticosteroids, Local anesthetics and nutritional supplements. *Bioinformation*, 16, 992 - 998. https://doi.org/10.6026/97320630016992.

Prescott, L. F., Balali-Mood, M., Critchley, J. A., Johnstone, A. F., & Proudfoot, A. (1982). Diuresis or urinary alkalinisation for salicylate poisoning? *BMJ (Clinical Research Ed.), 285*(6352), 1383–1386.

Preshaw, P. M., Alba, A. L., Herrera, D., Jepsen, S., Konstantinidis, A., Makrilakis, K., & Taylor, R. (2012). Periodontitis and diabetes: A two-way relationship. *Diabetologia*, 55(1), 21–31. https://doi.org/10.1007/s00125-011-2342-y.

Preshaw, P., Hefti, A., Jepsen, S., Etienne, D., Walker, C., & Bradshaw, M. (2004). Subantimicrobial dose doxycycline as adjunctive treatment for periodontitis: A review. *Journal of Clinical Periodontology, 31*(9), 697–707. https://doi.org/10.1111/J.1600-051X.2004.00558.X.

Prince, R., & Villar, L. (1983). Side-effect profiles of newer-generation cephalosporins. *Drug Intelligence & Clinical Pharmacy, 17*, 656–657. https://doi.org/10.1177/106002808301700917.

Proctor, R., Kumar, N., Stein, A., Moles, D., & Porter, S. (2005). Oral and dental aspects of chronic renal failure. Journal of Dental Research, 84(3), 199–208. https://doi.org/10.1177/154405910508400301.

Proudfoot, A. T., Krenzelok, E. P., Vale, J. A., Bradberry, S. M., Harrison, W., & Watt, B. E. (2002). AACT/EAPCCT position paper on urine alkalinization. *Journal of Toxicology. Clinical Toxicology, 40*, 310–312.

Pudakalkatti, P., Baheti, A., Hattarki, S., & Kambali, S. (2017). Personalized medicine in dentistry. *Journal of Orofacial Sciences*, 9(1), 3–6. https://doi.org/10.4103/0975-8844.164307.

Pulate, A., Shendge, R., Pandit, S., Sonyabapu, P., S., & V. (2021). *Design and development of clindamycin film for periodontal disease.*

Punnapurath, S., Vijayakumar, P., Platty, P., Krishna, S., & Thomas, T. (2021). A study of medication compliance in geriatric patients with chronic illness. *Journal of Family Medicine and Primary Care*, 10, 1644–1648. https://doi.org/10.4103/jfmpc.jfmpc_1302_20.

Pyle, M., & Tolbert, S. (1994). Pharmacologic considerations in geriatric dentistry. *Dental Clinics of North America*, 38(4), 755–767. https://doi.org/10.1016/s0011-8532(22)00188-4.

Qadir, M., Bashir, H., & Ahmad, M. (2023). Human oropharyngeal candidiasis: From etiology to current treatment. *Critical Reviews in Immunology, 43*(3), 15–24. https://doi.org/10.1615/critrevimmunol.2023049730.

Qian, L., Chen, L., & Lin, Y. (2024). Rapid alleviation of perioperative airway obstruction through positional adjustments in a patient with a giant anterior mediastinal mass: A case report. *Medicine: Case Reports and Study Protocols*. https://doi.org/10.1097/md9.0000000000000335.

Qiao-Ling, H. (2007). Overview on toxicological research on iodophors. *Chinese Journal of Veterinary Drug, 41*(2), 123–130.

Qiu, Y., Xu, J., Xu, Y., Shi, Z., Wang, Y., Zhang, L., & Fu, B. (2023). Disinfection efficacy of sodium hypochlorite and glutaraldehyde and their effects on the dimensional stability and surface properties of dental impressions: A systematic review. *PeerJ, 11*, e14868. https://doi.org/10.7717/peerj.14868.

Quick, J. D., Hogerzeil, H. V., Rankin, J. R., Dukes, M. N. G., Laing, R., Garnett, A., O'Connor, R. W., Health, M. S. for, & Drugs, W. A. P. on E. (1997). *Managing drug supply: The selection, procurement, distribution, and use of pharmaceuticals*. Kumarian Press. https://iris.who.int/handle/10665/41908.

Radu, C., Radu, C., Bochiş, S., Arbănaşi, E., Lucan, A., Murvai, V., & Zaha, D. (2023). Revisiting the therapeutic effects of essential oils on the oral microbiome. *Pharmacy, 11*(1), Article 33. https://doi.org/10.3390/pharmacy11010033.

Rahman, M., Abdullah-Al-Shoeb, M., Huq, S., & Azad, M. (2019). Assessment of antibacterial efficacy of Lugol's iodine compared with commercial hand sanitizers of Bangladesh. *Journal of World's Poultry Research, 9*(2), 123–130. https://doi.org/10.36380/scil.2019.jlsb21.

Rajadurai, S., Maharajan, M., Veettil, S., & Gopinath, D. (2021). Comparative efficacy of antifungal agents used in the treatment of oropharyngeal candidiasis among HIV-infected adults: A systematic review and network meta-analysis. *Journal of Fungi, 7*(8), 637. https://doi.org/10.3390/jof7080637.

Ralph, E., Clarke, J., Libke, R., Luthy, R., & Kirby, W. (1974). Pharmacokinetics of metronidazole as determined by bioassay. *Antimicrobial Agents and Chemotherapy, 6*, 691–696. https://doi.org/10.1128/AAC.6.6.691.

Ramanauskaite, E., Sakalauskaitė, U., & Machiulskiene, V. (2020). The efficacy of adjunctive aids in periodontal maintenance therapy: A systematic literature review and meta-analysis. *Oral Health & Preventive Dentistry, 18*. https://doi.org/10.3290/j.ohpd.a45406.

Ramanathan, R., Lee, J., Dalton, J., Lin, R., Lee, I., Gonzalez, C., Shaw, J., Schroeder, G., Kepler, C., Spitnale, M., Vaccaro, A., Gabrielli, A., & Wawrose, R. (2025). GLP-1 receptor agonists in orthopaedic surgery: Implications for perioperative care and outcomes. *The Journal of Bone and Joint Surgery. American Volume*, *107*, 1879–1886. https://doi.org/10.2106/jbjs.24.01287

Ramussen, J. C. (1976). Erythema multiforme in children. Response to treatment with systemic steroids. *British Journal of Dermatology, 95*, 181-186.

Rana, M., Bonasera, L., & Bordelon, G. (2017). Pharmacologic Considerations of Anesthetic Agents in Geriatric Patients. *Anesthesiology clinics*, 35 2, 259-271. https://doi.org/10.1016/j.anclin.2017.01.011.

Randall, C., & Dhar, V. (2023). Pediatric dentists' use of nonpharmacological behavior guidance techniques and experiences with parent/caregiver acceptance: A national survey. *Pediatric Dentistry, 45*(5), 418–424.

Rasool, G. (2019). Emerging trends in dentistry. Journal of Khyber College of Dentistry, 9(4). https://doi.org/10.33279/jkcd.v9i04.448.

Rautamo, M., Kvarnström, K., Sivén, M., Airaksinen, M., Lahdenne, P., & Sandler, N. (2020). A focus group study about oral drug administration practices at hospital wards—Aspects to consider in drug development of age-appropriate formulations for children. *Pharmaceutics, 12*(2), Article 119. https://doi.org/10.3390/pharmaceutics12020109.

Reda, B., Dudek, J., Martínez-Hernández, M., & Hannig, M. (2021). Effects of octenidine on the formation and disruption of dental biofilms: An exploratory in situ study in healthy subjects. *Journal of Dental Research, 100*, 950–959. https://doi.org/10.1177/0022034521999044.

Reddy, M., Shetty, S., & Vannala, V. (2019). Embracing personalized medicine in dentistry. *Journal of Pharmacy & Bioallied Sciences*, 11(Suppl 2), S92–S96. https://doi.org/10.4103/JPBS.JPBS_297_18.

Reeve, J., Maden, M., Hill, R., Turk, A., Mahtani, K., Wong, G., Lasserson, D., Krska, J., Mangin, D., Byng, R., Wallace, E., & Ranson, E. (2022). Deprescribing medicines in older people living with multimorbidity and polypharmacy: The TAILOR evidence synthesis. *Health Technology Assessment, 26*(32), 1–148. https://doi.org/10.3310/AAFO2475.

Refaey, M. S., Abosalem, E. F., El-Basyouni, R. Y., Elsheriri, S. E., Elbehary, S. H., & Fayed, M. A. (2024). Exploring the therapeutic potential of medicinal plants and their active principles in dental care: A comprehensive review. Heliyon, 10(18). https://doi.org/10.1016/j.heliyon.2024.e37641.

Reidenberg, M. M. (2011). Drug discontinuation effects are part of the pharmacology of a drug. *Journal of Pharmacology and Experimental Therapeutics, 339*(2), 324–328.

Rekatsina, M., Paladini, A., Myrcik, D., Viswanath, O., Urits, I., Pergolizzi, J., Breve, F., & Varrassi, G. (2021). Opioids in the elderly patients with cognitive impairment: A narrative review. *Pain and Therapy, 11*, 381–394. https://doi.org/10.1007/s40122-022-00376-y.

Renton, T. (2011). Dental (odontogenic) pain. *Reviews in Pain, 5*(1), 2–7. https://doi.org/10.1177/204946371100500102.

Reuss-Lamky, H. (2007). Administering dental nerve blocks.. *Journal of the American Animal Hospital Association,* 43 5, 298-305 . https://doi.org/10.5326/0430298.

Richard, P., Autret, E., Bardol, J., et al., (1991). The use of flumazenil in a neonate. *Journal of Toxicology: Clinical Toxicology, 29*(1), 137–140.

Rieken, S. E., & Terezhalmy, G. T. (2006). The pregnant and breastfeeding patient. *Quintessence International, 37*(6), 455–468.

Rim, H. S., Byun, J. Y., Kim, S. H., & Yeo, S. G. (2023). Optimal Bell's palsy treatment: Steroids, antivirals, and a timely and personalized approach. *Journal of Clinical Medicine, 13*(1), 51.

Rindal, D., Gryczynski, J., Asche, S., Truitt, A., Kane, S., Worley, D., & Mitchell, S. (2023). De-implementing opioid prescribing in a dental group practice: Lessons learned. *Community Dentistry and Oral Epidemiology*, 51(2), 123–130. https://doi.org/10.1111/cdoe.12820.

Rissanen, A., & Rissanen, M. (2023). *Health informatics and patient safety in pharmacotherapy* (pp. 366–374). https://doi.org/10.1007/978-981-99-7108-4_31.

Rivetti, S., Romano, A., Mastrangelo, S., Attina,' G., Maurizi, P., & Ruggiero, A. (2023). Aminoglycosides-related ototoxicity: Mechanisms, risk factors, and prevention in pediatric patients. *Pharmaceuticals, 16*, Article 1353. https://doi.org/10.3390/ph16101353.

Robertson, D. (2017). First pass metabolism. *Nurse Prescribing, 15*, 303–305. https://doi.org/10.12968/npre.2017.15.6.303.

Roden, D. M., Wilke, R. A., Kroemer, H. K., & Stein, C. M. (2011). Pharmacogenomics: The genetics of variable drug responses. *Circulation, 123*(15), 1661–1670.

Rodríguez-Fernández, A., Vázquez-Cancela, O., Piñeiro-Lamas, M., Herdeiro, M. T., Figueiras, A., & Zapata-Cachafeiro, M. (2023). Magnitude and determinants of inappropriate prescribing of antibiotics in dentistry: A nation-wide study. *Antimicrobial Resistance and Infection Control, 12*(1), 20. https://doi.org/10.1186/s13756-023-01225-z.

Roganović, J., & Barać, M. (2024). Rational antibiotic prescribing is underpinned by dental ethics principles: Survey on postgraduate and undergraduate dental students' perceptions. *Antibiotics, 13*(5), 460. https://doi.org/10.3390/antibiotics13050460.

Rokaya, D., Jaghsi, A., Jagtap, R., & Srimaneepong, V. (2024). Artificial intelligence in dentistry and dental biomaterials. *Frontiers in Dental Medicine*, 5. https://doi.org/10.3389/fdmed.2024.1525505.

Romain, K., Cheng, J., Kim, S., Watters, K., & Theodoraki, A. (2025). Perioperative prevention of euglycaemic diabetic ketoacidosis in people living with type 2 diabetes established on sodium-glucose transport-2 inhibitors – a cross-site multi-cycle audit. *Clinical Medicine*, *25*, 100502. https://doi.org/10.1016/j.clinme.2025.100502

Romano, A., Gaeta, F., Poves, M., & Valluzzi, R. (2016). Cross-reactivity among beta-lactams. *Current Allergy and Asthma Reports, 16*, 1–12. https://doi.org/10.1007/s11882-016-0594-9.

Romskaug, R., Skovlund, E., Straand, J., Molden, E., Kersten, H., Pitkala, K., Lundqvist, C., & Wyller, T. (2020). Effect of clinical geriatric assessments and collaborative medication reviews by geriatrician and family physician for improving health-related quality of life in home-dwelling older patients receiving polypharmacy: A cluster randomized clinical trial. *JAMA Internal Medicine*. https://doi.org/10.1001/jamainternmed.2019.5096.

Rosenbaum, M., Clemmensen, L., Bredt, D., Bettler, B., & Strømgaard, K. (2020). Targeting receptor complexes: A new dimension in drug discovery. *Nature Reviews Drug Discovery, 19*, 884–901. https://doi.org/10.1038/s41573-020-0086-4.

Rostoft, S., Van Den Bos, F., Pedersen, R., & Hamaker, M. (2020). Shared decision-making in older patients with cancer: What does the patient want? *Journal of Geriatric Oncology*. https://doi.org/10.1016/j.jgo.2020.08.001.

Rowe, H., Baker, T., & Hale, T. (2013). Maternal medication, drug use, and breastfeeding. *Pediatric Clinics of North America, 60*(1), 275–294. https://doi.org/10.1016/j.pcl.2012.10.009.

Rowland, A. S., Baird, D. D., Weinberg, C. R., et al., (1992). Reduced fertility among women employed as dental assistants exposed to high levels of nitrous oxide. *New England Journal of Medicine, 327*(14), 993–997.

Roy, A., & Somasundaram, J. (2020). Novel trends in drug delivery and application of curcumin in dentistry. *Indian Journal of Forensic Medicine & Toxicology*. https://doi.org/10.37506/ijfmt.v14i4.12400.

Ruggiero, A., Ariano, A., Triarico, S., Capozza, M. A., Ferrara, P., & Attinà, G. (2019). Neonatal pharmacology and clinical implications. *Drugs in Context, 8*.

Ruiz, M. E., & Scioli-Montoto, S. (2024). Routes of drug administration. In *ADME processes in pharmaceutical sciences: dosage, design, and pharmacotherapy* (pp. 129-172). Cham: Springer Nature Switzerland.

Russell, A., & W., R. (1990). Bacterial spores and chemical sporicidal agents. *Clinical Microbiology Reviews, 3*, 99–119. https://doi.org/10.1128/CMR.3.2.99.

Rutala, W., & Weber, D. (2016). Disinfection, sterilization, and antisepsis: An overview. *American Journal of Infection Control, 44*(5 Suppl), e1–e6. https://doi.org/10.1016/j.ajic.2015.10.038.

Rybak, M. J., & McGrath, B. J. (1996). Combination antimicrobial therapy for bacterial infections: Guidelines for the clinician. *Drugs, 52*(3), 390–405.

Rybak, M. J., Le, J., Lodise, T. P., Levine, D. P., Bradley, J. S., Liu, C., ... & Lomaestro, B. M. (2020). Therapeutic monitoring of vancomycin for serious methicillin-resistant Staphylococcus aureus infections: A revised consensus guideline and review by the American Society of Health-System Pharmacists, the Infectious Diseases Society of America, the Pediatric Infectious Diseases Society, and the Society of Infectious Diseases Pharmacists. *American Journal of Health-System Pharmacy, 77*(11), 835–864.

Sabanceva, E., Dmitrieva, N., Avramenko, E., Ivanova, E., Ezhova, E., & Pochivalin, V. (2021). Evaluation of effectiveness of a mouthwash containing antiseptic octenidine dihydrochloride. *Stomatologiia, 100*(2), 32–39. https://doi.org/10.17116/stomat202110002132.

Sachs, H. (2013). The transfer of drugs and therapeutics into human breast milk: An update on selected topics. *Pediatrics, 132*(4), e796–e809. https://doi.org/10.1542/peds.2013-1985.

Sadanandan, S., S., S., Venugopal, S., & Karur, K. (2021). Comparative evaluation of 0.1% octenidine mouthwash with 0.2% chlorhexidine mouthwash in prevention of plaque and gingivitis – A clinicomicrobiological study. *RGUHS Journal of Dental Sciences, 13*(3), Article 9. https://doi.org/10.26715/rjds.13_3_9.

Sadler, T. W. (2017). Establishing the embryonic axes: Prime time for teratogenic insults. *Journal of Cardiovascular Development and Disease, 4*(3), 15. https://doi.org/10.3390/jcdd4030015.

Safra, J. M., & Oakley, G. P., Jr. (1975). Association between cleft lip with or without cleft palate and prenatal exposure to diazepam. *Lancet, 2*(7933), 478–480.

Saginur, R., Hawley, C. R., & Bartlett, J. G. (1980). Colitis associated with metronidazole therapy. *The Journal of Infectious Diseases, 141*(6), 772–774. https://doi.org/10.1093/infdis/141.6.772.

Saguil, A., Kane, S., Lauters, R., & Mercado, M. (2019). Hand-foot-and-mouth disease: Rapid evidence review. *American Family Physician*, 100(7), 408–414.

Saha, M., Ryan, K., & Amir, L. (2015). Postpartum women's use of medicines and breastfeeding practices: A systematic review. *International Breastfeeding Journal, 10*, Article 53. https://doi.org/10.1186/s13006-015-0053-6.

Sahadevan, N. (2021). Drug interactions of azole antifungals. *Journal of Skin and Sexually Transmitted Diseases, 3*(2), 139–144. https://doi.org/10.25259/jsstd_61_2021.

Sahinovic, M., Struys, M., & Absalom, A. (2018). Clinical Pharmacokinetics and Pharmacodynamics of Propofol. *Clinical Pharmacokinetics*, 57, 1539 - 1558. https://doi.org/10.1007/s40262-018-0672-3.

Sahney, T. (2022). Herbs: The natural alternative to treat periodontal diseases. *International Journal of Advanced Research*. https://doi.org/10.21474/ijar01/14899.

Sainz, Á., García-Sancho, M., Rodríguez-Franco, F., Andres, M., Rodríguez, C., De Lucas, J., Andrés, M., Agulla, B., & Villaescusa, A. (2021). Effect of chemically modified tetracycline-8 (CMT-8) on hematology, blood chemistry, cytokines and peripheral blood lymphocyte subsets of healthy dogs. *Research in Veterinary Science, 136*, 200–208. https://doi.org/10.1016/j.rvsc.2021.02.022.

Saleem, K., Ahmad, P., Asif, J. A., Karobari, M. I., & Noorani, T. Y. (2021). The impact of drug therapy on minor oral surgery procedures. *Dental Update, 48*(11), 957–964. https://doi.org/10.12968/denu.2021.48.11.957.

Salvadori, M., Audino, E., Venturi, G., Garo, M. L., & Salgarello, S. (2019). Antibiotic prescribing for endodontic infections: A survey of dental students in Italy. *International Endodontic Journal, 52*(9), 1388–1396. https://doi.org/10.1111/iej.13126.

Salvi, G., Stähli, A., Schmidt, J., Ramseier, C., Sculean, A., & Walter, C. (2019). Adjunctive laser or antimicrobial photodynamic therapy to non-surgical mechanical instrumentation in patients with untreated periodontitis: A systematic review and meta-analysis. *Journal of Clinical Periodontology*. https://doi.org/10.1111/jcpe.13236.

Sampaio, M. M., Santos, M. L. C., Marques, H. S., de Souza Gonçalves, V. L., Araújo, G. R. L., Lopes, L. W., ... & de Melo, F. F. (2021). Chronic myeloid leukemia—from the Philadelphia chromosome to specific target drugs: A literature review. *World Journal of Clinical Oncology, 12*(2), 69.

Samuel, M. (2023). American Geriatrics Society 2023 updated AGS Beers Criteria® for potentially inappropriate medication use in older adults. *Journal of the American Geriatrics Society, 71*, 2052–2081. https://doi.org/10.1111/jgs.18372.

Sánchez-Guzmán, M., Loyola-Cruz, M., López-Ornelas, A., Cruz-Cruz, C., Durán-Manuel, E., & Bello-López, J. (2023). In situ and in vitro evaluation of two antiseptics for blood bank based on chlorhexidine gluconate/isopropyl alcohol and povidone-iodine. *Transfusion and Apheresis Science, 62*, 103854. https://doi.org/10.1016/j.transci.2023.103854.

Săndulescu, O., Preoțescu, L., Streinu-Cercel, A., Şahin, G., & Săndulescu, M. (2024). Antibiotic prescribing in dental medicine—Best practices for successful implementation. *Tropical Medicine and Infectious Disease*, 9(2), 31. https://doi.org/10.3390/tropicalmed9020031.

Santini, A. (2025). Research abstracts: General dentistry. *Primary Dental Journal, 14*, 43–45. https://doi.org/10.1177/20501684251331784.

Santos-Paul, M., Neves, I., Neves, R., & Ramires, J. (2015). Local anesthesia with epinephrine is safe and effective for oral surgery in patients with type 2 diabetes mellitus and coronary disease: a prospective randomized study. *Clinics*, 70, 185 - 189. https://doi.org/10.6061/clinics/2015(03)06.

Santos, M., De Almeida Aquino, S., De Souza, L., Peixoto, B., Da Rocha Taranto, M., Borges, R., Neto, M., & Madalena, I. (2024). Management of the epileptic patient in the dental office: A clinical case report and brief literature review. *Brazilian Journal of Health Review*. https://doi.org/10.34119/bjhrv7n2-212.

Santos, M., De Campos, W., Esteves, C., Santos-Paul, M., De Carvalho, C., Montano, T., Neves, I., Neves, R., & Lemos, C. (2019). Sedation with oral benzodiazepines in dental practice in cardiac patients. *Clinical and Laboratorial Research in Dentistry*. https://doi.org/10.11606/ISSN.2357-8041.CLRD.2019.151351.

Sanz, M., Bäumer, A., Buduneli, N., Dommisch, H., Farina, R., Kononen, E., ... & Winkel, E. (2015). Effect of professional mechanical plaque removal on secondary prevention of periodontitis and the complications of gingival and periodontal preventive measures: Consensus report of group 4 of the 11th European Workshop on Periodontology on effective prevention of periodontal and peri-implant diseases. *Journal of Clinical Periodontology, 42*, S214–S220. https://doi.org/10.1111/jcpe.12367.

Saravanan, T., Subha, M., Prem, P., & Venkatesh, A. (2014). Corticosteroids-its role in oral mucosal lesions. *International Journal of Pharmacy and Bio Sciences, 5*(4), 439-446.

Sarı, S., Kumar, J., & Turan, A. (2021). New peripheral nerve blocks and local anesthetics. *Current Opinion in Critical Care*, 27, 733 - 742. https://doi.org/10.1097/MCC.0000000000000873.

Sato, M., Yamana, H., Ono, S., Ishimaru, M., Matsui, H., & Yasunaga, H. (2022). Amoxicillin vs third-generation cephalosporin for infection prophylaxis after third molar extraction. *Oral Diseases*. https://doi.org/10.1111/odi.14421.

Satpathi, S., Rathod, Y. V., Rajpari, K. N., Kandlikar, R., Kumar, Y. R., Gachake, A., & Surana, P. (2024). Application of corticosteroids in dentistry: A review. *Journal of Pharmacy and Bioallied Sciences, 16*(Suppl 4), S3034-S3036.

Sbricoli, L., Grisolia, G., Stellini, E., Bacci, C., Annunziata, M., & Bressan, E. (2024). Antibiotic-prescribing habits in dentistry: A questionnaire-based study. *Antibiotics, 13*, Article 189. https://doi.org/10.3390/antibiotics13020189.

Scheme PB. (2020, February 13). Recommendations made by the PBAC – December 2019. Australian Government Department of Health. http://www.pbs.gov.au/info/industry/listing/elements/pbac-meetings/pbac-outcomes/recommendations-made-by-the-pbac-december-2019.

Scheuerle, A. E., & Aylsworth, A. S. (2016). Birth defects and neonatal morbidity caused by teratogen exposure after the embryonic period. *Birth Defects Research Part A: Clinical and Molecular Teratology, 106*(11), 935–939. https://doi.org/10.1002/bdra.23555.

Schierz, O., Hirsch, C., Krey, K., Ganss, C., Kämmerer, P., & Schlenz, M. (2023). Digital dentistry and its impact on oral health-related quality of life. *The Journal of Evidence-Based Dental Practice*, 24(1S), 101946. https://doi.org/10.1016/j.jebdp.2023.101946.

Schildkraut, J., Pennings, L., Ruth, M., De Brouwer, A., Wertheim, H., Hoefsloot, W., Jong, A., & Ingen, J. (2019). The differential effect of clarithromycin and azithromycin on induction of macrolide resistance in Mycobacterium abscessus. *Future Microbiology*. https://doi.org/10.2217/fmb-2018-0310.

Schjerning, A., McGettigan, P., & Gislason, G. (2020). Cardiovascular effects and safety of (non-aspirin) NSAIDs. *Nature Reviews Cardiology, 17*, 574–584. https://doi.org/10.1038/s41569-020-0366-z.

Schmader, K., Gnann Jr, J. W., & Watson, C. P. (2008). The epidemiological, clinical, and pathological rationale for the herpes zoster vaccine. *The Journal of Infectious Diseases, 197*(Supplement_2), S207-S215.

Schnappinger;, D., & Hillen, W. (1996). Tetracyclines: Antibiotic action, uptake, and resistance mechanisms. *Archives of Microbiology, 165*(6), 359–369. https://doi.org/10.1007/s002030050339.

Schoenfeld, A., Bary, M., Merlob, P., & Ovadia, Y. (1992). NSAIDs: Maternal and fetal considerations. *American Journal of Reproductive Immunology, 28*(3–4), 141–147.

Schoenfeld, A., Munigala, S., Gong, J., Schoenfeld, R., Banaag, A., Coles, C., & Koehlmoos, T. (2024). Reductions in sustained prescription opioid use within the US between 2017 and 2021. *Scientific Reports, 14*. https://doi.org/10.1038/s41598-024-52032-4.

Scholz, A. (2002). Mechanisms of (local) anaesthetics on voltage-gated sodium and other ion channels. *British Journal Of Anaesthesia*, 89 1, 52-61. https://doi.org/10.1093/BJA/AEF163.

Schraag, S., Pradelli, L., Alsaleh, A., Bellone, M., Ghetti, G., Chung, T., Westphal, M., & Rehberg, S. (2018). Propofol vs. inhalational agents to maintain general anaesthesia in ambulatory and in-patient surgery: a systematic review and meta-analysis. *BMC Anesthesiology*, 18. https://doi.org/10.1186/s12871-018-0632-3.

Schroeck, J., Ford, J., Conway, E., Kurtzhalts, K., Gee, M., Vollmer, K., & Mergenhagen, K. (2016). Review of Safety and Efficacy of Sleep Medicines in Older Adults. *Clinical therapeutics*, 38 11, 2340-2372. https://doi.org/10.1016/j.clinthera.2016.09.010.

Schroeder, A. R., Dehghan, M., Newman, T. B., Bentley, J. P., & Park, K. T. (2019). Association of opioid prescriptions from dental clinicians for US adolescents and young adults with subsequent opioid use and abuse. *JAMA Internal Medicine, 179*(2), 145–152. https://doi.org/10.1001/jamainternmed.2018.5419.

Schuijt, H., Smeeing, D., Verberne, W., Groenwold, R., Van Delden, J., Leenen, L., & Van Der Velde, D. (2023). Perspective; recommendations for improved patient participation in decision-making for geriatric patients in acute surgical settings. *Injury*, Article 110823. https://doi.org/10.1016/j.injury.2023.05.054.

Schulz-Weidner, N., Gruber, M., Schraml, E., Wöstmann, B., Krämer, N., & Schlenz, M. (2024). Improving the communication of dental findings in pediatric dentistry by using intraoral scans as a visual aid: A randomized clinical trial. *Dentistry Journal, 12*, Article 15. https://doi.org/10.3390/dj12010015.

Schwendicke, F., & Krois, J. (2022). Precision dentistry—what it is, where it fails (yet), and how to get there. *Clinical Oral Investigations, 26*, 3395–3403. https://doi.org/10.1007/s00784-022-04420-1.

Schwendicke, F., Samek, W., & Krois, J. (2020). Artificial intelligence in dentistry: Chances and challenges. *Journal of Dental Research*, 99, 769–774. https://doi.org/10.1177/0022034520915714.

Sefton, A. M. (1999). Macrolides and changes in the oral flora. *International Journal of Antimicrobial Agents, 11* Suppl 1, S23–S32. https://doi.org/10.1016/s0924-8579(98)00100-9.

Segura-Egea, J. J., Martín-González, J., del Carmen Jiménez-Sánchez, M., Crespo-Gallardo, I., Saúco-Márquez, J. J., & Velasco-Ortega, E. (2017). Worldwide pattern of antibiotic prescription in endodontic infections. *International Dental Journal, 67*(4), 197–205. https://doi.org/10.1111/idj.12287.

Segura-Egea, J., Gould, K., Şen, B., Jonasson, P., Cotti, E., Mazzoni, A., Sunay, H., Tjäderhane, L., & Dummer, P. (2017). Antibiotics in endodontics: A review. *International Endodontic Journal, 50*, 1169–1184. https://doi.org/10.1111/iej.12741.

Segura-Egea, J. J., Gould, K., Hakan Şen, B., Jonasson, P., Cotti, E., Mazzoni, A., ... & Dummer, P. M. H. (2018). European Society of Endodontology position statement: The use of antibiotics in endodontics. *International Endodontic Journal, 51*(1), 20–25. https://doi.org/10.1111/iej.12781.

Segura-Egea, J. J., Gould, K., Şen, B. H., Jonasson, P., Cotti, E., Mazzoni, A., ... & Dummer, P. M. H. (2017). Antibiotics in endodontics: A review. *International Endodontic Journal, 50*(12), 1169–1184. https://doi.org/10.1111/iej.12741.

Seidman, A. D., Berry, D., Cirrincione, C., Harris, L., Muss, H., Marcom, P. K., ... & Hudis, C. (2008). Randomized phase III trial of weekly compared with every-3-weeks paclitaxel for metastatic breast cancer, with trastuzumab for all HER-2 overexpressors and random assignment to trastuzumab or not in HER-2 nonoverexpressors: Final results of Cancer and Leukemia Group B protocol 9840. *Journal of Clinical Oncology, 26*(10), 1642–1649.

Serrano, D. R., Luciano, F. C., Anaya, B. J., Ongoren, B., Kara, A., Molina, G., Ramirez, B. I., Sánchez-Guirales, S. A., Simon, J. A., Tomietto, G., Rapti, C., Ruiz, H. K., Rawat, S., Kumar, D., & Lalatsa, A. (2024). Artificial Intelligence (AI) Applications in Drug Discovery and Drug Delivery: Revolutionizing Personalized Medicine. *Pharmaceutics, 16*(10), 1328. https://doi.org/10.3390/pharmaceutics16101328.

Serrano, J., Escribano, M., Roldan, S., Martin, C., & Herrera, D. (2015). Efficacy of adjunctive anti-plaque chemical agents in managing gingivitis: A systematic review and meta-analysis. *Journal of Clinical Periodontology, 42*, S106–S138. https://doi.org/10.1111/jcpe.12331.

Setiawatie, E., Valentina, R., & Meiliana, R. (2023). Effectiveness of cetylpyridinium chloride in reducing the growth of bacteria that cause periodontal disease. *e-GiGi, 11*(2), 44510. https://doi.org/10.35790/eg.v11i2.44510.

Seymour, R. A., & Heasman, P. A. (1995). Tetracyclines in the management of periodontal diseases: A review. *Journal of Clinical Periodontology, 22*(1), 22–35. https://doi.org/10.1111/J.1600-051X.1995.TB01767.X.

Sgolastra, F., Petrucci, A., Gatto, R., Giannoni, M., & Monaco, A. (2011). Long-term efficacy of subantimicrobial-dose doxycycline as an adjunctive treatment to scaling and root planing: A systematic review and meta-analysis. *Journal of Periodontology, 82*(11), 1570–1581. https://doi.org/10.1902/jop.2011.110026.

Shaat, M., Bakry, N., Elshafie, A., & Talaat, D. (2021). Intranasal versus sublingual route of dexmedetomidine sedation in pediatric dentistry: A randomized controlled clinical trial. *International Journal of Paediatric Dentistry, 31*(2), 128–135. https://doi.org/10.1111/ipd.12848.

Shan, T., Tay, F., & Gu, L. (2020). Application of artificial intelligence in dentistry. *Journal of Dental Research*, 100, 232–244. https://doi.org/10.1177/0022034520969115.

Shanbhag, V. K. L. (2015). Medical management of oral submucous fibrosis. *Asia-Pacific Journal of Oncology Nursing, 2*(1), 51. https://doi.org/10.4103/2347-5625.143766.

Shankar, S., Gopinath, P., & Roja, E. (2022). Role of spices and herbs in controlling dental problems. *Research Journal of Pharmacology and Pharmacodynamics, 14*(1), 23–28. https://doi.org/10.52711/2321-5836.2022.00004.

Sharma, V., & Kadu, A. (2024). Technology shaping the future of dentistry. *Medical Journal*, Armed Forces India, 80(4), 375–377. https://doi.org/10.1016/j.mjafi.2024.05.019.

Sharon, V., & Fazel, N. (2010). Oral candidiasis and angular cheilitis. *Dermatologic Therapy, 23*(3), 230–242. https://doi.org/10.1111/j.1529-8019.2010.01320.x.

Shay, K., Truhlar, M. R., & Renner, R. P. (1997). Oropharyngeal candidosis in the older patient. *Journal of the American Geriatrics Society, 45*(7), 863–870. https://doi.org/10.1111/j.1532-5415.1997.tb01517.x.

Shehabi, Z., Doshi, M., Liu, S., & Geddis-Regan, A. (2025). General anaesthesia in special care dentistry. Part 2: delivering dental care. *Dental Update*. https://doi.org/10.12968/denu.2025.52.1.35.

Shen, M., Manna, R., Banerjee, S., Nelson, C., Alexander, K., Alici, Y., Gangai, N., Parker, P., & Korc-Grodzicki, B. (2020). Incorporating shared decision making into communication with older adults with cancer and their caregivers: Development and evaluation of a geriatric shared decision-making communication skills training module. *Patient Education and Counseling*. https://doi.org/10.1016/j.pec.2020.04.032

Shenoy, N., Mallya, L., Shenoy, N., & Shenoy, A. (2016). Pharmacology in endodontics: A review article. *Research Journal of Pharmaceutical, Biological and Chemical Sciences, 7*, 2481–2485.

Sheshaprasad, R., & Pai, A. (2020). A comprehensive review of therapeutic agents used in the treatment of recurrent aphthous ulcer and oral ulcers in Bechet's syndrome. *Indian Journal of Pharmacy and Pharmacology*. https://doi.org/10.18231/2393-9087.2018.0012.

Shetti, A., Bhavar, T., & Khunt, M. (2025). Geriatric anaesthesia: Challenges and recent updates – A review. *Annals of Geriatric Education and Medical Sciences*. https://doi.org/10.18231/j.agems.2024.009.

Shijith, K. (2021). A review on cetylpyridinium chloride. *International Journal of Research, 8*, 439–445. https://doi.org/10.52403/IJRR.20210453.

Shin, S. W. (2014). Medications in treatment of postherpetic neuralgia. *Korean Journal of Pain, 27*(1), 1-2. https://doi.org/10.3344/kjp.2014.27.1.1.

Sim, I. K., Davis, T. M., & Ilett, K. F. (2005). Effects of a high-fat meal on the relative oral bioavailability of piperaquine. *Antimicrobial Agents and Chemotherapy, 49*(6), 2407–2411.

Simon, C., Bozenhardt, E., Celluzzi, C., Dobnik, D., Grant, M., Lakshmipathy, U., ... & Vessillier, S. (2024). Mechanism of action, potency and efficacy: Considerations for cell therapies. *Journal of Translational Medicine, 22*. https://doi.org/10.1186/s12967-024-05179-7.

Simonini, A., Brogi, E., Cascella, M., & Vittori, A. (2022). Advantages of ketamine in pediatric anesthesia. *Open Medicine*, 17, 1134-1147. https://doi.org/10.1515/med-2022-0509.

Singgih, M., Achmad, H., Sukmana, B., Carmelita, A., Putra, A., Ramadhany, S., & Putri, A. (2020). A review of nonsteroidal anti-inflammatory drugs (NSAIDs) medications in dentistry: Uses and side effects. *Systematic Reviews in Pharmacy, 11*, 293-298. https://doi.org/10.31838/srp.2020.5.43.

Sinicropi, M., Iacopetta, D., Ceramella, J., Catalano, A., Mariconda, A., Pellegrino, M., Saturnino, C., Longo, P., & Aquaro, S. (2022). Triclosan: A small molecule with controversial roles. *Antibiotics, 11*(6), Article 735. https://doi.org/10.3390/antibiotics 11060735.

Sionov, R., & Steinberg, D. (2022). Targeting the holy triangle of quorum sensing, biofilm formation, and antibiotic resistance in pathogenic bacteria. *Microorganisms, 10*. https://doi.org/10.3390/microorganisms10061239.

Siqueira, J. F., Jr., & Rôças, I. N. (2013). Microbiology and treatment of acute apical abscesses. *Clinical Microbiology Reviews, 26*(2), 255–273. https://doi.org/10.1128/CMR.00082-12.

Şitilci, T., Demirgan, S., Akçay, Ç., Kahraman, N., Köseoğlu, B., Erdem, M., & Cankaya, A. (2017). Comparison of patients with and without intellectual disability under general anesthesia: A retrospective study. *Nigerian Journal of Clinical Practice*, 20, 438 - 444. https://doi.org/10.4103/1119-3077.204372.

Sivilotti, M. L. (2016). Flumazenil, naloxone and the 'coma cocktail.' British Journal of Clinical Pharmacology, 81(3), 428-436.

Sivrikaya, E., Yılmaz, O., & Sivrikaya, P. (2021). Dentist-patient communication on dental anxiety using the social media: A randomized controlled trial. *Scandinavian Journal of Psychology*. https://doi.org/10.1111/sjop.12769.

Śliwa, P., Dziurzyńska, M., Kurczab, R., & Kucwaj-Brysz, K. (2024). The pivotal distinction between antagonists' and agonists' binding into dopamine D4 receptor—MD and FMO/PIEDA studies. *International Journal of Molecular Sciences, 25*. https://doi.org/10.3390/ijms25020746.

Slot, D. E., Valkenburg, C., & Van der Weijden, G. A. (2020). Mechanical plaque removal of periodontal maintenance patients: A systematic review and network meta-analysis. *Journal of Clinical Periodontology, 47*, 107–124. https://doi.org/10.1111/jcpe.13275.

Slots, J., & Rosling, B. (1983). Suppression of the periodontopathic microflora in localized juvenile periodontitis by systemic tetracycline. *Journal of Clinical Periodontology, 10*(5), 465–486. https://doi.org/10.1111/J.1600-051X.1983.TB02179.X.

Slots, J., Bragd, L., Wikstrom, M., & Dahlén, G. (1986). The occurrence of Actinobacillus actinomycetemcomitans, Bacteroides gingivalis and Bacteroides intermedius in destructive periodontal disease in adults. *Journal of Clinical Periodontology, 13*(6), 570–577. https://doi.org/10.1111/j.1600-051x.1986.tb00849.x.

Slots, J., Saygun, I., Sabeti, M., & Kubar, A. (2006). Epstein-Barr virus in oral diseases. *Journal of Periodontal Research*, 41(4), 235–244. https://doi.org/10.1111/j.1600-0765.2006.00865.x.

Smith, R., & Alexander, A. (1992). Serious professional misconduct arising out of dental anaesthesia and sedation. *British Dental Journal*, 173, 161-165. https://doi.org/10.1038/sj.bdj.4807984.

Soar, J., Standing, J., Courtenay, M., & Griffiths, M. (2009). Parenteral drug administration. In *Medication Safety: An Essential Guide* (pp. 97–112). Cambridge University Press.

Soares, A., & Sokumbi, O. (2021). Recent updates in the treatment of erythema multiforme. *Medicina, 57*(9), 921. https://doi.org/10.3390/medicina57090921

Sokumbi, O., & Wetter, D. A. (2012). Clinical features, diagnosis, and treatment of erythema multiforme: A review for the practicing dermatologist. *International Journal of Dermatology, 51*(8), 889-902.

Soldin, O. P., & Mattison, D. R. (2009). Sex differences in pharmacokinetics and pharmacodynamics. *Clinical Pharmacokinetics, 48*(3), 143–157.

Soman, H., Kumar, M., Kumar, N., Radhakrishnan, K., Loganathan, D., & Kaul, R. (2021). Does the effect of adrenaline on intraoral 2% lidocaine contribute to haemodynamic instability?: A prospective, randomized double blinded study. *Oral Surgery*. https://doi.org/10.1111/ORS.12637.

Spencer, J., Thomas, S., & Pawlowski, R. (2022). Medication safety in breastfeeding. *American Family Physician, 106*(6), 638–644.

Sperotto, F., France, K., Gobbo, M., Bindakhil, M., Pimolbutr, K., Holmes, H., ... & Edefonti, V. (2024). Antibiotic prophylaxis and infective endocarditis incidence following invasive dental procedures: A systematic review and meta-analysis. *JAMA Cardiology, 9*(7), 599–610.

Sperotto, F., France, K., Gobbo, M., Bindakhil, M., Pimolbutr, K., Holmes, H., Monteiro, L., Graham, L., Hong, C., Sollecito, T., Lodi, G., Lockhart, P., Thornhill, M., Dios, P., Turati, F., & Edefonti, V. (2024). Antibiotic prophylaxis and infective endocarditis incidence following invasive dental procedures: A systematic review and meta-analysis. *JAMA Cardiology*. https://doi.org/10.1001/jamacardio.2024.0873.

Spielman, A. (2024). Dental education and practice: Past, present, and future trends. *Frontiers in Oral Health*, 5, Article 1368121. https://doi.org/10.3389/froh.2024.1368121.

Spížek, J., & Řezanka, T. (2017). Lincosamides: Chemical structure, biosynthesis, mechanism of action, resistance, and applications. *Biochemical Pharmacology, 133*, 20–28. https://doi.org/10.1016/j.bcp.2016.12.001.

Srivastava, R., Tangade, P., & Priyadarshi, S. (2023). Transforming public health dentistry: Exploring the digital foothold for improved oral healthcare. *International Dental Journal of Student's Research*. https://doi.org/10.18231/j.idjsr.2023.013.

Stana, O. L., Lile, I. E., Freiman, P., Vaida, L., Popovici, R. A., Oalriu, I., ... & Hosszu, T. (2023). Dynamic strategies for mechanical dental plaque removal. *Medicine in Evolution, 29*(4), 582–589. https://doi.org/10.70921/medev.v29i4.989.

Steigmann, L., Kačarević, Ž., Khoury, J., Nagy, K., & Feres, M. (2024). Integration of precision medicine into the dental care setting. *Frontiers in Dental Medicine, 5*. https://doi.org/10.3389/fdmed.2024.1398897.

Stein, K., Farmer, J., Singhal, S., Marra, F., Sutherland, S., & Quiñonez, C. (2018). The use and misuse of antibiotics in dentistry: A scoping review. *Journal of the American Dental Association, 149*(10), 869–884.e5. https://doi.org/10.1016/j.adaj.2018.05.034.

Stewart, B., Shibli, J., Araújo, M., Figueiredo, L., Panagakos, F., Matarazzo, F., Mairink, R., Onuma, T., Faveri, M., Retamal-Valdes, B., & Feres, M. (2020). Effects of a toothpaste containing 0.3% triclosan on periodontal parameters of subjects enrolled in a regular maintenance program: A secondary analysis of a 2-year randomized clinical trial. *Journal of Periodontology, 91*(4), 456–464. https://doi.org/10.1002/JPER.18-0501.

Strappa, E. M., Memè, L., Cerea, M., Roy, M., & Bambini, F. (2022). Custom-made additively manufactured subperiosteal implant. *Minerva Dental and Oral Science, 71*, 353–360. https://doi.org/10.23736/S2724-6329.22.04640-X.

Stuart, M. J., Gross, S. J., Elrad, H., & Graeber, J. E. (1982). Effects of acetylsalicylic acid ingestion on maternal and neonatal hemostasis. *New England Journal of Medicine, 307*(15), 909–912.

Sturaro, M., Araújo, R., Aniceto, L., De Medeiros, G., De Almeida De Souza, G., & Simionatto, S. (2025). Cephalosporin-based combination therapies for combating ESKAPE pathogens: A patent review. *Journal of Applied Microbiology*. https://doi.org/10.1093/jambio/lxaf107.

Sturgill, M. G., & Rapp, R. P. (1992). Clarithromycin: Review of a new macrolide antibiotic with improved microbiologic spectrum and favorable pharmacokinetic and adverse effect profiles. *The Annals of Pharmacotherapy, 26*(9), 1099–1108. https://doi.org/10.1177/106002809202600912.

Su, N., Liu, Y., Yang, X., Shi, Z., & Huang, Y. (2014). Efficacy and safety of mepivacaine compared with lidocaine in local anaesthesia in dentistry: a meta-analysis of randomised controlled trials. *International Dental Journal*, 64 2, 96-107. https://doi.org/10.1111/idj.12087.

Subapriya, R., & Nagini, S. (2005). Medicinal properties of neem leaves: A review. *Current Medicinal Chemistry – Anti-Cancer Agents, 5*(2), 149–156.

Subasi, N. (2020). Formaldehyde advantages and disadvantages: Usage areas and harmful effects on human beings. In *Biochemical Toxicology - Heavy Metals and Nanomaterials* (pp. 123–134). IntechOpen. https://doi.org/10.5772/intechopen.89299.

Subtil, D., Brabant, G., Tilloy, E., Devos, P., Canis, F., Fruchart, A., Bissinger, M., Dugimont, J., Nolf, C., Hacot, C., Gautier, S., Chantrel, J., Jousse, M., Desseauve, D., Plennevaux, J., Delaeter, C., Deghilage, S., Personne, A., Joyez, E., ... Dessein, R. (2018). Early clindamycin for bacterial vaginosis in pregnancy (PREMEVA): A multicentre, double-blind, randomised controlled trial. *The Lancet, 392*, 2171–2179. https://doi.org/10.1016/S0140-6736(18)31617-9.

Suda, K. J., Zhou, J., Rowan, S. A., McGregor, J. C., Perez, R. I., Evans, C. T., Gellad, W. F., & Calip, G. S. (2020). Overprescribing of opioids to adults by dentists in the U.S., 2011–2015. *American Journal of Preventive Medicine, 58*(4), 473–486. https://doi.org/10.1016/j.amepre.2019.11.006.

Suehs, C., Menzies-Gow, A., Price, D., Bleecker, E., Canonica, G., Gurnell, M., & Bourdin, A. (2020). Expert Consensus on the Tapering of Oral Corticosteroids for the Treatment of Asthma: A Delphi Study.. *American journal of respiratory and critical care medicine*. https://doi.org/10.1164/rccm.202007-2721oc.

Sugiarta, A., Lessang, R., & N. (2019). Effect of herbal toothpaste containing neem leaves extract (Azadirachta indica) against gingivitis: A clinical study. *International Journal of Applied Pharmaceutics*. https://doi.org/10.22159/IJAP.2019.V11S1.AR173.

Suharyani, I., Mohammed, A., Muchtaridi, M., Wathoni, N., & Abdassah, M. (2021). Evolution of Drug Delivery Systems for Recurrent Aphthous Stomatitis. Drug Design, Development and Therapy, 15, 4071 - 4089. https://doi.org/10.2147/DDDT.S328371.

Sun, L., Fan, Y., Wang, X., & Zheng, H. (2020). Pharmacodynamic elucidation of glutamate & dopamine in ketamine-induced anaesthesia. *Chemico-biological interactions*, 109164. https://doi.org/10.1016/j.cbi.2020.109164.

Sun, L., Liang, S., Sa, Y., Wang, Z., X., Jiang, T., & Wang, Y. (2011). Surface alteration of human tooth enamel subjected to acidic and neutral 30% hydrogen peroxide. *Journal of Dentistry, 39*(10), 686–692. https://doi.org/10.1016/j.jdent.2011.07.011.

Suresh, S., & Suresh, R. (2023). Medication adherence in elderly patients with chronic diseases: A review. *Journal of Geriatric Care and Research*, 10(1), 1–7. https://doi.org/10.5005/jp-journals-10005-2516.

Suri, N., Kalra, G., Kumar, M., Avasthi, A., Kalra, T., & Singh, R. (2022). A literature review on various complications associated with administration of local anesthesia in dentistry. *IP International Journal of Maxillofacial Imaging*. https://doi.org/10.18231/j.ijmi.2022.015.

Svetlakova, E., Ginkel, D., Brusnitsyna, E., Kotikova, A., Nersesyan, P., Legkih, A., & Ivashov, A. (2025). General state of the issue: Dental status of incurable pediatric patients. Actual Problems in Dentistry. https://doi.org/10.18481/2077-7566-2025-21-1-165-171.

Svsg, N., & Degala, S. (2020). Dental concerns and management of children with epilepsy: An overview. *Dental, Oral and Maxillofacial Research*. https://doi.org/10.15761/DOMR.1000356.

Swamy, D. N., Sanivarapu, S., Moogla, S., & Kapalavai, V. (2015). Chemically modified tetracyclines: The novel host modulating agents. *Journal of Indian Society of Periodontology, 19*(4), 370–374. https://doi.org/10.4103/0972-124X.149934.

Sweeney, C., & Gilden, D. (2001). Ramsay Hunt syndrome. *Journal of Neurology, Neurosurgery & Psychiatry*, 71(2), 149–154. https://doi.org/10.1136/jnnp.71.2.149.

Świeboda, P., Filip, R., Prystupa, A., & Drozd, M. (2013). Assessment of pain: Types, mechanism and treatment. *Pain, 2*(7), 2-7.

Sykara, M., Maniatakos, P., Tentolouris, A., Karoussis, I. K., & Tentolouris, N. (2022). The necessity of administrating antibiotic prophylaxis to patients with diabetes mellitus prior to oral surgical procedures: A systematic review. *Diabetes & Metabolic Syndrome: Clinical Research & Reviews, 16*(10), 102621. https://doi.org/10.1016/j.dsx.2022.102621.

Szefczyk, M., Szulc, N., Bystranowska, D., Szczepańska, A., Pérez, J., Dudek, A., Pawlak, A., Ożyhar, A., & Berlicki, Ł. (2025). Construction and cytotoxicity evaluation of peptide nanocarriers based on coiledcoil structures with a cyclic βamino acid at the knobintohole interaction site. *Journal of Materials Chemistry B*. https://doi.org/10.1039/d5tb00752f.

Szoszkiewicz, M., Deskur-Śmielecka, E., Styszyński, A., Urbańska, Z., Neumann-Podczaska, A., & Wieczorowska-Tobis, K. (2024). Potentially inappropriate prescribing identified using STOPP/START version 3 in geriatric patients and comparison with version 2: A cross-sectional study. *Journal of Clinical Medicine*, 13, Article 6043. https://doi.org/10.3390/jcm13206043.

Tabari, M., Poźniak, B., Youssefi, M., Sarvandani, M., & Giorgi, M. (2021). Comparative pharmacokinetics of metronidazole in healthy and *Trichomonas gallinae* infected pigeons (*Columba livia*, var. domestica). *British Poultry Science, 62*, 485–491. https://doi.org/10.1080/00071668.2021.1881043.

Taekman, J., & Bonakdar, R. (2018). Integrative pain management must include diet considerations. *Anesthesia & Analgesia*. https://doi.org/10.1213/ANE.0000000000003347.

Taheri, J., Azimi, S., Rafieian, N., & Zanjani, H. (2011). Herbs in dentistry. *International Dental Journal, 61*(6), 287–296. https://doi.org/10.1111/j.1875-595X.2011.00064.x.

Takeda, D., Kurita, H., Kashima, Y., Hasegawa, T., Miyakoshi, M., Yamada, S. I., ... & Soutome, S. (2023). Is withdrawal of antiresorptive agents necessary before and after tooth extraction? A systematic review. *Clinical Oral Investigations, 28*(1), 38. https://doi.org/10.1007/s00784-023-05462-9.

Talbot, B. (2018). Improving patient medication education. *Nursing*, 48, 58–60. https://doi.org/10.1097/01.NURSE.0000531909.68714.85.

Tally, F., Jacobus, N., Bartlett, J., & Gorbach, S. (1975). Susceptibility of anaerobes to cefoxitin and other cephalosporins. *Antimicrobial Agents and Chemotherapy, 7*, 128–132. https://doi.org/10.1128/AAC.7.2.128.

Tam, Y. (1993). Individual variation in first-pass metabolism. *Clinical Pharmacokinetics, 25*, 300–328. https://doi.org/10.2165/00003088-199325040-00005.

Tan, S. J., Baharin, B., Mohd, N., & Nabil, S. (2022). Effect of anti-diabetic medications on dental implants: A scoping review of animal studies and their relevance to humans. *Pharmaceuticals, 15*(12), 1518. https://doi.org/10.3390/ph15121518.

Tan, Y., Neo, E., & Wee, T. (2022). Ultrasound-guided Genicular Nerve Blockade With Pharmacological Agents for Chronic Knee Osteoarthritis: A Systematic Review. *Pain Physician*, 25 4, E489-E502 .

Tang, L., & Varma, M. (2025). Hepatic impairment and the differential effects on drug clearance mechanisms: Analysis of pharmacokinetic changes in disease state. Clinical Pharmacology & Therapeutics. https://doi.org/10.1002/cpt.3643.

Tariq, M., Jalli, V., Dhurubatha, J., Medhi, R., Malawat, K., Gowdar, I., & Arya, S. (2023). Clinical efficacy of topical Kenacort and aloe vera gel in minor aphthous stomatitis: A comparative study. *Journal of Pharmacy & Bioallied Sciences, 16*, S570–S573. https://doi.org/10.4103/jpbs.jpbs_868_23.

Tatch, W. (2019). Opioid prescribing can be reduced in oral and maxillofacial surgery practice. *Journal of Oral and Maxillofacial Surgery, 77*(9), 1771–1775. https://doi.org/10.1016/J.JOMS.2019.03.009.

Tatullo, M., Marrelli, B., Facente, A., Paduano, F., & Qutachi, O. (2024). Novel biopolymer spray formulation for drug delivery in precision dentistry. *Heliyon, 10*. https://doi.org/10.1016/j.heliyon.2024.e36038.

Taylor, R., Neville, Q., Mullin, C., Mekhail, N., Kallewaard, J., Hayek, S., Pope, J., Hunter, C., Costandi, S., Kapural, L., Gilmore, C., Petersen, E., Patel, K., Eldabe, S., Levy, R., Gilligan, C., Durbhakula, S., Abd-Elsayed, A., Bedder, M., ... Nurmikko, T. (2024). Validation of a holistic composite outcome measure for the evaluation of chronic pain interventions. *Pain Reports, 9*. https://doi.org/10.1097/PR9.0000000000001202.

Tedesco, F. (2020). Clindamycin-associated colitis. *The American Journal of Digestive Diseases, 21*, 26–32. https://doi.org/10.1007/BF01074135.

Teoh, L. (2020). Opioid prescribing in dentistry–is there a problem? *Australian Prescriber, 43*(5), 144.

Teoh, L., Hollingworth, S., Marino, R., & McCullough, M. J. (2020). Dental opioid prescribing rates after the up-scheduling of codeine in Australia. *Scientific Reports, 10*(1), 8463.

Teoh, L., Löffler, C., Mun, M., Agnihotry, A., Kaur, H., Born, K., & Thompson, W. (2025). A systematic review of dental antibiotic stewardship interventions. *Community Dentistry and Oral Epidemiology, 53*(3), 245–255.

Teoh, L., Moses, G., & McCullough, M. (2020). A review of drugs that contribute to bleeding risk in general dental practice. *Australian dental journal.* https://doi.org/10.1111/adj.12751.

Teoh, L., Stewart, K., Marino, R. J., & McCullough, M. J. (2021). Improvement of dental prescribing practices using education and a prescribing tool: A pilot intervention study. *British Journal of Clinical Pharmacology, 87*(1), 152–162.

Terzi, O., & Yilmaz, F. (2021). The rational drug use of dentists in a university hospital. *Annals of Medical Research, 28*(3), 496. https://doi.org/10.5455/annalsmedres.2020.02.089.

Teughels, W., Feres, M., Oud, V., Martín, C., Matesanz, P., & Herrera, D. (2020). Adjunctive effect of systemic antimicrobials in periodontitis therapy: A systematic review and meta-analysis. *Journal of Clinical Periodontology.* https://doi.org/10.1111/jcpe.13264.

Thabit, A., Fatani, D., Bamakhrama, M., Barnawi, O., Basudan, L., & Alhejaili, S. (2019). Antibiotic penetration into bone and joints: An updated review. *International Journal of Infectious Diseases, 81*, 128–136. https://doi.org/10.1016/j.ijid.2019.02.005.

Thangavelu, A., Kaspar, S., Kathirvelu, R., Srinivasan, B., Srinivasan, S., & Sundram, R. (2020). Chlorhexidine: An elixir for periodontics. *Journal of Pharmacy & Bioallied Sciences, 12*(S57–S59). https://doi.org/10.4103/jpbs.jpbs_162_20.

Theodorou, M., Tsiantou, V., Pavlakis, A., Maniadakis, N., Fragoulakis, V., Pavi, E., & Kyriopoulos, J. (2009). Factors influencing prescribing behaviour of physicians in Greece and Cyprus: Results from a questionnaire based survey. *BMC Health Services Research, 9*(1), 150. https://doi.org/10.1186/1472-6963-9-150.

Thomas, B. (1941). Penetration of phenol in tooth structure. *Journal of Dental Research, 20*, 435–445. https://doi.org/10.1177/00220345410200050601.

Thomas, R., & Thomas, B. (2019). A systematic review of studies of the STOPP/START 2015 and American Geriatric Society Beers 2015 criteria. Current Aging Science. https://doi.org/10.2174/1874609812666190516093742.

Thompson, W., Teoh, L., Hubbard, C. C., Marra, F., Patrick, D. M., Mamun, A., Campbell, A., & Suda, K. J. (2022). Patterns of dental antibiotic prescribing in 2017: Australia, England, United States, and British Columbia (Canada). *Infection Control & Hospital Epidemiology, 43*(2), 191–198. https://doi.org/10.1017/ice.2021.87.

Thornhill, M. H., Suda, K. J., Durkin, M. J., & Lockhart, P. B. (2019). Is it time US dentistry ended its opioid dependence? *Journal of the American Dental Association, 150*(10), 883–889. https://doi.org/10.1016/j.adaj.2019.07.003.

Thornhill, M., Dayer, M., Prendergast, B., Baddour, L., Jones, S., & Lockhart, P. (2015). Incidence and nature of adverse reactions to antibiotics used as endocarditis prophylaxis. *The Journal of Antimicrobial Chemotherapy, 70*(8), 2382–2388. https://doi.org/10.1093/jac/dkv115.

Thornhill, M., Prendergast, B., Dayer, M., Frisby, A., Lockhart, P., & Baddour, L. M. (2024). Prevention of infective endocarditis in at-risk patients: How should dentists proceed in 2024? *British Dental Journal, 236*(9), 709–716.

Thornsberry, C. (1985). Review of in vitro activity of third-generation cephalosporins and other newer beta-lactam antibiotics against clinically important bacteria. *The American Journal of Medicine, 79*(2A), 14–20. https://doi.org/10.1016/0002-9343(85)90255-4.

Thosar, N., Basak, S., Bahadure, R., & Rajurkar, M. (2013). Antimicrobial efficacy of five essential oils against oral pathogens: An in vitro study. *European Journal of Dentistry, 7*(S71–S77). https://doi.org/10.4103/1305-7456.119078.

Thürmann, P. (2019). Pharmacodynamics and pharmacokinetics in older adults. *Current Opinion in Anaesthesiology*. https://doi.org/10.1097/ACO.0000000000000814.

Tiemstra, J. D., & Khatkhate, N. (2007). Bell's palsy: Diagnosis and management. *American Family Physician, 76*(7), 997-1002.

Tilakaratne, W. M., Ekanayaka, R. P., Herath, M., Jayasinghe, R. D., Sitheeque, M., & Amarasinghe, H. (2016). Intralesional corticosteroids as a treatment for restricted mouth opening in oral submucous fibrosis. *Oral Surgery, Oral Medicine, Oral Pathology and Oral Radiology, 122*(2), 224-231. https://doi.org/10.1016/j.oooo.2015.11.023.

Tilotta, F., Folliguet, M., & Radoï, L. (2023). Preserving the oral health of patients on antiresorptive drugs. *La Revue du Praticien, 73*(4), 421–429.

Tily, F., & Thomas, S. (2007). Glycemic effect of administration of epinephrine-containing local anaesthesia in patients undergoing dental extraction, a comparison between healthy and diabetic patients. *International Dental Journal*, 57 2, 77-83. https://doi.org/10.1111/J.1875-595X.2007.TB00442.X.

Tindall, T., McColl, E., Curl, C., & Miller, D. (2025). Managing patients with epilepsy in primary care: An update. *Dental Update*. https://doi.org/10.12968/denu.2025.52.3.186.

Tobias, G., & Spanier, A. (2020). Developing a mobile app (iGAM) to promote gingival health by professional monitoring of dental selfies: User-centered design approach. JMIR mHealth and uHealth, 8. https://doi.org/10.2196/19433.

Tobias, G., SganCohen, H., Spanier, A., & Mann, J. (2020). Perceptions and attitudes toward the use of a mobile health app for remote monitoring of gingivitis and willingness to pay for mobile health apps (Part 3): Mixed methods study. *JMIR Formative Research, 5*. https://doi.org/10.2196/26125.

Tole, N., & Neeli, A. (2024). Evaluation of the efficacy of buffered local anesthetic in extraction of infected teeth-randomized double-blind study. *Oral And Maxillofacial Surgery*. https://doi.org/10.1007/s10006-024-01206-5.

Toma, M., Radu, F., Ciochindă, G., Mihai, C., Popescu, S., Perieanu, V., Cristache, C., Costache, M., Eftene, O., Dina, M., Malita, M., Babiuc, I., Costea, R., Costea, R., Marcov, E., Per, S., Sava, V., & Perieanu, M. (2020). The follow-up care process in pediatric dentistry – part II. *Romanian Journal of Medical Practice*. https://doi.org/10.37897/rjmp.2020.4.10.

Tong, D. C., & Rothwell, B. R. (2000). Antibiotic prophylaxis in dentistry: A review and practice recommendations. *Journal of the American Dental Association, 131*(3), 366–374.

Torrent Rodríguez, A., Font I Barceló, A., Barrantes González, M., Echeverria Esnal, D., Soy Muner, D., Martínez, J. A., & Tuset Creus, M. (2024). Clinically important pharmacokinetic drug-drug interactions with antibacterial agents. *Revista espanola de quimioterapia : publicacion oficial de la Sociedad Espanola de Quimioterapia, 37*(4), 299–322. https://doi.org/10.37201/req/037.2024.

Torres, J., & Jewtuchowicz, V. (2025). Clinical update on oropharyngeal candidiasis in HIV patients. *Odontología (Montevideo)*. https://doi.org/10.62486/agodonto2025193.

Townsend, T., Cerdá, M., Bohnert, A., Lagisetty, P., & Haffajee, R. (2021). CDC guideline for opioid prescribing associated with reduced dispensing to certain patients with chronic pain. *Health Affairs, 40*(11), 1766-1775. https://doi.org/10.1377/hlthaff.2021.00135.

Tran, T. H., Smith, C., & Mangione, R. A. (2013). Drug absorption in celiac disease. *American Journal of Health-System Pharmacy, 70*(24), 2199–2206.

Trapani, G., Altomare, C., Sanna, E., Biggio, G., & Liso, G. (2000). Propofol in anesthesia. Mechanism of action, structure-activity relationships, and drug delivery.. *Current medicinal chemistry*, 7 2, 249-71. https://doi.org/10.2174/0929867003375335.

Tredwin, C. J., Scully, C., & Bagan-Sebastian, J. V. (2005). Drug-induced disorders of teeth. *Journal of Dental Research*, 84(7), 596–602.

Treede, R. D., Rief, W., Barke, A., Aziz, Q., Bennett, M. I., Benoliel, R., ... & Wang, S. J. (2015). A classification of chronic pain for ICD-11. *Pain, 156*(6), 1003-1007.

Trescot, A., Datta, S., Lee, M., & Hansen, H. (2008). Opioid pharmacology. *Pain physician*, 11 2 Suppl, S133-53.

Trombelli, L., Franceschetti, G., & Farina, R. (2015). Effect of professional mechanical plaque removal performed on a long-term, routine basis in the secondary prevention of periodontitis: A systematic review. *Journal of Clinical Periodontology, 42*, S221–S236. https://doi.org/10.1111/jcpe.12339.

Tucker, G., & Mather, L. (1979). Clinical Pharmacokinetics of Local Anaesthetics. Clinical Pharmacokinetics, 4, 241-278. https://doi.org/10.2165/00003088-197904040-00001.

Turnidge, J. (2012). Pharmacokinetics and pharmacodynamics of fluoroquinolones. *Drugs, 58*, 29–36. https://doi.org/10.2165/00003495-199958002-00006.

U.S. Food and Drug Administration. (2014). *Pregnancy and lactation labeling resources.* https://www.fda.gov/drugs/labeling-information-drug-products/pregnancy-and-lactation-labeling-resources.

Udhnawala, H. J., Chaudhari, H. B., & Gor, A. (2024). Amoxicillin+clavulanic acid induced toxic epidermal necrolysis (TEN). *Journal of Health Sciences and Professions Education, 4*(1), 59.

Umapathy, V. R., Swamikannu, B., Jones, S., Kiran, M., Lell, T., Mayasa, V., & Govindaraj, J. (2022). Effects of turmeric (*Curcuma longa*) on oral health. *Bioinformation, 18*(6), 538–542. https://doi.org/10.6026/97320630018538.

Usman, N., & Annamaraju, P. (2023). Type III Hypersensitivity Reaction. In StatPearls. StatPearls Publishing.

UStün, Y., Erdogan, O., Esen, E., & Karsli, E. D. (2003). Comparison of the effects of 2 doses of methylprednisolone on pain, swelling, and trismus after third molar surgery. *Oral Surgery, Oral Medicine, Oral Pathology, Oral Radiology, and Endodontics, 96*(5), 535–539. https://doi.org/10.1016/S1079210403004645.

Vaishnani, D., Vekaria, P., Patel, R., White, M., Vaishnani, M., & Raiyani, T. (2019). Amoxicillin-clavulanate related mixed cholestatic-hepatocellular injury. *American Journal of Gastroenterology*. https://doi.org/10.14309/01.ajg.0000602216.07733.1d.

Valdez, N. (2020). *Preparing the Patient for Anesthesia*. 7-14. https://doi.org/10.1201/9781351012911-2.

Vallance, P., & Smart, T. G. (2006). The future of pharmacology. *British Journal of Pharmacology, 147*(Suppl 1), S304–S307. https://doi.org/10.1038/sj.bjp.0706454.

Vambheim, S., Kyllo, T., Hegland, S., & Bystad, M. (2021). Relaxation techniques as an intervention for chronic pain: A systematic review of randomized controlled trials. *Heliyon, 7*. https://doi.org/10.1016/j.heliyon.2021.e07837.

Van Amsterdam, J., & Van Den Brink, W. (2022). Nitrous oxide–induced reproductive risks: Should recreational nitrous oxide users worry? *Journal of Psychopharmacology*, 36, 951–955. https://doi.org/10.1177/02698811221077194.

Van Der Jagt, É. (2018). The Sedation Continuum. *The Pediatric Procedural Sedation Handbook*. https://doi.org/10.1093/med/9780190659110.003.0003.

Van der Weijden, G. A., & Hioe, K. P. K. (2005). A systematic review of the effectiveness of self-performed mechanical plaque removal in adults with gingivitis using a manual toothbrush. *Journal of Clinical Periodontology, 32*, 214–228. https://doi.org/10.1111/J.1600-051X.2005.00795.X.

Van der Weijden, G. A., & van Loveren, C. (2023). Mechanical plaque removal in step-1 of care. *Periodontology 2000*. https://doi.org/10.1111/prd.12541.

Vanreppelen, G., Wuyts, J., Van Dijck, P., & Vandecruys, P. (2023). Sources of antifungal drugs. *Journal of Fungi, 9*(2), 171. https://doi.org/10.3390/jof9020171.

Varughese, S., & Ahmed, R. (2021). Environmental and Occupational Considerations of Anesthesia: A Narrative Review and Update. *Anesthesia and Analgesia*, 133, 826 - 835. https://doi.org/10.1213/ane.0000000000005504.

Velioglu, O., Çalış, A., Koca, H., & Velioğlu, E. (2020). Bupivacaine vs. lidocaine: a comparison of local anesthetic efficacy in impacted third molar surgery. Clinical Oral Investigations, 24, 3539 - 3546. https://doi.org/10.1007/s00784-020-03224-5.

Venkatesh, E., Bagewadi, A., Keluskar, V., & Shetti, A. (2010). Role of corticosteroids in dentistry. *Archives of Dental Sciences, 1*(1), 03-11.

Verbeeck, R. K., Blackburn, J. L., & Loewen, G. R. (1983). Clinical pharmacokinetics of non-steroidal anti-inflammatory drugs. *Clinical Pharmacokinetics, 8*(4), 297–331. https://doi.org/10.2165/00003088-198308040-00003.

Verhulst, M., Loos, B., Gerdes, V., & Teeuw, W. (2019). Evaluating all potential oral complications of diabetes mellitus. *Frontiers in Endocrinology*, 10. https://doi.org/10.3389/fendo.2019.00056

Verma, R., Sindgi, R., Gavarraju, D., Manasa, P., Bakkuri, P., Dubey, A., & Ravula, S. (2024). Effectiveness of different behavior management techniques in pediatric dentistry. *Journal of Pharmacy & Bioallied Sciences*, 16, S2434–S2436. https://doi.org/10.4103/jpbs.jpbs_262_24.

Verma, T., Grover, N., & Malhotra, S. (2023). Various applications of chlorhexidine as an antimicrobial agent in dentistry: A review. *International Dental Journal of Student's Research, 11*(2), 11. https://doi.org/10.18231/j.idjsr.2023.011.

Verna, C., Hartig, L. E., Kalia, S., & Melsen, B. (2006). Influence of steroid drugs on orthodontically induced root resorption. *Orthodontics & Craniofacial Research, 9*(1), 57-62. https://doi.org/10.1111/j.1601-6343.2006.00342.x.

Vesell, E. S. (1991). Genetic and environmental factors causing variation in drug response. *Mutation Research/Fundamental and Molecular Mechanisms of Mutagenesis, 247*(2), 241–257.

Vidović Juras, D., Škrinjar, I., Križnik, T., Andabak Rogulj, A., Lončar Brzak, B., Gabrić, D., ... & Ivanišević, A. (2024). Antibiotic prophylaxis prior to dental procedures. *Dentistry Journal, 12*(11), 364.

Vidovic, B., Gusic, I., Tamas, I., Mihajlović, D., Mitić, V., Obradović, R., Radovanović, M., & Brkić, S. (2019). The effect of the octenidine-based oral antiseptic on the structure of microbial communities and periodontal status in patients with fixed orthodontic treatments. *European Review for Medical and Pharmacological Sciences, 23*(19), 8598–8605. https://doi.org/10.26355/eurrev_201910_19176.

Viola, K., Coaguila-Llerena, H., Rodrigues, E., Santos, C., Chávez-Andrade, G., Magro, M., Tanomaru-Filho, M., Guerreiro-Tanomaru, J., & Faria, G. (2022). Different formulations of peracetic acid: Effects on smear layer removal, dentine erosion, cytotoxicity and antibiofilm activity. *Journal of Applied Oral Science, 30*, Article e20210575. https://doi.org/10.1590/1678-7757-2021-0575.

Visvanathan, T., Kluger, T., Webb, R., Westhorpe, R., & Runciman, P. (2005). Crisis management during anaesthesia: obstruction of the natural airway. *Quality and Safety in Health Care*, 14, e2 - e2. https://doi.org/10.1136/qshc.2002.004325.

Volkow, N. D., Jones, E. B., Einstein, E. B., & Wargo, E. M. (2019). Prevention and treatment of opioid misuse and addiction: A review. *JAMA Psychiatry, 76*(2), 208–216. https://doi.org/10.1001/jamapsychiatry.2018.3126.

Volpe, C., De Melo, E., De Aguiar, L., Pinho, D., & Stival, M. (2016). Risk factors for medication errors in the electronic and manual prescription 1. *Revista Latino-Americana de Enfermagem*, 24. https://doi.org/10.1590/1518-8345.0642.2742.

Wahl, M. J. (2014). Dental surgery and antiplatelet agents: Bleed or die. *American Journal of Medicine, 127*(4), 260–267. https://doi.org/10.1016/j.amjmed.2013.11.013.

Wallace, C., Schofield, C., Burbridge, L., & O'Donnell, K. (2021). Role of teledentistry in paediatric dentistry. *British Dental Journal*, 1–6. https://doi.org/10.1038/s41415-021-3015-y.

Walsh, D., Horgan, A., O'Driscoll, M., Hannan, M., Goggin, C., & Sahm, L. (2024). Reducing potentially inappropriate medication use and patient harm in a dedicated geriatric oncology clinic: A cross-sectional study. *International Journal of Pharmacy Practice*. https://doi.org/10.1093/ijpp/riae013.024.

Walsh, L., Ford, P., McGuire, T., Van Driel, M., & Hollingworth, S. (2021). Trends in Australian dental prescribing of antibiotics: 2005–2016. *Australian Dental Journal, 66*(S1). https://doi.org/10.1111/adj.12846.

Wan-Jun, D. (2008). Research progress of antibiotic use during pregnancy and lactation.

Wang, H., Lv, X., Wu, L., F., Wang, L., Wang, Y., Wang, X., & Li, Y. (2025). The effect of neuromuscular blocking reversal agents on perioperative neurocognitive function after general anaesthesia: a systematic review and meta-analysis. *BMC Anesthesiology*, 25. https://doi.org/10.1186/s12871-025-03019-9.

Wang, J., Cheng, Z., & Li, Y. (2024). Medication management difficulty, medication nonadherence, and risk of hospitalization among cognitively impaired older Americans: A nationally representative study. *Journal of Applied Gerontology*, 44, 27–34. https://doi.org/10.1177/07334648241262940.

Wang, J., Wang, B., Liu, Y., Luo, Y., Wu, Y., Xiang, L., Yang, X., Qu, Y., Tian, T., & Man, Y. (2024). Recent advances in digital technology in implant dentistry. *Journal of Dental Research*, 103, 787–799. https://doi.org/10.1177/00220345241253794.

Wang, L., Lin, H., Lin, C., Chen, Y., & Lin, H. (2010). Increased risk of adverse pregnancy outcomes in women receiving zolpidem during pregnancy. *Clinical Pharmacology & Therapeutics*, 88. https://doi.org/10.1038/clpt.2010.97.

Wang, L., Shen, J., Ge, L., Arango, M., Tang, X., Moodie, J., McConnell, B., Cheng, D., & Martin, J. (2019). Dexmedetomidine for craniotomy under general anesthesia: A systematic review and meta-analysis of randomized clinical trials.. *Journal of clinical anesthesia*, 54, 114-125. https://doi.org/10.1016/j.jclinane.2018.11.001.

Wang, P., Sun, F., & Ling, X. (2024). Effectiveness of photodynamic therapy as an adjunctive treatment for periodontitis: A systematic review and meta-analysis. *Journal of Stomatology, Oral and Maxillofacial Surgery*, 102036. https://doi.org/10.1016/j.jormas.2024.102036.

Wang, Y., Lin, I., Huang, C., & Fan, S. (201s2). Dental anesthesia for patients with special needs.. *Acta anaesthesiologica Taiwanica : official journal of the Taiwan Society of Anesthesiologists*, 50 3, 122-5 . https://doi.org/10.1016/j.aat.2012.08.009.

Wang, Y., Zheng, K., Guo, H., Tian, L., He, Y., Wang, X., Zhu, T., Sun, P., & Liu, Y. (2022). Potassium permanganate-based advanced oxidation processes for wastewater decontamination and sludge treatment: A review. *Chemical Engineering Journal, 427*, 139529. https://doi.org/10.1016/j.cej.2022.139529.

Wang, Z., Shen, Y., & Haapasalo, M. (2020). Dynamics of dissolution, killing, and inhibition of dental plaque biofilm. *Frontiers in Microbiology, 11*. https://doi.org/10.3389/fmicb.2020.00964.

Wänman, A., & Marklund, S. (2019). Treatment outcome of supervised exercise, home exercise and bite splint therapy, respectively, in patients with symptomatic disc displacement with reduction: A randomised clinical trial. *Journal of Oral Rehabilitation, 47*, 143–149. https://doi.org/10.1111/joor.12888.

Warner, A., Hathaway-Schrader, J., Lubker, R., Davies, C., & Novince, C. (2022). Tetracyclines and bone: Unclear actions with potentially lasting effects. *Bone*, 116377. https://doi.org/10.1016/j.bone.2022.116377.

Warrington, R., & Silviu-Dan, F. (2011). Drug allergy. *Allergy, asthma, and clinical immunology : official journal of the Canadian Society of Allergy and Clinical Immunology, 7 Suppl 1*(Suppl 1), S10. https://doi.org/10.1186/1710-1492-7-S1-S10.

Watanabe, H., Nagano, N., Tsuji, Y., Noto, N., Ayusawa, M., & Morioka, I. (2023). Challenges of pediatric pharmacotherapy: A narrative review of pharmacokinetics, pharmacodynamics, and pharmacogenetics. European Journal of Clinical Pharmacology, 79(5), 681–693. https://doi.org/10.1007/s00228-023-03598-x.

Waxman, D. J., & Strominger, J. L. (1983). Penicillin-binding proteins and the mechanism of action of beta-lactam antibiotics. *Annual Review of Biochemistry, 52*, 825–869. https://doi.org/10.1146/annurev.bi.52.070183.004141.

Weaver, J. (2019). The History of the Specialty of Dental Anesthesiology. *Anesthesia progress*, 66 2, 61-68 . https://doi.org/10.2344/anpr-66-02-12.

Webb, D. J., Muirhead, G. J., Wulff, M., Sutton, J. A., Levi, R., & Dinsmore, W. W. (2000). Sildenafil citrate potentiates the hypotensive effects of nitric oxide donor drugs in male patients with stable angina. *Journal of the American College of Cardiology, 36*(1), 25–31.

Weber, J., Bonn, E., Auer, D., Kirschneck, C., Buchalla, W., Scholz, K., & Cieplik, F. (2023). Preprocedural mouthwashes for infection control in dentistry—an update. *Clinical Oral Investigations, 27*, 33–44. https://doi.org/10.1007/s00784-023-04953-z.

Wehling, M., Burkhardt, H., Kuhn-Thiel, A., Pazan, F., Throm, C., Weiss, C., & Frohnhofen, H. (2016). VALFORTA: A randomised trial to validate the FORTA (Fit fOR The Aged) classification. *Age and Ageing*, 45(2), 262–267. https://doi.org/10.1093/ageing/afv200.

Wei, Y., Deng, Y., Ma, S., Ran, M., Jia, Y., Meng, J., ... & Tang, X. (2021). Local drug delivery systems as therapeutic strategies against periodontitis: A systematic review. *Journal of Controlled Release, 333*, 269–282. https://doi.org/10.1016/j.jconrel.2021.03.041.

Weibel, S., Schaefer, M., Raj, D., Rücker, G., Pace, N., Schlesinger, T., Meybohm, P., Kienbaum, P., Eberhart, L., & Kranke, P. (2020). Drugs for preventing postoperative nausea and vomiting in adults after general anaesthesia: an abridged Cochrane network meta-analysis. *Anaesthesia*, 76. https://doi.org/10.1111/anae.15295.

Weiner, S. G., Griggs, C. A., Langlois, B. K., Mitchell, P. M., Nelson, K. P., Friedman, F. D., & Feldman, J. A. (2015). Characteristics of emergency department "doctor shoppers." *The Journal of Emergency Medicine, 48*(4), 424-431.

Weisfeld, C., Turner, J., Dunleavy, K., Ko, A., Bowen, J., Roelk, B., Eissa, R., Benfield, E., & Robertson, K. (2021). Dealing with anxious patients: A systematic review of the literature on nonpharmaceutical interventions to reduce anxiety in patients undergoing medical or dental procedures. *Journal of Alternative and Complementary Medicine*. https://doi.org/10.1089/acm.2020.0504.

Wellner, F., & Goettel, N. (2020). Geriatric Anesthesia: An Issue of Anesthesiology Clinics.. *Anesthesia & Analgesia*. https://doi.org/10.1213/ane.0000000000004732.

Westfelt, E. (1996). Rationale of mechanical plaque control. *Journal of Clinical Periodontology, 23*(3), 263–267. https://doi.org/10.1111/J.1600-051X.1996.TB02086.X.

WHO. (1972). International drug monitoring: The role of national centres. *Tech Rep Ser WHO*, No. 498.

Wiemer, S., Nathan, J., Heggestad, B., Fillmore, W., Viozzi, C., Van Ess, J., Arce, K., & Ettinger, K. (2020). Safety of Outpatient Procedural Sedation Administered by Oral and Maxillofacial Surgeons: The Mayo Clinic Experience in 17,634 Sedations (2004 to 2019). *Journal of oral and maxillofacial surgery : official journal of the American*

Association of Oral and Maxillofacial Surgeons. https://doi.org/10.1016/j.joms.2020.12.002.

Wierzbiński, P., Hubska, J., Henzler, M., Kucharski, B., Bieś, R., & Krzystanek, M. (2023). Depressive and other adverse CNS effects of fluoroquinolones. *Pharmaceuticals, 16*, Article 1105. https://doi.org/10.3390/ph16081105.

Wiesner, A., Zagrodzki, P., Gawalska, A., & Paśko, P. (2024). Clinically important interactions of macrolides and tetracyclines with dietary interventions—a systematic review with meta-analyses. *Journal of Antimicrobial Chemotherapy, 79*, 2762–2791. https://doi.org/10.1093/jac/dkae315.

William, W. M. (2015). Drug interactions, analgesic protocols and their consequences, and analgesic drug antagonism. In J. S. Gaynor & W. W. Muir (Eds.), *Handbook of Veterinary Pain Management* (3rd ed., pp. 335–355). Mosby. https://doi.org/10.1016/B978-0-323-08935-7.00016-8.

William, W. M., & Sams, R. A. (2009). Pharmacologic principles and pain: Pharmacokinetics and pharmacodynamics. In J. S. Gaynor & W. W. Muir (Eds.), *Handbook of Veterinary Pain Management* (2nd ed., pp. 113–140). Mosby. https://doi.org/10.1016/B978-032304679-4.10007-3.

Williams, J., Naber, K., Bryskier, A., Høby, N., Gould, I., Periti, P., Giamarellou, H., & Rouveix, B. (2001). Classification of oral cephalosporins: A matter for debate. *International Journal of Antimicrobial Agents, 17*(6), 443–450. https://doi.org/10.1016/S0924-8579(01)00309-0.

Wilson, T. D., McNeil, D. W., Kyle, B. N., Weaver, B. D., & Graves, R. W. (2014). Effects of conscious sedation on patient recall of anxiety and pain after oral surgery. *Oral Surgery, Oral Medicine, Oral Pathology, Oral Radiology, 117*(3), 277–282.

Wise, J. (2023). Maternity care: Entonox is withdrawn from some hospitals because of risk to staff from high exposure. BMJ, 380. https://doi.org/10.1136/bmj.p212.

Wnuk-Kłosińska, A., Jenerowicz, D., Bowszyc-Dmochowska, M., Pietrzak-Kaczmarek, H., & Adamski, Z. (2020). Melkersson-Rosenthal syndrome – a therapeutically challenging disease. *Postępy Dermatologii i Alergologii, 38*(3), 533-536. https://doi.org/10.5114/ada.2020.92569.

Wolfson, J., & Hooper, D. (1991). Overview of fluoroquinolone safety. *The American Journal of Medicine, 91*(6A), 153S–161S. https://doi.org/10.1016/0002-9343(91)90330-Z.

Wołowiec, Ł., Grześk, G., Osiak, J., Wijata, A., Mędlewska, M., Gaborek, P., Banach, J., Wołowiec, A., & Głowacka, M. (2023). Beta-blockers in cardiac arrhythmias-Clinical pharmacologist's point of view. *Frontiers in pharmacology, 13*, 1043714. https://doi.org/10.3389/fphar.2022.1043714.

Wong, F., Zhang, L., & Wang, Z. (2021). Sedation and analgesia for HIFU ablation. In *High-Intensity Focused Ultrasound (HIFU) Ablation* (pp. 13–21). https://doi.org/10.1007/978-981-16-0939-8_2.

Wong, M. (2022). Reversal Agents in Sedation and Anesthesia Practice for Dentistry. Anesthesia progress, 69 1, 49-58 . https://doi.org/10.2344/anpr-69-01-09.

Wongpakorn, P., Chantarangsu, S., & Prapinjumrune, C. (2024). Factors involved in the remission of oral lichen planus treated with topical corticosteroids. *BDJ Open, 10*, 34. https://doi.org/10.1038/s41405-024-00217-4.

Wongrakpanich, S., Wongrakpanich, A., Melhado, K., & Rangaswami, J. (2018). A comprehensive review of non-steroidal anti-inflammatory drug use in the elderly. *Aging and Disease, 9*(1), 143–150. https://doi.org/10.14336/AD.2017.0306.

Woodroffe, A., Weldon, M., Meadows, R., & Lawrence, J. (1975). Acute interstitial nephritis following ampicillin hypersensitivity. *Medical Journal of Australia, 1*. https://doi.org/10.5694/j.1326-5377.1975.tb111234.x.

Workowski, K. A., Bachmann, L. H., Chan, P. A., et al., (2021). Sexually transmitted infections treatment guidelines, 2021. *MMWR Recommendations and Reports, 70*(4), 1–187. https://doi.org/10.15585/mmwr.rr7004a1.

World Health Organization (WHO). (2002). Breastfeeding and maternal medication, recommendations for drugs in the Eleventh WHO Model List of Essential Drugs. http://apps.who.int/iris/bitstream/handle/10665/62435/55732.pdf;jsessionid=6B47B933AC2796FD49DA7C70B703CFA9?sequence=1.

World Health Organization. (1993). *How to investigate drug use in health facilities: Selected drug use indicators*. WHO.

World Health Organization. (1994). *Guide to good prescribing: A practical manual*. World Health Organization. https://apps.who.int/iris/handle/10665/59001.

World Health Organization. (2002a). *Promoting rational use of medicines: Core components—WHO policy perspectives on medicines*.

World Health Organization. (2002b). *The world health report 2002: Reducing risks, promoting healthy life*.

World Health Organization. (2010). *The world medicines situation: Chapter 8, rational use of medicines*. WHO. http://apps.who.int/medicinedocs/en/d/JS/6160e/10.html.

World Health Organization. (2014). Congenital anomalies (Fact Sheet No. 370). Geneva, Switzerland: Author. http://www.who.int/mediacentre/factsheets/fs370/en/.

Wu, M., Cai, J., Yu, Y., Hu, S., Wang, Y., & Wu, M. (2021). Therapeutic agents for the treatment of temporomandibular joint disorders: Progress and perspective. *Frontiers in Pharmacology, 11*, 596099. https://doi.org/10.3389/fphar.2020.596099.

Wu, X., Al-Abedalla, K., Eimar, H., Arekunnath Madathil, S., Abi-Nader, S., Daniel, N. G., ... & Tamimi, F. (2016). Antihypertensive medications and the survival rate of osseointegrated dental implants: A cohort study. *Clinical Implant Dentistry and Related Research, 18*(6), 1171–1182. https://doi.org/10.1111/cid.12414.

Wulifan, J. K., Brenner, S., Jahn, A., & De Allegri, M. (2016). A scoping review on determinants of unmet need for family planning among women of reproductive age in low and middle income countries. *BMC Women's Health, 16*, 2. https://doi.org/10.1186/s12905-015-0281-3.

Xie, Y., Choi, T., & Al-Aly, Z. (2025). Mapping the effectiveness and risks of GLP-1 receptor agonists. Nature Medicine. https://doi.org/10.1038/s41591-024-03412-w.

Xu, W., Wang, L., Yuan, X., Wang, T., Li, W., Qu, W., Hong, Z., & Huang, Z. (2019). Sevoflurane depresses neurons in the medial parabrachial nucleus by potentiating postsynaptic GABAA receptors and background potassium channels. *Neuropharmacology*, 181. https://doi.org/10.1016/j.sleep.2019.11.1195.

Xu, X., Gu, Z., Chen, X., Shi, C., Liu, C., Liu, M., ... & Sun, H. (2019). An injectable and thermosensitive hydrogel: Promoting periodontal regeneration by controlled-release of aspirin and erythropoietin. *Acta Biomaterialia, 86*, 235–246. https://doi.org/10.1016/j.actbio.2019.01.001.

Yaacob, N., Loganathan, M., Hisham, N., Kamaruzzaman, H., Isa, K., Ibrahim, M., & Ng, K. (2024). The impact of pharmacist medication reviews on geriatric patients: A scoping review. *Korean Journal of Family Medicine*, 45, 125–133. https://doi.org/10.4082/kjfm.23.0220.

Yadav, J., Tangade, P., Jain, A., Agrahari, P., & Chaudhary, V. (2021). Dental herbs: Ethnomedicinal plants in dentistry. *International Journal of Applied Dental Sciences*. https://doi.org/10.22271/oral.2021.v7.i3b.1290.

Yang, Y., Liao, B., Deng, R., Ren, L., Sun, Y., Xiong, S., & Wu, X. (2024). Comparison of anaesthesia strategies on postoperative nausea and vomiting in laparoscopic sleeve gastrectomy: a randomised controlled trial. *BMC Anesthesiology*, 24. https://doi.org/10.1186/s12871-024-02577-8.

Yasui, N., Otani, K., Kaneko, S., Ohkubo, T., Osanai, T., Sugawara, K., ... & Ishizaki, T. (1996). A kinetic and dynamic study of oral alprazolam with and without erythromycin in humans: In vivo evidence for the involvement of CYP3A4 in alprazolam metabolism. *Clinical Pharmacology & Therapeutics, 59*(5), 514–519.

Yeo, X., Gillway, D., Kahatab, A., Doshi, M., Shehabi, Z., & Geddis-Regan, A. (2025). General anaesthesia in special care dentistry: Part 3. case series. *Dental Update*. https://doi.org/10.12968/denu.2025.52.2.93.

Yoon, S., Kim, P., Jang, S., Choi, S., Kim, K., & Kim, H. (2022). Ceftriaxone- and cephalexin-induced acute reversible encephalopathy. *Journal of the Korean Neurological Association*. https://doi.org/10.17340/jkna.2022.4.5.

Yordanova, I., Toneva, R., Petkova, N., & Dimova, E. (2018). Tetracycline-related pigmentation in children's dentition: A literature review. *SSVS, 2*, 69. https://doi.org/10.14748/SSVS.V2I0.4735.

Young, J., Dasgupta, N., Chidgey, B., Stürmer, T., Pate, V., Hudgens, M., & Funk, M. (2021). Impacts of Initial Prescription Length and Prescribing Limits on Risk of Prolonged Postsurgical Opioid Use. *Medical Care*, 60, 75 - 82. https://doi.org/10.1097/mlr.0000000000001663.

Yousef, N., Aljoujou, A., Mashlah, A., & Hajeer, M. (2022). Assessment of the effectiveness of aloe vera versus amlexanox in the treatment of recurrent aphthous ulcers: A three-arm placebo-controlled randomized clinical trial. *Cureus, 14*. https://doi.org/10.7759/cureus.30693.

Yu, D., Shen, X., Lai, L., Chen, Y., Liu, K., & Shen, Q. (2023). Application of Dexmedetomidine as an Opioid Substitute in Opioid-Free Anesthesia: A Systematic Review and Meta-analysis. *Pain physician*, 26 6, E635-E649. https://doi.org/10.36076/ppj.2023.26.e635.

Zabiszak, M., Frymark, J., Ogawa, K., Skrobańska, M., Nowak, M., Jastrzab, R., & Kaczmarek, M. T. (2023). Complexes of β-lactam antibiotics and their Schiff-base derivatives as a weapon in the fight against bacterial resistance. *Coordination Chemistry Reviews, 493*, 215326.

Zaccara, G., & Franco, V. (2022). Pharmacokinetic interactions between antiseizure and psychiatric medications. *Current Neuropharmacology, 21*, 1666–1690. https://doi.org/10.2174/1570159X20666220524121645.

Zazzara, M. B., Palmer, K., Vetrano, D. L., Carfì, A., & Graziano, O. (2021). Adverse drug reactions in older adults: A narrative review of the literature. *European Geriatric Medicine, 12*, 463–473.

Zhanel, G. G., Homenuik, K., Nichol, K., Noreddin, A., Vercaigne, L., Embil, J., Gin, A., Karlowsky, J. A., & Hoban, D. J. (2004). The glycylcyclines: A comparative review with the tetracyclines. *Drugs, 64*(1), 63–88. https://doi.org/10.2165/00003495-200464010-00005

Zhang, D., Wei, C., Hop, C., Wright, M., Hu, M., Lai, Y., Khojasteh, S., & Humphreys, W. (2021). Intestinal excretion, intestinal recirculation, and renal tubule reabsorption are underappreciated mechanisms that drive the distribution and pharmacokinetic behavior of small molecule drugs. *Journal of Medicinal Chemistry*. https://doi.org/10.1021/acs.jmedchem.0c01720.

Zhang, G. F., Liu, X., Zhang, S., Pan, B., & Liu, M. L. (2018). Ciprofloxacin derivatives and their antibacterial activities. *European Journal of Medicinal Chemistry, 146*, 599–612. https://doi.org/10.1016/j.ejmech.2018.01.078.

Zhang, J., Qin, Z., Lou, C., Huang, J., & Xiong, Y. (2021). The efficacy of vaccination to prevent human papilloma viruses infection at anal and oral: A systematic review and meta-analysis. *Public Health*, 196, 165–171. https://doi.org/10.1016/j.puhe.2021.05.012.

Zhang, L., Zhang, Y., Zhou, Y., An, S., Zhou, Y., & Cheng, J. (2002). Response of gene expression in *Saccharomyces cerevisiae* to amphotericin B and nystatin measured by microarrays. *The Journal of Antimicrobial Chemotherapy, 49*(6), 905–915. https://doi.org/10.1093/jac/dkf001.

Zhang, Y., He, S., Nie, B., Li, X., & Wang, D. (2020). Emergence delirium is associated with increased postoperative delirium in elderly: a prospective observational study. *Journal of Anesthesia*, 34, 675 - 687. https://doi.org/10.1007/s00540-020-02805-8.

Zheng, L., Fang, T., Zhang, W., Zhang, X., Ren, Z., Qin, W., Liang, W., , Q., & Yin, N. (2024). Beneficial Effects of Low-Dose Intravenous Dexmedetomidine Premedication in Patient Undergoing Laparoscopic Cholecystectomy Under General Anesthesia: A Prospective, Double-Blind, Randomized Controlled Trial. *Drug Design, Development and Therapy*, 18, 443 - 452. https://doi.org/10.2147/DDDT.S452077.

Zhou, J., Peng, G., Liang, W., Chen, Z., Liu, Y., Guo, M., Deng, Y., Ye, J., Zhong, M., & Wang, L. (2023). Recent advances in the study of anesthesia-and analgesia-related mechanisms of S-ketamine. *Frontiers in Pharmacology*, 14. https://doi.org/10.3389/fphar.2023.1228895.

Zhou, X., Zhong, Y., Pan, Z., Zhang, J., & Pan, J. (2023). Physiology of pregnancy and oral local anesthesia considerations. PeerJ, 11. https://doi.org/10.7717/peerj.15585.

Zhu, W. Y., Yang, W. F., Wang, L., Lan, X., Tao, Z. Y., Guo, J., ... & Su, Y. X. (2023). The effect of drug holiday on preventing medication-related osteonecrosis of the jaw in osteoporotic rat model. *Journal of Orthopaedic Translation, 39*, 55–62. https://doi.org/10.1016/j.jot.2022.12.006.

Zou, H., Liu, Z., Wang, Z., & Fang, J. (2022). Effects of aloe vera in the treatment of oral ulcers: A systematic review and meta-analysis of randomised controlled trials. *Oral Health & Preventive Dentistry, 20*. https://doi.org/10.3290/j.ohpd.b3666483.

Appendices

Frequently used drugs in dentistry, possible interactions and recommendations:

Drug Group	Example Drugs	Possible Interactions	Lexicomp Recommendation / Warning
Antibiotics	Amoxicillin, Clindamycin	Oral contraceptives, Anticoagulants	Oral contraceptive efficacy may decrease, bleeding risk may increase. Alternative contraception may be recommended if needed (controversial).
NSAIDs	Ibuprofen, Diclofenac	Anticoagulants, Antihypertensives, Lithium	Increased bleeding risk, reduced antihypertensive efficacy, risk of lithium toxicity. Short-term and low-dose use is recommended.
Local Anesthetics	Lidocaine, Articaine	Beta blockers, Antiarrhythmics, Antidepressants	Cardiac side effects may increase. Avoid epinephrine-containing anesthetics especially with tricyclic antidepressants.
Analgesics	Paracetamol, Tramadol	Alcohol, Anticonvulsants	Risk of hepatotoxicity with paracetamol, increased sedation with tramadol. Pay attention to dose and duration.
Antifungals	Nystatin, Fluconazole	Warfarin, Oral hypoglycemics, Statins	Fluconazole increases bleeding risk with warfarin, risk of rhabdomyolysis with statins. Monitor INR.
Corticosteroids	Prednisolone, Dexamethasone	NSAIDs, Antidiabetics	Risk of ulcer, impaired glucose regulation. Use with NSAIDs cautiously.

Conversion tables for dosage calculations in dentistry:

Weight and Volume Conversions	
Unit	Equivalent
1 kg	1000 grams (g)
1 g	1000 milligrams (mg)
1 mg	1000 micrograms (mcg)
1 L	1000 milliliters (mL)
1 mL	1 cubic centimeter (cc)

Concentration Conversions	
Percentage (%)	mg/mL
1%	10 mg/mL
2%	20 mg/mL
0.5%	5 mg/mL

Example: 2% lidocaine = 20 mg/mL

Local anesthetic maximum dose calculations:

Local Anesthetic	Max Dose (mg/kg)	Max Total Dose (mg)
Lidocaine (w/ epi)	7 mg/kg	500 mg
Articaine	7 mg/kg	500 mg
Mepivacaine	6.6 mg/kg	400 mg
Prilocaine	8 mg/kg	600 mg

Common Abbreviations:

Abbreviation	Meaning	Explanation
qd (not recommended)	Once daily	Take once every day
bid	Twice daily	Take two times a day
tid	Three times daily	Take three times a day
qid	Four times daily	Take four times a day
qh	Every hour	Take every hour
q4h	Every 4 hours	Take every 4 hours
q6h	Every 6 hours	Take every 6 hours
q8h	Every 8 hours	Take every 8 hours
q12h	Every 12 hours	Take every 12 hours
prn	As needed	Take only when necessary

Pediatric dosage calculations:

Clark's Rule: Child dose = (Weight (kg) / 70) × Adult dose

Young's Rule: Child dose = (Age (years) / (Age + 12)) × Adult dose

About the Author

Associate Professor Dr. Nilay Aksoy is a distinguished academic and clinical pharmacist with extensive expertise in pharmacotherapy, rational drug use, and patient-centered care. She holds a PhD in Clinical Pharmacy from Marmara University and has served in leading academic roles at several universities in Istanbul, Türkiye, including Altınbaş University, Istanbul Medipol University, Nişantaşı University, and Istanbul Health and Technology University. Dr. Aksoy's research spans clinical pharmacy, oncology, medication adherence, and the rational use of medicines, digital health with numerous publications and book chapters to her name. She is an active member of the European Society of Clinical Pharmacy, the American Pharmacists Association and the Multinational Association of Supportive Care in Cancer. Dr. Aksoy is dedicated to advancing education in pharmacotherapy and rational drug use, teaching pharmacotherapy to both pharmacy and dentistry students at undergraduate and postgraduate levels. Her commitment to interdisciplinary education and evidence-based practice has made her a respected figure in both pharmacy and dental education, inspiring future healthcare professionals to prioritize safe and effective medication management.

Index

A

B

C

D

E

G

R

S

T